The Nursing Home Survival Guide

2014

l.e. green

Copyright © 2014 l.e. green

ISBN-13:

978-1463592608

ISBN-10:

1463592604

DEDICATION

To C.L, Jack, Marjorie, Freddy & Edna

l.e. green

THE NURSING HOME SURVIVAL GUIDE

Table of Contents

l.e. green

Introduction

One of the most important decisions you'll make for your parent is the nursing home where he'll be spending the final days of his life. Whether he's being admitted for short-term rehabilitation or long-term care, the patient or his family has the right to participate in the choice as to which facility will serve him. It's often difficult for family members to find the time to choose a nursing home when they've just been told that their parent will be discharged from the hospital within a day or two. At that point, people are often told where their family member will be sent – not asked.

Because people don't plan ahead for nursing home placement, they'll probably end up spending more time picking out a new television than they do choosing a nursing home for a family member. Unfortunately, families trust that the system will work in their favor and that the patient will be sent to the best place available. Nothing could be farther from the truth – patients are usually sent to whichever nursing home is the first to accept them, or the one that holds a contract with their insurance provider. If the provider chooses the nursing home, it rarely has anything to do with the quality of care that the patient will receive.

Whether or not they're run for profit, every nursing home is competing for your insurance dollars. Their marketers (often paid on commission) display professionally designed brochures that refer to their "community," evoking feelings of happy people enjoying their final years in beautiful surroundings. The brochures include photos of smiling residents in tastefully decorated private rooms with beautiful, relaxed staff members attending to them. When you take a tour of the nursing home, the staff will be smiling and on their best behavior because all of the staff has been alerted that you're a potential customer.

Once your mother has been admitted, you might find that there are probably no private rooms available and those happy, relaxed employees have been replaced by stressed and overworked staff members. The food is bland and the part of the facility where patients live look nothing at all like the photos in the brochure. The administrator's "open-door policy" might not make him any more available to you, and the admissions representative who was so attentive while she was trying to get your mother admitted no longer has any time to spend discussing your concerns.

No one looks forward to nursing home placement, but sometimes people have no other caregiving options available to them. At that point, a hospital staff member is insisting that your parent needs to leave the hospital as son as possible and time is of the essence. Families will rely upon the doctor or a discharge planner to advise them as to which facility is best for their parent, not realizing that the recommended facility might be the one that brought the biggest gift basket for Christmas, or brings pens & notepads on a regular basis. The discharge planner might "owe" the facility for having accepted a difficult patient, and so they offer up your family member to appease the nursing home. There are many reasons that patients are referred to certain nursing homes (such as the referring physician being part owner or otherwise affiliated with the nursing home), but one thing is certain; referrals rarely have anything to do with a nursing home's quality of care or its ability to meet the specific needs of the patient.

When researching nursing homes for your family member, don't rely on the advertising materials, which use certain buzz words:

- Excellence.
- Dedicated to providing the highest quality of life in a home-like setting.
- The "Premiere Facility" in the community.
- Experienced, caring staff members.
- Individualized plans of care.
- Recipient of President's Five-Star Award for Excellence.

All of these claims are marketing magic that sound great, but actually mean very little. My personal favorite is a certificate that was prominently displayed in the front lobby of a nursing home where I once worked, proclaiming that the facility had been awarded "the president's five-star award for excellence." This award had been bestowed upon the facility by its parent corporation in the hopes that it would be confused with the Medicare ratings system. Ironically, every nursing home that particular corporation owned was awarded with the exact same rating. The dirty little secret is that many companies frequently give themselves awards that look pretty hanging on the wall, as well as to garner free publicity when the award is posted in their local newspaper's business announcement section.

Even the Medicare five-star rating might not be what it seems, because nursing homes are rated in several areas. The five-star rating that's most desired is the inspection results, but those are often too low to use in their advertisements. Instead, the nursing home might display the ratings for the ratio of staff members to patient, intimating that this information is a reflection of the care provided. Staffing ratios can be misleading because the nursing home is able to use the hours of licensed administrative staff members to skew the numbers and make it appear as though they have a higher ratio of medical staff to patients. The director of nursing might rarely leave her office, but her hours count toward staffing ratios anyway – as do the hours of the staff development coordinator and other office positions. While they're not lying when they post these ratings, nursing homes most certainly are manipulating the information for marketing purposes.

Not every nursing home can be the premiere facility in its particular area, but all of their brochures will claim this honor. Their claims of having experienced staff members might be true, but chances are there are some inexperienced nurses caring for patients because they all have to start *somewhere*. The nursing home might very well provide an excellent long-term mentoring program for new nurses – but it's also possible that they provided a week of orientation after which the nurse was on her own. It's possible that the nurse caring for your mother is a LPN who just graduated from a one-year course after working as a nursing aide for a couple of years, which is not exactly the experience you'd hope for when it comes to your family member. Nurses aren't always supportive of one another, which can make it difficult to ask for help from coworkers. In fact, there's a common saying: "nurses eat their young," which refers to the lack of support and direction new nurses often receive from more experienced nurses. If this is the atmosphere in which your family member resides, the care isn't exactly of the quality the brochure presents it to be. The consumer might never know the difference, and the patients can suffer.

It's laughable when nursing homes advertise that they provide personalized care, considering that the federal government requires that every nursing home develop individualized care plans designed to meet the specific needs of each of their patients. Even though it looks good in the brochure, this little tidbit actually applies to every nursing home across the country.

Sometimes a family would like their family member to be admitted to a specific facility, but that nursing home isn't willing to accept the patient. Nursing homes aren't required to accept every patient that's referred to them; there could be any number of reasons that a patient might be denied admissions. Nursing homes have to evaluate the needs of each patient and ensure that the facility can properly care for him; if the patient appears to require too much staff attention the nursing home might issue a denial. The nursing home is responsible to meet the needs of the patient from the moment that he's admitted, and if there's any question as to whether the patient will require more help than the nursing home is able to offer he won't be admitted in the first place.

For example, if the patient is constantly getting out of bed on his own and falling, he will probably require that a staff member sit with him at all times to ensure his safety. Even if the family has promised to stay with him all day, the nursing home must be prepared to provide a sitter for him; this type of patient is often too expensive for the nursing home to accept. In fact, finances are the reason that most patients are denied admission to a nursing home. Whether the patient has no source of payment or his treatments will cost too much, each nursing home is a business and must weigh the costs of caring for him when considering his admission.

If there's a potential problem with the patient's ability to pay, he will probably be denied entry. Patients being admitted for long-term care must have a verifiable payment source in place; the nursing home won't be willing to accept the patient of he can't pay for his care. They don't usually *say* this, instead they'll say that there are no beds available, which can be code for "we're afraid we won't get paid," or "we already have too many patients waiting for their Medicaid to be approved."

Patients who are being admitted for rehabilitation under the Medicare benefit might be denied because the patient's care is too expensive. It's illegal for the patient to be charged extra fees if Medicare is footing the bill, so if the patient is receiving expensive medications or treatments (such as radiation) the family's choice of nursing home will be severely limited. Nearly every town has one nursing home that will accept every patient that's referred; once the patient has been admitted, they'll call the doctor and request less expensive treatments or medications in order to break even. Sometimes the doctor is willing to change the treatment orders to accommodate the nursing home's bottom line, while other times the doctor will refuse to accommodate the nursing home's demands. In these cases, the nursing home's medical director will surely be giving that physician a call in an attempt to pressure him into changing the patient's treatment plan. In every case, the nursing home has to weigh the benefits of accepting the patient against the costs of his treatment, because once the patient is admitted the orders must be followed no matter how much money the nursing home will lose on the deal.

Finances aren't the only reason a patient is denied entry. There's always the dreaded excuse, "We're not able to meet his needs." That *could* mean that they can't meet the patient's complex medical needs, but it usually means that the family or patient is more trouble than they're worth. It's hard to believe that someone could be that difficult to work with – but it happens more often than you think. Dealing with all of the related issues when a family member is critically ill can be stressful, and people are usually not at their best. There's also "family dynamics," meaning that the separate family members aren't able to agree on the patient's care and it's creating a problem for the nursing staff. Families don't realize that their actions and the way that they've treated the hospital staff is dutifully recorded in the patient's medical record – and that this information is related to the nursing home before they make a decision as to whether or not they'll accept the patient.

If you become upset and have a meltdown in the waiting room, it's written in the chart. If you yell at the nurse and demand the doctor's personal cell phone number, it's written in the chart. If you refuse to sign consents on behalf of the patient, make too many requests, demand changes of medication or additional tests, or otherwise interfere with the patient's treatment, it's all recorded in the medical chart. It doesn't matter whether the patient intends to go to the nursing home for short-term rehabilitation services (the highest insurance reimbursement) or long-term care, all that matters is that there are problems that far outweigh the financial benefits to the nursing home. Staff members are used to dealing with some issues, but you'd be amazed at the ways that people mistreat the medical staff.

And so, the dreaded denial is issued. I've seen families so dysfunctional that psychiatrists and social workers are called in to deal with *them* (not the patient) – DENIED! Or those who read about the patient's diagnosis on the internet and become pseudo-experts, demanding certain tests or medications – DENIED! Even the passive-aggressive patients or family members who complain about the hospital's care when the nursing home's liaison is evaluating the patient – DENIED! Families who refuse to provide information to help complete a Medicaid application – DENIED! Family members who are so unhappy with the current nursing home that they request a patient be transferred to another had better have a good reason (such as that nursing home being closer to their home) or the patient's not going anywhere – DENIED! Facilities carefully review the social service and nursing notes, which detail the problems the family or patient has caused.

It doesn't seem fair. A family member once told me that the nursing home for which I worked had a bad reputation and we were the last choice for her aunt; she complained that her first choice had told her that they "weren't able to meet her needs." She demanded that we transfer her aunt to another nursing home, but unfortunately they too "weren't able to meet her needs." A few weeks later, her father became ill and we wouldn't accept him because she was so difficult to work with. The rest of the family was upset and demanded to meet with the administrator, who explained exactly why we wouldn't accept him. This one person took up too much of the staff's time, and her constant threats of suing the nursing home resulted in her father being admitted to a nursing home over 30 miles away. She spent her time driving between facilities, visiting her family members.

Those patients who are admitted to the nursing home and later found to be difficult are dealt with differently; the nursing home can't just discharge them, so they'll wait for their chance to get rid of the patient. If and when he requires hospitalization, the nursing home will pack up his items and refuse to accept him back. The chances of another nursing home being willing to accept this patient are pretty slim, as they too have read the hospital chart that includes the discussions with the nursing home that is refusing to take the patient back.

When attempting to discharge a problem patient, the first thing the hospital will do is to attempt to bully the nursing home from which he was admitted into accepting the patient back by threatening to withhold future admissions. These are fairly empty threats, but the hospital discharge planners will do their best to find a way to punish the nursing home because the way that hospitals view it, the nursing home is obligated to take the patient back. Even if the patient was only in the nursing home for one day, the hospital feels that the nursing home "owns" him forever. The nursing home is painfully aware that by refusing to take the patient back, it won't be getting the "choice" patients for awhile – so it will increase its marketing campaign. The discharge planners will receive more lunches and giveaway items; it's all part of the game.

It's possible that the nursing home will eventually cave in and accept the patient back (and the floor staff will be stuck dealing with the situation), but if not there's usually one nursing home somewhere (often referred to as the "patient dumping grounds") that will accept any patient that's referred. This nursing home probably won't be located in the immediate area, and might have a history of providing such poor patient care that it can't be picky about the patients it receives. In such a case, the patient will be sent to that facility whether or not it's convenient to his family unless they get their lawyers involved. In that case it's possible that the patient will remain in the hospital for months on end while an equitable solution can be found. During that time, the patient will incur hundreds of thousands of dollars in medical costs, which will never be paid.

It's possible that the patient's family isn't the only problem; if the patient himself is rude or demanding, chances are he'll have a difficult time getting into the nursing home. For some reason, people often believe the way to get what they want is to yell and make unreasonable demands; the truth is that the louder you yell, the slower the staff responds. If you demand that the doctor call you, chances are it'll never happen. If you disrespect the staff – especially the nurse manager, physical therapist or social worker – you'll have a tough time coming back from that. It doesn't feel good when you are accused of being incompetent; why would you do that to someone who is responsible for your mother's healthcare? Threatening the staff members with their jobs isn't exactly the most effective method of communication.

The doctor is ultimately in charge of the patient's care; if you don't like the doctor assigned to your family member, you can fire him and get another. Don't yell at the nurses if the doctor doesn't call you back, because the doctor will be yelling at the nurse for giving you his number. Nursing homes aren't hospitals; they rarely have in-house doctors and often must send the patients out of the facility to be seen. This isn't the nurse's fault, but she's the one the family yells at. This makes her grumpy and hard to deal with; a grumpy nurse will turn around and yell at the aides who are providing the personal care services. Nobody wins in this situation, especially the patient.

When questioning staff members about your mother's care, listen carefully to their response. If you are asking a nursing aide what type of medication your mother is taking and they ask you to speak with the nurse – speak with the nurse. The aide's job doesn't include medication management or treatments, and you'll only upset them if you yell at them about something that is out of the scope of their practice.

Many family members are quiet, kind, thoughtful, and bring their concerns to the staff in a positive manner. Those are the ones that are most appreciated. The staff believes that they're providing good care or they wouldn't work there, and it doesn't help to have a demanding family member taking up the majority of their time. They don't have a lot of time to deal with you because they're busy caring for your family member and at least fifteen other residents; please remember this when you're placed on hold as you call the nursing home to inquire how your mother is doing.

This doesn't mean that you can't visit the patient; the staff appreciates family members who are actively involved with patients. But staying all day, interfering with physical therapy and demanding personal service for your family member can create an adversarial relationship with the staff. Nobody wants that.

The caregiving staff isn't the billing office; if you have a problem with the nursing home's billing practices or the way that your insurance is paying, don't yell at the nurses or social workers. Every nursing home watches the bottom line whether or not they're operated for-profit. It's not their fault that your parents don't qualify for Medicaid, or that you can't afford to live without mom's income. Especially in these tough economic times, I've seen many people who can't make it without their parent's financial assistance – but at some point the patient will either be forced to pay for his care or leave. Yelling at the nurses and asking them how many illegal aliens are receiving free care in the nursing home doesn't do anything but make you look like a jerk.

I'm constantly amazed at how people will listen to some random person they met in line in the grocery store when it comes to Medicare and Medicaid, but refuse to speak with a professional about these issues. Random strangers are the last people you should listen to because they don't know what the hell they're talking about. They often have a horror story about how Medicaid threw some old person out on the street. Why someone would accept the advice of a total stranger over a professional is beyond me – but it happens all the time. When that person turns out to be wrong and the nursing home sends you a bill for thousands of dollars, you'll wish you'd never listened to them. If you have questions about the payment, discuss it with the billing office, a social worker, or meet with an elder law attorney – but please don't take it out on the nursing home staff members who are physically caring for your parent. They have no control over such issues.

For the most part, nursing homes are filled with dedicated staff members who like their jobs and want to be there. They want everyone to feel welcome and hope that there will be little conflict with patients and families. Many patients are satisfied with their placement and some nursing homes are truly recognized for their excellence by legitimate organizations.

I've found that many nursing home staff members aren't even aware when the companies they work for settled a wrongful death lawsuit in the millions of dollars or that their most recent state inspection results were below average (or worse). These are things that the administrator and parent company don't share with the floor staff. It's difficult – but possible – to verify a nursing home's claims of excellence, although most people don't have a clue where to start. Use this book as a guide to choosing a nursing home, do your homework and it is possible to make your search for a nursing home a positive experience.

I've worked in nursing homes and hospitals for many years and can tell you from personal experience that no one is ever truly prepared for a family member to be placed in a nursing home. People don't live their lives in anticipation of the day they'll need to apply for Medicaid, their finances are in disarray and the application process can be difficult to understand. There are many issues involved, and people simply don't understand how nursing homes operate. It's difficult for family members to help a patient maneuver through the system that they don't understand themselves, and their questions are often met with a wall of silence from the staff.

Most nursing home employees only know the part of the facility that affects their job, and they might not be able to help you maneuver through the system. The office manager you are trusting to provide professional advice might be a new hire with no practical experience at all. In one nursing home where I worked, the office manager had no clue as to the different payment sources and yet she gave out advice as if she had written the rules. If there is any question as to how your family member will pay for his placement, it's worth the cost of hiring a professional to help understand how the nursing home payment system will affect you and the patient.

The main lesson that I hope people learn about nursing homes from this book is that there are many ways to ensure that your family member receives the best care possible. Talk to the charge nurse, social worker, administrator, complain to the parent corporation, call the ombudsman, or complain to the state licensing bureau. Start small and work your way up, but don't give up if you believe that there is a problem that needs to be addressed. Nursing homes are no longer horrible, awful places where people go to die. They are now places where people go to receive therapy or to live their final days, treated with dignity and respect while they receive necessary medical care.

I've seen so many examples of both good and bad treatment that I wanted to give customers the opportunity to understand how nursing homes operate and allow them to easily maneuver through the system. With the information contained in *The Nursing Home Survival Guide*, you'll have the ability to form a partnership with the nursing home and it will be a less stressful experience for everyone.

Nursing Home Placement – An Overview

It used to be that people rarely strayed from the geographical area where they were raised. It was common to have multiple generations living under one roof, sharing chores and expenses, or at least living nearby. With so much family support available there wasn't a great need for nursing homes. This began to change when the highway system made it easier to travel across the country in a reasonable amount of time and air travel became accessible to the average person. Jobs became more centralized and the workers followed; people moved far away from their families, knowing that they could stay in touch by telephone (and more recently, using email or text messaging). These days a person can be reached almost anywhere in the world, making our planet a much smaller place – satellite calls have even been made from the top of Mt. Everest.

As people began to move further away from their families, they often lost the feeling of connection with their extended family members. The concept of family members caring for one another was difficult to accomplish when people lived hundreds, if not thousands, of miles apart. Caring for a senior became impossible when none of the adult children wanted to move back home and the senior wasn't interested in moving away.

Distance wasn't the only reason that people weren't able to care for frail family members. Women began working outside of the home and there wasn't anyone around during the day to care for a senior, not to mention that the layout of the home might not be conducive to caregiving. Housing lots grew smaller, creating the need for two-story homes that are less accessible to frail seniors who are no longer able to climb stairs.

The type of assistance that a patient receives in a nursing home or other setting when he can't safely live alone is called ***custodial care*** or ***long-term care***. Long-term care became the only option available to an elderly person without family members living nearby to ensure that he received appropriate care. There have always been board & care homes that provide limited assistance to seniors who aren't able to live alone, but when a patient requires personal care it might become difficult for the board & care home to continue to meet his needs. For this reason formal nursing homes began to spring up in many communities – and an entire industry was born. It became part of a natural progression for the elderly to go to a nursing home when they were no longer able to live independently.

At first, a patient's ability to pay determined which nursing home would accept him. There were horror stories about nursing homes and the care they provided to patients who had little or no money, and much of the time the stories were true. Nursing homes were notorious for dumping patients out on the street after they ran out of money, and there wasn't much oversight to ensure that patients received the care that they needed. After the ***Medicaid*** program was created in 1965, nursing homes were able to count on getting paid for most of their patients after they ran out of money. The Medicaid program also implemented regulations and policies that assured patients were treated with dignity and respect. Things weren't perfect; many nursing homes segregated their patients according to payment source, and they were treated differently depending upon who was footing their bill. But it *was* progress, and people who had gone broke paying for nursing home placement no longer had to worry about being placed out on the curb. At first it wasn't difficult to get a Medicaid application approved – the system accepted anyone with little proof of their financial status. Patients were approved even if they gave away (**gifted**) their assets to family members in order to meet the eligibility criteria.

The Medicaid program has changed dramatically over the past 45 years, and so has its rules and the oversight it provides. It's not only much harder to qualify for Medicaid, it's now illegal for a nursing home to discriminate on the basis of payment source. A patient whose room & board are paid by the Medicaid program might be sharing a room with a patient who is paying privately, with both receiving exactly the same quality of care. Medicaid payments to nursing homes have increased over the years, but they often don't cover the entire cost of caring for patients. As a result, nursing home corporations are always looking for ways to increase their revenue.

These days, nearly every nursing home in the United States accepts Medicaid as a payment source; not because the owners are kind-hearted folks, but because there's a guaranteed payment source for those patients who run out of money after paying the nursing home privately for years. Some nursing homes limit the number of Medicaid patients that they will accept because they can charge more for patients with other sources of payment. It's legal for the nursing home to do so, and is the reason many Medicaid patients are placed on waiting lists for admission. However, nursing homes receive most of their patient referrals from hospitals, and they will often accept a patient whose payment is Medicaid in order to also receive referrals for patients with higher payment sources.

As the laws have evolved, it's become increasingly difficult for nursing homes to discharge a problem patient once he's been admitted. Family members are wising up, and are doing their best to manipulate the system in their favor. They can get a patient in the door by promising to pay privately for his room & board, only to apply for Medicaid as soon as he gets there. Although nursing homes attempt to fight this strategy they still must follow all of the applicable laws regarding discharge. One method that nursing homes is to require that the family sign forms accepting financial responsibility for the patient's stay; however, in many cases this paperwork isn't presented to the family until a week or more after the patient has been admitted. At that point the family can refuse to sign the form and there might be nothing that the nursing home can do to force them (refer to the section entitled *Determining the Payment Source: "Free" Nursing Home Placement* for additional information about financial responsibility). Those patients who don't qualify for Medicaid or other types of payment for indigent patients might very well remain in the nursing home for free until an appropriate discharge plan can be developed. Of course, the nursing home won't tell you this – it's something that they would rather you not know.

Nursing homes have other ways of generating revenue besides providing general long-term care services; they're often able to bill Medicare and Medicaid for extra (called *ancillary*) services such as rehabilitation, skilled nursing care, and behavior management programs that generate much of the profits in the nursing home industry. In the early days of those programs, nursing homes could bill for pretty much any type of service because there wasn't a lot of government oversight. *The Centers for Medicare and Medicaid Services (CMS)* has since made it more complicated for nursing homes to bill for ancillary services, forcing the nursing home to justify every charge that's submitted. However, these extra services continue to remain vital to the nursing home's financial bottom line.

Nursing homes used to be more concerned about the amount that they'd receive on a per patient basis, because Medicaid paid a higher daily rate for those patients who required more care. The amount of care that a patient requires is called his *acuity*; the higher the acuity, the greater the revenue the nursing home could expect. Patients with a higher acuity would be admitted directly from the hospital, with the nursing home counting on being paid handsomely for the first 100 days under the Medicare benefit. After the Medicare benefit had been exhausted, the nursing home would "roll them over" to Medicaid as a payment source and continue to charge separately for each service it provided. Most of the time nursing homes weren't required to justify the amounts for which they were billing; the system was easy to manipulate in order to receive the maximum amount of revenue.

Nowadays, nursing homes aren't as concerned about admitting patients with higher acuities. In most areas, Medicaid payments to nursing homes are calculated based on the average acuity of all of their patients, rather than paying a different amount for each patient. Nursing homes aren't as concerned about the amount of care each patient requires as they are about the total amount they'll ultimately be paid, and their ability to hold down costs. Nursing homes are no longer able to charge extra for each service they provide to their patients, and must eat the cost of treatments such as feeding tubes, IV's, wound care and equipment such as specialty hospital beds and wheelchairs.

The practice of admitting a patient following a hospital admission is still quite common; in fact, it's the easiest and best way for a patient to become admitted into a facility. Most patients qualify for Medicare to pay for skilled nursing care or physical therapy after a hospital discharge. However, Medicare regulations are much harder for the nursing home to manipulate, and there's no longer a guarantee that the patient will qualify to receive the full 100 days of services covered by the Medicare Part A benefit. Before accepting the patient, many nursing homes estimate the amount of time the patient will be paid via Medicare; if it doesn't appear that the patient will qualify long enough for the nursing home to turn a profit the patient will be denied entry.

A patient's payment source, both long and short-term, is extremely important to the nursing home and is often the reason that a patient is denied. Medicaid patients are often placed on a waiting list in the hopes that they will give up and eventually find another facility. Even though federal law states that a person can't be discriminated against because of his payment source, placing a patient on a waiting list isn't illegal and discrimination is difficult to prove. All of this can be confusing to those people whose parents require care that can no longer be provided at home; they're simply looking for a place to send their parents in the final stages of their lives. But just because they can't provide care for their parent, it doesn't mean that a nursing home is the most appropriate place for the patient to be.

There are minimum physical requirements that patients must meet in order to qualify for nursing home placement, and those who don't meet the level of care criteria set by CMS won't be approved for nursing home placement regardless of their ability to pay. Patients must require assistance with certain *activities of daily living (ADL's)* such as eating, bathing, and toileting themselves, or require medical treatments that can't easily be provided in another setting.

If the patient doesn't meet the level of care required for nursing home placement, he will need to utilize other caregiving options available. These options include hiring in-home care or being admitted to an *assisted living facility (ALF)*. An inability to afford other types of care doesn't make a patient appropriate for nursing home placement; the patient must present a physical need or he won't be allowed to remain in a nursing home. Although Medicaid pays for 24-hour care in a nursing home, the program rarely pays for enough care to help a senior remain in his own home. Unfortunately, low-income patients are usually forced to go to a nursing home rather than to have enough care provided at a lesser cost in their home.

Whether or not a patient can afford to pay for services out of his own pocket, he might be eligible to receive payment for additional services from a Medicaid Waiver program, the Veteran's Administration or via a *Long-term Care Insurance* policy. There are many different caregiving options, and often the doctor, a social worker or other professional can help to provide direction as you attempt to decide what might be best for your family member.

How to Determine the Patient's Needs

There are many different types, or levels, of care that can be provided to a patient. They vary from limited in-home care by a private caregiving agency to nursing home placement paid by public dollars (Medicaid). There are pros and cons to each type of care, many of which aren't covered by Medicaid or Medicare. The levels of care are all based on the patient's ability to perform *activities of daily living (ADL's)* which include bathing, eating, dressing, walking, toileting and bed mobility, or *instrumental activities of daily living (IADL's)* which include shopping, managing finances, meal preparation, performing housework, using a telephone, and administering his own medications or treatments (such as insulin injections for diabetes).

Patients often require nursing home placement, but they're not ready to accept that they're no longer able to maintain their independence. A good way to gauge the level of care that the patient requires is to evaluate the amount of ADL's that he is able to perform. If the patient is able to remain independent except for some assistance with shopping and meal preparation, he's obviously able to remain at home. However, if he's unable to walk, dress, take his medications, do his laundry and cook his meals, he's probably (physically) ready for nursing home placement. Hopefully he'll be willing to accept the assistance.

It's common for hospitalized patients to suddenly be told they're being discharged to a nursing home, having been provided with no warning at all. Many discharges occur late on Friday afternoon and if patients refuse to leave, they or their families might be threatened with having to pay huge amounts out of their own pocket. Patients often feel bullied into accepting whichever facility is presented to them as the next step in their recovery and trust that the nursing home was carefully chosen to meet the patient's specific needs. There could be any number of reasons that particular nursing home was chosen, but it's doubtful that the facility's superior record and ability to meet that patient's needs will be a factor. Chances are that it was the first nursing home to accept the patient, or it might be the only one that works with the patient's insurance plan. Medicare Advantage plans develop contracts with nursing homes that are willing to accept rock-bottom prices, and it's possible that the quality of care suffers in turn.

Once the patient and his family have been told which facility will be serving him after he's discharged, they'll be presented with forms that clearly state they were offered a choice of provider and that they chose that specific nursing home. These "patient choice" forms are designed to protect the hospital from claims of steering patients toward specific facilities, because it's illegal for hospitals to funnel all of their patients to one nursing home. Family members often feel pressured to sign the forms, which are part of the discharge instructions, but they don't have to sign anything they don't want to. If they felt railroaded into accepting a certain facility, they can write that on the form – or simply refuse to sign it. Nothing bad will happen to them if they choose not to sign the Patient Choice form.

Don't just accept it when the case managers tell you that a specific nursing home is the best facility for your family member. Ask why, and feel free to visit the new facility to see what it's like. Ask around, and review the nursing home's caregiving record on the Medicare and state department of health websites. The nursing home that the hospital chose for the patient might not be convenient to the family, might not be highly rated and might very well have the worst reputation in town. The accepting facility might have been chosen because it recently brought lunch to the case managers, or might be affiliated with the hospital in some way. In other words, the nursing home might meet the hospital's needs – not the patient's.

Patients and their families aren't aware that they have the right to refuse a transfer or discharge until they've had the opportunity to research their next step; all that they know is that the hospital case manager is rushing them and can be very intimidating in these instances. The hospital administration is pressuring the case manager to get the patient out and the family is stuck in the middle. At that point it's possible that the social worker or case manager will attempt to send the patient to any facility that will accept him. It's intimidating when a case manager informs a family member that their father will be discharged at 3:00pm; this notice is often provided by phone and the family feels powerless. The hospital staff won't tell you that late afternoon is the worst time for a patient to be admitted to a nursing home (see the chapter "*Admissions Day*.")

To ensure that that patients don't feel railroaded into a nursing home admission, family members should begin researching facilities in the area from the day that the patient is admitted to the hospital. It's best to make an informed choice ahead of time rather than to wait to be told that this will be the next step in the recovery process. Hospitals, nursing homes and other healthcare providers don't like it getting out that patients have the right to delay a discharge; the only way the patient can truly be forced to move is if the hospital legally evicts the patient (a lengthy legal process). Healthcare providers don't want you to know how little power they actually have and they definitely don't want the state regulatory agency intervening with their patients. Threatening to call the state is often all the patient needs to do in order to buy enough time to choose a nursing home or rehabilitation center.

Patients are often steered toward certain agencies even if they're being discharged home with services; hospital corporations often require that their staff members refer to the home or hospice providers affiliated with the hospital. If the doctor works for the hospital corporation, it's highly probable he will recommend the company-owned provider because that's what the hospital administration wants. It's also possible that the doctor will refer the patient to a home health company (or outpatient physical therapy clinic) in which he has a financial interest. This is just a

14

thinly veiled attempt on the hospital's or doctor's behalf to create more revenue for their preferred corporation *and is illegal*. Patients and their families have the right to choose who will provide their care and the hospital has to honor the request, with the only exception being whether or not the patient's insurance is contracted with the provider of their choosing.

In an attempt to justify the referral, staff members might claim that the providers affiliated with the hospital will have more complete access to the patient's information. What they're not telling you is that the hospital is required to provide the exact same information to whichever agency or nursing home that the patient requests. Affiliation with the hospital doesn't necessarily translate into better care for the patient; in fact, because these companies are guaranteed the majority of referrals from that hospital it's possible that the care provided isn't as good as the care provided by other agencies in the area. These other agencies have to work harder and receive their referrals based on their service and reputation. One thing is certain – the hospital would prefer that it benefit financially in every way possible, regardless of the patient's preference. Hospital staff members often have to meet with members of administration to justify why they aren't referring more patients to company-affiliated home health and hospice providers. A hospital for which I worked required these rather uncomfortable meetings every two weeks, where a member of administration yelled at us and questioned our professional ethics. It was loads of fun.

Regardless of which facility is discharging them, patients have the right to choose their service provider. It isn't up to the discharging facility to limit patient choice – in fact, it's illegal. I worked for a nursing home where the administrator severely limited patient's choice of home health providers and rarely allowed hospice referrals. She instructed the staff to tell patients that this was because her favored agencies provided the best care (she privately bragged that these agencies always referred back to her, which is considered to be an "in-kind referral" and is prohibited under Medicare rules.) Patients were told that they must, at the very least, allow the agencies to perform an initial in-home evaluation (for which Medicare paid handsomely). Patients and their families didn't realize that they were being exploited. I was present when this administrator ordered her staff to find out who was informing patients they had a right to choose their company; she stated that they were interfering with her referrals and intended to fire them. This administrator was later fired for her actions, but remains employed in the industry.

Patients not only have the right to choose their providers, they also have the right to refuse treatment or even to remain at home without services if they wish. This is true even if it appears to be a poor choice on their part. As long as they are competent to make decisions, people have the right to make poor choices. The best that can be done is for the medical provider to present the information, explain how the patient can benefit from the offered services, and to document the encounter. Facilities must help the patient choose the agency (or facility) that is able to provide the level of care that would best suit his needs within the amounts that he is able to pay. Patients can't be forced to accept assistance as long as they are able to make informed choices.

Home Health Care

A patient might qualify for services in his home after he has been discharged from a healthcare facility, or might qualify for services in his home whether or not he has recently been discharged from a healthcare facility. A referral can be made as long as his primary doctor believes he requires medical care. Medicare, Medicaid and most insurance companies will pay for a patient to receive *home health care* from a licensed nursing agency if as the patient requires intermittent services that must be provided by registered nurses, physical therapists, occupational and speech therapists. These services are referred to as *skilled services*. Depending upon his needs, the patient might also qualify for a nurse's aide to help with bathing and personal care.

In addition to his presenting a medical need, the patient must be home-bound, meaning that he must be confined to his home except for medical appointments or other necessary trips. The definition of homebound can be somewhat murky, but essentially the patient must not be able to leave the house except for medical appointments or to access necessary treatments. A quick trip to the grocery store to pick up a few food items while accessing the pharmacy is okay, but for the most part, if the patient is able to leave the house to go grocery shopping he is also able to access outpatient services. It doesn't matter that a patient doesn't have a car, or that there's no taxi or medical transportation available in the area; a lack of transportation doesn't render a patient homebound. If the patient is able to freely come and go, he is able to go to an outpatient clinic or rehabilitation facility to obtain necessary treatments and doesn't qualify for home health care.

The services provided by home healthcare agencies are limited to visits for specific reasons, such as an hour or so for the nurse to change a dressing, or for a physical therapist to provide therapy in the patient's home. If the patient appears to need community referrals, they might be referred to an agency social worker. However, these services are designed to be for specific medical purposes only, not to provide supervision while the primary caregiver is out of the house. It is not custodial care.

Home health care services are designed to rehabilitate the patient back to his former level of functioning, and to ensure his safety in his home or in an assisted living. The care is generally short-term in nature, for a month or two, although this service might be provided as long as the patient demonstrates a need for the skilled care. As soon as the patient has recovered to the point that he can access care on an outpatient basis, the home health care is no longer necessary. There are generally no out-of-pocket costs to the patient for home health care, although there are copayments and/or deductibles charged for medical equipment and miscellaneous supplies.

The length and amount of services provided is based on a complicated formula provided by Medicare or by the patient's insurance company. The patient's diagnosis, prior medical treatments and estimated ability to participate in therapies are entered into a computer program, and the program authorizes a certain amount of visits. As the patient's status changes, the information is updated and the length of treatment is adjusted. Those patients whose bills are paid by private insurance generally follow the same rules as Medicare, although they're often monitored by a case manager whose responsibility is to hold down costs. If the patient or family believes that the patient requires additional medical care for which the insurance won't pay, they're able to appeal a denial of services. They are also welcome to pay privately for the service, although this can be extremely expensive.

Most communities offer several home health care agencies from which to choose, and whether or not they're run for-profit they still operate in the same manner. Just like other medical providers, these agencies send out professional marketers to healthcare providers in the hopes of obtaining patient referrals. A physician who refers to one agency might truly believe that agency is better than the others, or he might be responding to their marketing tactics. It's also possible that physician is the medical director for the home health agency, and that he's steering patients to the agency because his payment is based on the number of patients served. This behavior is not only highly unethical, it's also illegal. Unfortunately, people out in the community don't understand the laws or know how to complain, and the behavior often goes unreported. Most of the time, patients trust that their doctor has their best interests in mind when referring to an agency, but isps possible that he's rewarding the sales representative who brings him the nicest pens or the best lunches.

It's also fairly common for hospital administrators to attempt to limit referrals to agencies owned by the facility's parent corporation; staff members are often afraid to report such unethical behaviors because they can easily lose their jobs. Hospitals can make it difficult for outside agencies to serve their patients by insisting that they only enter the hospital if invited; they must sign in at the front desk and the hospitals limit their access to patients and their charts. At the same time, they are providing an office for the affiliated agency liaison and providing him with open access to patient medical records. The nurses and social workers are pushing their agencies to the patients and families, and the doctors are instructed to write orders referring patients to the corporate-owned entities. The patient choice forms often offer the hospital-preferred entity as the first option, and if the patient says that they have no preference the agency affiliated with the hospital will receive the referral.

Just as with all other medical providers, patients don't appear to realize that in most cases they have the right to choose which agency they want, and that the referring doctor, hospital or nursing home is required to honor their decision without coercion. It's illegal to limit a patient's choices; hospitals and other providers who do so can lose their ability to participate in the Medicare & Medicaid programs. If it can be proven that a healthcare provider is receiving incentives or has been promised that the agency will return the favor at some point in the future, they can actually be sentenced to jail time. Of course, this is extremely hard to prove and usually goes unreported.

Even if the allegations aren't able to be substantiated, it's possible that an investigation will stop such behaviors in the future. A quick call to the Medicare fraud hotline at *1-800-Medicare* will start an investigation; for more information go to www.Medicare.gov and search the website using "report fraud." In addition to reporting suspected fraud to Medicare, there are state agencies that are contracted with Medicare to investigate these issues. These agencies include the nursing home Ombudsman, or the Area Agency on Aging.

Patients with private insurance or HMO's/PPO's might not have as many providers from which to choose; they will be required to use an agency or nursing home that contracts with the insurance company. In most cases, patients will still have a choice of providers but this choice might be limited to a few companies. It's also possible that the company that a patient prefers is able to negotiate a one-time contract in order to serve that patient, although this is a rare occurrence.

The competition for patients is fierce: a common practice for home health agencies is to attempt to "lay claim" to a patient who is in a nursing home or hospital by obtaining the names of potential patients from a staff member. The marketer will then tape his business card on the front of the patient chart, and then "follow" the patient throughout the hospital and the rehabilitation center. When the patient is finally ready to be discharged home, the patient will be referred to that agency without anyone asking questions. In most cases, the patient won't be offered a choice of provider, as it is assumed that the agency has a prior relationship with him. Marketers will also "claim" former patients and insist that they receive the referral upon the patient's discharge; essentially they'll use whatever tactic necessary in order to gain as many referrals as possible for their agency.

Regardless of which agency the hospital recommends or who is attempting to claim him, a patient and/or his family members nearly always have the option of choosing the home health care agency they prefer (unless that agency doesn't accept the patient's insurance plan or operates out of the patient's service area). All that they have to do is tell a staff member which company they want and the facility is required to make a referral. If the facility refuses to refer to your agency of choice, feel free to call the home health agency yourself. They'll take it from there.

Hospice Care

Hospice Care, which is also called *Palliative Care* or *Terminal Care*, is a type of medical care designed to make a patient comfortable by providing medications, supplies, nursing, counseling and assistance with personal care as they progress through the dying process. A patient who has been diagnosed with a terminal condition might qualify to receive hospice care as long as he meets certain clinical criteria that indicates he has a prognosis of six months or less. This is a decision that a physician makes with the patient, and the patient has to be willing to stop receiving aggressive treatment and to accept comfort care.

The most common payment source for hospice is Medicare, although Medicaid, the Veteran's Administration and private insurance plans also pay for hospice care. Most hospices will provide free care for patients who don't have the ability to pay, although charity care is generally provided on a case-by-case basis. Many hospice companies also offer a charitable foundation that can be used to help fund the care that they provide to patients who aren't able to pay for the services. These funds can also be used to help with specialty items not usually provided by the hospice, such as the rental of a motorized wheelchair. In most cases, payment for hospice care usually follows the Medicare model; the hospice receives a daily rate and must provide hospice care to the patient regardless of the actual costs. Hospices make their profits based on patient volume and their ability to hold down costs.

It's important to understand that hospice is not a place; it is a type of care that can be provided in a patient's home or that of a family member, a group home, an assisted living facility, a nursing home, or just about anywhere. The hospice benefit is designed to supplement the care in the home, although it doesn't replace the need for a primary caregiver. Hospice patients who live alone are encouraged to develop a caregiving plan so that their needs can be met as they continue to decline.

Hospice care provides for light homemaking, personal care, skilled nursing, social services, spiritual care and delivery of medications to the patient's home. It also provides medical equipment and supplies such as gloves, wipes, and incontinence briefs. The care is usually limited to about an hour each day; hospice programs do not provide 24-hour (custodial) care in the home. A hospice social worker can help to coordinate in-home caregiving, but the hospice itself doesn't provide this service. Unlike home health care services, hospice patients don't have to be homebound to receive hospice care; in fact, patients are encouraged to leave the house if at all possible.

For those patients who aren't able to remain at home, many communities offer small privately owned homes that offer 24-hour care to hospice patients. These homes often aren't required to be licensed in the same manner as larger facilities, although they generally must meet state guidelines of some type. Additionally, hospices with stand-alone inpatient units might possibly hold out a couple of rooms for long-term patients. For the most part, though, patients receive hospice care wherever they live.

Under the Medicare benefit, hospices are required to offer a five-day "respite," which allows caregivers to take a much needed break. These respite admissions are generally provided in nursing homes, although they can also be provided in hospice inpatient units. Many private insurance companies don't provide payment to hospices for respite admissions because they are designed to help the caregiver and not the patient. It's up to each individual hospice as to whether it will provide for respite care if the insurance carrier isn't willing to provide reimbursement.

Hospices also provide a higher level of care for patients whose symptoms need to be managed by nurses (and doctors) for a short period of time. This level of care is called *General Inpatient Care* or *G.I.P.*, and it must be provided in a facility that is staffed by registered nurses who are present 24-hours per day. This requirement limits the environment to a skilled nursing facility, hospice inpatient unit or hospital. Regardless of whether the patient is admitted to a facility for respite or inpatient services, at the time he is ready for discharge he will be sent to his home or wherever he lived before he entered the facility unless other arrangements have been made.

The services that hospices provide aren't as limited as the services that are provided by home health agencies; hospices must develop a plan of care depending upon patient need. If the patient requires daily personal care (bathing, changing briefs, etc), a nurse's aide will be scheduled every day. If the patient refuses to allow an aide to assist with bathing, no aide will be scheduled. Nursing visits are scheduled according to the patient's needs as well; they might vary from bi-weekly visits to daily visits depending upon the patient's physical needs. Social workers, chaplains and volunteers are sent into the home to provide extra support for hospice patients according to the patient's schedule. Hospices must be flexible in the care they provide, and must have nurses available 24-hours per day to answer questions and to make home visits.

In most cases hospice programs don't order or pay for laboratory tests, x-rays, MRI's or other tests mainly because the patient's treatment plan won't change regardless of the test results. The goal is for the patient to remain as comfortable as possible by providing all of the services that he needs. Because the hospice is able to provide for their medical needs, patients aren't able to go to the hospital – even the emergency room – without prior authorization. If a patient decides to seek treatment without first coordinating with the hospice, he will have to pay for these services out-of-pocket or revoke the hospice benefit in order to receive the treatment.

Hospices employ professional marketers who use the same sales practices as do home health care agencies, and their medical directors often refer their private practice patients to the hospice without allowing the patient any other choices. Hospital corporations that own hospice and home health care agencies strongly encourage their staff members to keep their referrals in-house, and often require an explanation when referrals are made to outside agencies. Nursing homes and assisted living facilities often attempt to limit their patients' choice of providers to ones that they favor. This is highly unethical and might even be illegal, yet it continues. The Medicare program rarely monitors agency referrals; abuses are difficult to prove and the competition is fierce for every patient signed onto service.

If you or your family member is referred to a hospice program, you have the right to choose any program that serves your geographical area – although if you are a resident of a nursing home, the hospice program that you choose must have a contract with that particular facility. Remember that every hospice operates in the same manner and must follow the same rules, whether or not the hospice is a non-profit or for-profit entity. A great method of choosing a hospice is to ask your friends and neighbors if they've had any experience with a local hospice, or to speak with a trusted family physician and asking for his input.

In-Home Care

In-Home Care is housekeeping and non-medical personal care assistance that is an excellent solution for patients who need help to remain in their homes, although it doesn't necessarily have to be *nursing* care. Private in-home caregiving agencies can be found in the nursing section of the yellow pages, although some Medicare accredited home health agencies provide this type of care in addition to their medical services. In-home care can be provided concurrently with other services such as home health care or hospice care. In-home care is also referred to as *Custodial Care.*

In-home care is generally paid out of the patient's pocket, although there are some Medicaid Waiver programs that will pay for extra services in the home. Long-term care policies might also cover some or all of the cost of in-home care, although every policy is different. This type of care is often considered to be non-medical, although many agencies provide nursing services as well. The majority of care is provided by homemakers, caregivers and certified nursing assistants. Most agencies will provide care at an hourly rate, usually with a two or four-hour minimum. Some agencies allow the caregiving hours to be split; for example, a worker from the agency can arrive for two hours in the morning to shower and provide for other personal care needs as well as to prepare the patient breakfast, while another worker arrives in the evening to help the patient to bed and do a load of laundry. It's up to each individual agency as to whether it will split caregiver hours because it depends on how far the workers will have to travel and how many caregivers they have available.

Along with the help of a personal alert button and a medication box that alarms to remind him when to take his medications, in-home caregiving can be an excellent way to ensure that the patient's needs are met at home either on a long-term basis or until he is able to get back on his feet as he recovers from a hospitalization.

Agencies that provide in-home care are usually professionally staffed, meaning that they perform background checks on their workers and generally provide their staff members with ongoing training. These agencies are licensed, bonded, and provide liability insurance as well as worker's compensation, which protects against lawsuits should the worker get hurt in the patient's home. Their insurance also protects the agency from liability if a patient is injured while receiving care.

There are rarely laws requiring that in-home care be provided by an agency, and some people choose to pay a family member or private party to provide caregiving services at a substantially lesser cost. Paying a private party – one arranged on your own, not through an agency – to stay with a patient can be a huge financial and personal liability. It's important to speak with your homeowner's insurance provider to make sure that household help is covered, in case the person is injured while caring for the patient (or steals from the home). There might also be tax implications for hiring household help without paying employment taxes. I've had people tell me that there's little chance that they'll be caught, only to attempt to write off the cost of the caregiver on their income taxes. The IRS has no sense of humor when it comes to these issues.

Hiring a private caregiver also means that there's no guarantee the person caring for the patient is properly trained to provide assistance, or that he'll be committed to the patient. If the caregiver leaves without notice, the patient is on his own. Family members should check in daily to ensure that the patient is receiving the promised care, and should remain alert to signs of abuse. It's also best to limit the caregiver's access to the patient's finances or valuable items. There have been many people financially exploited by a caregiver who has worked his way into a patient's life only to rob them blind. Hiring an agency helps to ensure that this doesn't happen to you or your family member.

The cost for in-home caregivers varies; it might be as little as $10 per hour in a smaller town to $30 per hour in a larger city. In-home care is rarely covered by a regular health insurance policy. Medicaid programs often pay for limited assistance in the home, but only from agencies with which they have a contract (this will limit the patient's ability to choose his provider). Some Medicaid programs even pay family members to provide assistance in the home, but in most cases there's a maximum amount of hours covered (generally 2-3 hours per day). Depending upon the state, this type of assistance might be immediate or there might be a lengthy waiting list before services are available. This type of care is intermittent and limited according to the amount of Medicaid financing available.

It is possible to pay a person or agency to provide 24-hour care in the patient's home, although this can be quite expensive. An in-home caregiving agency can cost $6,000 (or more) per month for a live-in caregiver, with a relief caregiver on the weekends. ~~The cost for 24-hour in-home care is usually more expensive than placement in the nicest assisted living facility or nursing home.~~ The benefit is that the patient is able to remain at home. The disadvantage is that a stranger is living in the patient's home, and the patient is fairly isolated to the caregiver or to those people who visit the patient's home. This opens up the possibility that the patient will be exploited financially or even physically abused without being discovered, which is why it's so important that the family remain involved and visit as often as possible. Those families that aren't able to visit should make arrangements for friends or even community professionals to visit the patient to ensure their safety and continued well-being.

Most private caregiving agencies are able to provide 24-hour caregivers if given enough notice. It can be difficult for an agency to find a worker who is able to start providing 24-hour care on an immediate basis. Again, the benefit to the patient is that he will be able to remain n his home, but the possibility remains that the worker will become sick or have to leave suddenly and the patient might possibly be left alone until other arrangements can be made. It's also possible that the caregiver can leave without notifying the family and the patient could be alone for hours or even days until someone discovers that the caregiver has left.

Many families attempt to save money by offering free room & board to a college student to stay with the senior, but it's important to remember that this person will be gone all day (or night) to attend college and enjoy a social life; he might spend much of his time at home studying instead of attending to the senior. A student might also need to work outside the home, which further limits the amount of assistance the senior will receive. There is also the possibility that "nice" student is stealing from the patient or is abusive, something that you won't know unless you visit frequently. If a stranger offers to move in with a senior, they probably are homeless and need a place to live. A person desperate for a place to live might not be the best person to provide care to your family member.

The Veteran's Administration will also pay a limited amount for veterans who require in-home care; if the patient is receiving assistance from the VA it's possible he can receive in-home care from that program. It's best to ask the VA doctor if this type of assistance is available.

There are non-profit agencies that provide immediate in-home care via the Veteran's Administration *Aid & Attendance* benefit; they apply on the patient's behalf, pay for the care the patient receives and are later reimbursed when the patient's benefit is awarded. They do not advance money; they only provide care in the home. This type of service isn't helpful when it comes to paying for nursing home room & board, but by sending in caregivers a veteran might be able to remain at home with his family. For more information on Aid & Attendance, refer to the section *"Other Veteran's Programs"* in the chapter entitled **Determining the Payment Source**.

You get what you pay for, and the patient deserves the best of care. There are good, honest people who are willing to provide care to the elderly, but if these people can't be easily located or the care can't be reasonably provided in the patient's home, it's best to look into alternative arrangements for the patient's care.

Adult Day Care Programs

As we age we often lose the ability to live independently. Many people choose to move a senior into their household, but providing 24-hour care can be a difficult endeavor. It isn't easy to care for a senior at home while attempting to run a busy household and, in many cases, hold down a full-time job. This is the reason that seniors are placed in alternative settings such as assisted living facilities or nursing homes. Even though this provides the care the senior requires, it also removes the senior from a familiar environment.

Another option is to utilize the services of an adult day care program. These programs cost anywhere from $50 to $150 per day, depending upon the location and the senior's physical needs. Much of the time the cost includes transportation to and from the program, and in many areas the care is provided on a 24-hour basis (a bonus for the family member who works the swing or graveyard shift). Some aging waiver programs pay for adult day care via Medicaid, or there are grant-funded programs that will help to pay for day care services. Unfortunately, with the current economic climate, Medicaid programs that provide day care are experiencing deep program cutbacks.

Adult Day Care programs can be a wonderful caregiving option, in that they provide a safe environment for seniors to spend the day or night. They offer organized activities, meals and the opportunity to socialize with others. Most don't offer medical care, and instead contract with home health agencies so that patients can receive their medications during the day as scheduled. Depending upon their licensing and the senior's ability to assist with administering his medications, it's possible that a senior with a condition such as Diabetes can be served in a day care program. Some programs also offer medical assistance such physical & occupational therapies, nursing assistance, etc. but the cost of this type of program is much higher than a program designed to offer socialization.

There are specific adult day care providers that serve seniors with Alzheimer's and other dementias; they offer fenced yards and activity programs designed specifically for these residents. Day care providers must be licensed and are subject to inspections and regulations just the same as many other facilities. For additional information about Adult Day care providers in your area, contact your Area Agency on Aging or contact the daycare providers directly.

Assisted Living Facilities (ALF)

A patient might not require 24-hour *nursing* care, yet still requires assistance with his ***independent activities of daily living (IADL's)***. These include supervision and monitoring to ensure his safety, grocery shopping and assistance with meal preparation, housekeeping and laundry services. This level of care might possibly be provided in an ***assisted living facility (ALF)***, which can be a small facility with a few beds (known as a ***group home***), or a large corporate-run facility with over a hundred private apartment units. An ALF typically saves the patient thousands of dollars per year over the cost of nursing home placement and is an excellent caregiving option for people who don't require 24-hour nursing care.

Some Assisted Living Facilities are able to offer a higher level of care to those patients who require assistance with their ***Activities of Daily Living (ADL's)***, which include bathing, transferring in/out of bed, toileting, eating and ambulating. The greater the patient's needs, the more the ALF will charge for the assistance provided. It depends upon the state and local rules as to the type of care an ALF is able to provide – sometimes the patient must be independent when they're first admitted with the care the ALF provides increasing as the patient declines. For answers to your questions as to the type of care your family member might need, contact your local Area Agency on Aging.

The most common form of payment for an assisted living facility is for the senior to pay privately from his own funds. Some long-term insurance policies pay for this level of care, and there are also Medicaid waiver programs that help to fund a patient in an ALF. Check with your Area Agency on Aging about Medicaid-based programs available where you live.

There are other benefits to ALF's than just financial considerations. In most instances, patients have private rooms or apartments that they are able to decorate with their own furniture and personal items. ALF's are considerably less restrictive than nursing homes; seniors are allowed to come and go as they please (unless they are in a locked unit for dementia), can choose to eat in the dining room or in their private room without staff interfering, and patients' medications can be self-administered if they are able to do so. ALF's usually provide transportation to medical appointments as well as to offer social outings and other activities.

It used to be that patients went to assisted living facilities until they declined to point that they couldn't walk; at that point patients were required to move to nursing homes. This was because the assisted living staff members weren't able to safely evacuate all of the patients in the event of a fire. However, buildings now must meet stricter fire codes and are safer environments for the elderly; it's now possible for a patient to remain in his home environment (the ALF) until his death.

Most ALF's don't provide nurses on-site; medications are generally passed to the residents by a nurse's aide or a specially trained medication aide. The larger

ALF's might have a nurse on staff who oversees the personal care and medications, as well as to assess patients prior to being admitted to the facility. Most of the smaller ALF's don't have nurses on staff, but will hire a nurse as a consultant if required. It's important to understand that nurses who work in ALF's generally don't provide hands-on care; if the patient requires nursing care it will generally be provided by a home-health agency.

A lack of professional medical staff in an ALF doesn't create a problem because the residents don't necessarily require medical care. The caregiving staff is trained in emergency procedures including CPR; if a patient appears to be in distress they'll call 911 and send the patient to the emergency room (it's important to note that this is the exact same protocol followed in a nursing home). Sometimes family members are afraid to send a patient to an ALF because the patient might fall and break a hip, but the truth is that a patient can just as easily fall and break a hip in a nursing home. Since ALF's often have carpeting, chances are that a fall will be less serious in an ALF than if it occurred in a nursing home (or hospital) with tile floors.

Patients who are frail and require a nurse to assess them on a regular basis might possibly be better served in a nursing home, although a home health agency, hospice, or private nursing service can provide this service to a resident of an ALF. Unless a higher level of medical care is required, patients are often happier in an ALF and enjoy the home-like atmosphere. Living in an ALF is often a happy medium between remaining at home and being admitted to a nursing home, if the payment issue can be worked out.

Most people follow the recommendations of their doctor, who responds to the marketing representatives that frequent medical offices and hospitals. This is the reason that a doctor will recommend a patient be placed in a nursing home even though the patient can be cared for at less than half the cost in an ALF. The doctor probably doesn't understand how much assistance the ALF can provide, nor does he have the time to personally check the facilities. An ALF is often a good alternative to nursing home placement when the patient's needs are able to be met in a less restrictive, less institutional environment; as long as the ALF is willing to accept the patient the doctor can't dictate where the patient lives. If your doctor refuses to discuss or "allow" your family member to be admitted to an ALF, it's worth the time and energy to speak with him about his concerns. The ultimate decision is up to the patient and the assisted living facility.

A resident of an ALF is able to receive physical therapy or nursing services from a home health agency in the same manner as if he were living in his own home. Many ALF's offer gyms and some have in-house contracts with physical therapy companies as well. Patients who live in ALF's may receive care from hospices just as if they lived at home and have the right to choose their provider; unlike nursing homes, hospices aren't required to have a contract with ALF's to provide services to their patients. The facility's administrator might attempt to steer you toward an agency that he prefers, although in most cases it has nothing to do with the care the hospice provides. The ALF might believe that the hospice provides excellent care, but it's also possible that the hospice is paying illegal kickbacks for the referrals.

If a patient prefers to live in an ALF and has the ability to pay, all that must be done to determine whether the ALF can meet his needs is to visit a facility and speak with the admissions clerk. The ALF will request medical information from the doctor and might schedule a nursing assessment to determine whether the facility is able to meet his needs. The facility will coordinate with the doctor and order medications to ensure the patient has a smooth transition into the facility.

The requirements for assisted living facilities vary from state to state, and they're monitored via annual inspections from the same agency that monitors nursing home care. If ALF's aren't able to provide the level of professional services that are required, they'll lose their licensure. Since most ALF's don't receive federal funding, the facility won't lose out financially but it will lose its ability to provide services. If that happens, it's likely that the facility will be closed. There are ways around the closure, as was discovered in Iowa in 2009.

> In 2009, an ALF in Iowa willingly surrendered its license after being fined a total of $16,500 for multiple violations that included having no hot water for three days, repeated medication errors, and failing to find a patient who had fallen and broken a hip for fifteen hours. The facility changed the way it operated; it stopped providing assistance and instead became a landlord. The ALF rented rooms to residents, and home health providers privately contracted to provide assistance. It's unclear as to whether the loophole in Iowa state law that the facility used to remain open for business exists in other states; before placing a family member in an ALF, licensure history most certainly should be a consideration.

If the ALF will not accept the patient, it's possible that nursing home placement is the best caregiving option available for him – but it's also possible that another facility will accept him. They'll usually tell you why the patient is being denied, and you always have the option of visiting other ALF's to see if they will accept the patient instead. Different facilities provide various levels of care, and a denial from one ALF doesn't always mean that nursing home placement is imminent. There are facilities that provide a secured environment to residents who have Alzheimer's disease or other dementias, as well as specialized programming to keep them busy.

Just like a nursing home, once a patient is admitted to an ALF it's considered to be his home. Even if he can't afford to pay his rent any longer, the facility can't evict him without arranging for a safe discharge, although many will try to do so. It's common for facilities to attempt to bully family members into paying or taking the patient home, but patients do have rights. If your family member receives an eviction from an assisted living facility, contact the Ombudsman for assistance. Your local Area Agency on Aging should be able to provide the contact information if the ALF refuses to provide it to you. You also have the right to contact an attorney for assistance in any rental situation.

Extended Care Facilities (ECF)

A patient who can no longer remain at home because he requires 24-hour nursing care and monitoring is often admitted to a nursing home for *long-term care*. A nursing home is also known as an *extended care facility (ECF)*. Nursing homes provide their patients with assistance for all of the activities of daily living in an institutional environment, and are professionally staffed with nurses, nurse's aides, social workers, dieticians, etc. These staff members are often able to provide specialty services and clinical care, as well as a formal activity program, although many of the services that they provide are compliance (Medicare paperwork) related.

The usual sources of payment in an ECF are Medicaid, private-pay or long-term care insurance. Medicare does not pay for long-term care. All of the care that is provided by extended care facilities is done at the direction of a physician and follows the guidelines set forth by the Centers for Medicare and Medicaid Services. These facilities undergo annual inspections and must follow the same laws and guidelines as skilled nursing facilities.

Extended care facilities that aren't combined with skilled nursing are able to provide 24-hour care from *Licensed Practical Nurses (LPN's)* or *Licensed Vocational Nurses (LVN's)* and nurse's aides, but they aren't required to provide a registered nurse 24-hours per day. These facilities might possibly be able to use the services of an outside agency to provide therapies or wound care.

Skilled Nursing Facilities (SNF)

A patient who is able to participate in therapy up to two hours per day, six days per week is often discharged from the hospital to a *skilled nursing facility (SNF)*, also referred to as a nursing home. SNF's provide services from physical therapists, occupational therapists and speech therapists on an inpatient basis. In addition to rehabilitation, residents who are newly fed by a feeding tube, require wound care or other services that must be provided by a registered nurse qualify for skilled services. Most skilled nursing facilities offer a combination of short-term therapy and the long-term care that's provided in an extended care facility, so that patients are able to remain after they've completed their therapy.

The most common payment for placement in a SNF is Medicare, and depending upon the type of care the patient requires, payment for the skilled services can last up to 100 days (the full Medicare skilled nursing benefit), although there are co-payments for days 21-100. This copayment can either be paid out of pocket or by a **Medigap** (Medicare supplemental) insurance policy. Medicare Advantage plans (also known as HMO's and PPO's) also pay for skilled services, although the copayments and deductibles vary according to the plan the senior has chosen. Other types of payment for skilled nursing include private insurance policies, TriCare, the Veteran's Administration and Medicaid. Skilled nursing facilities are subject to annual inspections and are required to follow federal and state laws regarding the types of care they provide.

Skilled nursing facilities generally aren't staffed with in-house physicians; if patients need to see a doctor they're either transported to his office or the doctor makes a special visit to see them. There are exceptions for specialty services; depending upon the type of care the patient receives it's possible that the doctors will regularly see them in-house. For example, a patient who requires special wound care services might be seen in the facility by the doctor who is treating him, or a ventilator patient will be seen in-house by a pulmonologist.

Some SNF's provide sub-acute services, such as ventilator assistance, for patients who no longer require a physician 24-hours each day but do require a higher level of care than that which is offered by most skilled nursing facilities. These SNF's provide respiratory therapists on-site to ensure the professional management of their ventilator patients, and they are licensed to bill Medicare and Medicaid at a substantially higher rate than a regular SNF.

Some SNF's do their best to limit their care to 20 days or less; they only accept patients who will appear to require therapy for 2-1/2 weeks. If it appears that a patient will require therapy for a longer period of time or he doesn't have anywhere to go after the 20 days are up, he won't be accepted in the first place. These facilities provide the exact same level of care as every other skilled nursing facility except that they discharge their patients before the need arises to begin billing Medigap policies.

There are SNF's that only provide skilled care (for the full 100 days if at all possible). They are able to provide extended care, but choose not to. The patient turnover in these facilities is often difficult for the staff to manage, with multiple patient admissions and discharges every day. Their goal is to get patients in, provide the maximum amount of billable services, and then get them out as quickly as possible. The reporting requirements for patients who are receiving skilled nursing or rehabilitation services under the Medicare benefit are so demanding that certain staff members, such as social workers and some nurses, often spend more time completing paperwork than providing patient care. Skilled nursing facilities are required to provide the same staffing ratios as do long-term care facilities, meaning that the patient needs are greater but the staffing might not be. Facilities such as this may tout their expertise in rehabilitation because of the volume they serve, but the nurses and therapists might be overwhelmed and the social workers are so busy filling out paperwork that they have no time to work with patients to ensure they have a safe discharge plan. Unless the facility has substantially increased their staffing, these facilities might not be the best place for your family member to receive rehabilitation. Staffing ratios can be verified on the Medicare website; please refer to the chapter _Checking The Nursing Home's Performance Ratings_.

As mentioned above, most SNF's combine long-term care with skilled nursing services, which enables them to admit patients from the hospital under the higher Medicare payment source and allow them to remain on a long-term basis. Once the patients have been rehabilitated, the nursing home is required to provide **restorative services** to ensure that they remain at their highest level of functioning. Specially trained certified nursing assistants walk with the patients and/or provide **range-of-motion** exercises in the patients' beds. The facility is not reimbursed by Medicare or other insurance, and is required to provide this service to its patients at no additional cost.

If the patient continues to decline in spite of the restorative care, he will receive physical therapy via the Medicare Part B benefit, which is less intense and shorter in duration than the services offered under Part A. These services are designed to keep patients functioning at their current level, the nursing home is required to do everything possible to keep patients at their current level or must justify why the patient is declining. Just like all Medicare-based therapies, Part B services contribute significantly to the nursing home's profits. Administrators often meet with the physical therapy department to review patients who might be able to participate in therapy, and will do everything possible to encourage the patients & families to accept the service. Since permission to provide therapy under the Medicare Part B benefit is often buried deep within the admission paperwork, families are often surprised to find that a patient is participating in therapy in the nursing home, especially when their notification is in the form of a bill for copayments of services they don't recall authorizing. Patients might not even understand that they're being billed for that nice therapist who walks them up & down the hall, which seems no different than the restorative aide who was walking them up & down the hall before.

Extended care facilities that are combined with skilled nursing are staffed with a registered nurse during the day and are able to care for medically complex patients such as those with feeding tubes or who require specialty nursing care. Nursing homes generally don't provide doctors on-staff; if a patient needs to see his doctor he will either be transported to his office or the doctor will make a special trip to see him (if the doctor has multiple patients in the nursing home, it might be easier for him to visit them in the nursing home).

Acute Rehabilitation Facilities (ARF)

An *Acute Rehabilitation Facility* is an excellent option for the patient who is ready to be discharged from the hospital and is able to participate in therapies at a higher level than can be provided in a nursing home (three or more hours per day). These facilities are staffed with doctors during the day and are often hospital-based, although they can be stand-alone facilities. The average length of stay in an acute rehabilitation facility is about two weeks; this care is paid out of the Medicare patient's acute hospital benefit and doesn't count toward the 100 day maximum skilled nursing benefit. Patients are usually discharged to nursing homes for skilled services or rehabilitation after they leave acute rehabilitation facilities.

It's possible that a patient will be discharged from the hospital directly to a skilled nursing facility for a week or two while he recovers from a surgery, at which point he'll be admitted to an ARF for more comprehensive therapy than the nursing home is able to provide. The nursing home can – and often will – do everything possible to block the patient from leaving, not wanting to lose the patient and the potential reimbursement from Medicare that he represents. In fact, I was present when a SNF administrator advised a patient's family that sending him to an ARF would use up all of the Medicare Part A rehabilitation benefit; when that didn't deter the family, she told them that the patient would require another a 3-day admission to the hospital before he would be eligible for admission to an ARF. None of this was true, but the family allowed the patient to remain in the nursing home rather than to take a chance. The patient would surely have benefitted from more comprehensive therapy in a facility with specialty equipment, rather than to remain in the nursing home.

The bottom line is that patients have options. It's the patient's choice as to whether he wants to receive a higher level of rehabilitation services in an ARF as long as the facility is willing to accept him. The patient can always return to that nursing home (or to another) after he's completed his treatment at the acute rehabilitation facility.

Long-Term Acute Care Hospitals (LTAC)

A Long-Term Acute Care Hospital is a regular hospital that's equipped to provide long-term hospitalization services for patients. LTAC's are able to hold down costs because they don't offer maternity wards, emergency rooms, etc, although they're staffed the same as a regular hospital. Medicare, Medicaid and private insurance pay for this level of care in the same manner that they pay for regular acute care hospitals.

LTAC's serve the most medically complex patients, such as those who are newly placed on a ventilator, or who might not be able to go to an acute rehabilitation facility or skilled nursing facility due to their requiring physicians on-site 24-hours a day. Regular acute hospitals aren't equipped to hold these patients for several months and so they're sent to an LTAC. LTAC's are common in larger cities, but in smaller towns they often don't make fiscal sense.

Acute Care Hospitals

An acute care facility is the hospital most people consider when thinking of hospitals; they're stand-alone facilities with emergency rooms and surgical units, ICU's and maternity wards. Some hospitals have skilled nursing beds, although most do not. These hospitals are designed to keep patients for a very short period of time and then discharge them to longer-term facilities.

Choosing a Nursing Home

As I've mentioned before, sometimes a patient and family have plenty of time to research and choose a nursing home, but that's not the norm. Most often, they're given little warning that the patient is ready to be discharged from the hospital. There might be only a few hours before the patient is forced to leave, and immediate bed availability of local nursing homes might narrow down the choices. If the patient and family are able to choose a facility beforehand, their preferred nursing home might be able to save a bed for the patient.

Discharge planners, physicians, social workers and nurses often steer the patient toward a certain facility rather than to allow the family the opportunity to choose. This isn't necessarily because it's the best facility for the patient; it's possible that the discharge planner works there part-time, the doctor owns an interest in that facility, or a close friend of the discharge planner or nurse works there. Although it isn't ethical for them to do so, discharge planners will have the patient sign a "provider choice" form that gives the appearance that the patient chose that facility. Patients or their family members will trust that the discharge planner is sending them to the best place in town and sign the form as a part of the discharge packet – and just like that the referral officially became the patient's choice.

There can be any number of reasons that one facility will be favored over others in the area; it isn't always favoritism on the part of the staff. It's possible that the facility is the only one with a bed available, or that the nursing home has a specialty program that is able to meet a patient's medical needs. It's also possible that the patient's physician prefers that nursing home because it's close to his office and he can visit the patient there rather than requiring that the patient come to his office for visits. The doctor might also have a financial interest in boosting the census of that particular nursing home; for example, he might be the facility medical director. Another possibility is that the nursing home is the only one that will accept the patient, whether it is because of the patient's physical needs (such as ventilator dependence) or the patient's/family's behaviors that were dutifully noted in the hospital medical record.

Patients and families do have the right to choose the nursing home they want, even after they've already been admitted to another facility. As long as the other facility is willing to accept the patient, they can request a transfer to another nursing home and both facilities are required to help with the transition. This transfer can happen at any time, whether the patient was admitted that day or has been there for over a year. It's possible that a nursing home will do everything possible to block the discharge. Medicare pays nursing homes a substantial amount of money to provide therapy and skilled nursing services, and in most cases a nursing home won't let a patient go without a fight.

I've seen discharges blocked by administrators who insist that patients attend a "discharge planning meeting" prior to leaving (setting the meeting a couple of weeks in the future). They'll use such excuses as "the doctor won't discharge," even though the doctor hasn't even been called. If your family member is in a nursing home and you believe that the discharge is being blocked, speak with the administrator. If you don't get the results you'd like, feel free to call the local ombudsman or the state regulatory agency and file a complaint. Don't trust that the staff is on your side, they work for the nursing home and their continued employment often depends upon cooperating in delaying your discharge. If there is a bed available in the new facility, a transfer should be able to occur within 3 days (at the most).

In the event that the patient's doctor truly won't agree to the transfer, it might be necessary to make an appointment with him to discuss the issue; in extreme cases, find another doctor. It is possible that the new nursing home will require a transfer summary that has been dictated by his physician, which could delay the discharge a day or two but it shouldn't take any longer than that (the dictation can be ordered "stat" no matter what the nursing home might say). Once a patient and family choose a facility, the accepting facility's admissions coordinator can help to have the patient transferred.

Of course, a transfer depends upon the patient being accepted by the preferred facility, which is their decision. They can refuse to accept the patient and there's nothing that the patient and family can do. I worked for one nursing home where the administrator blocked a patient's request to transfer by claiming to the new nursing home that there were vague "problems with Medicaid" (there were none, she just didn't want the census to drop, and the new nursing home believed her). In my experience, the most common reason that a patient won't be accepted is financial; if there's any chance the facility won't be paid or the patient requires expensive treatments, most nursing homes aren't willing to take a financial hit. The second most common reason a patient is refused is due to the patient's and family's behavioral issues, whether it's abusing the staff or being too demanding. It's important to remember that everything the patient and/or family says and does is recorded in the medical chart.

When looking for a nursing home, go to the Medicare site and print out a list of all of the facilities in the area – and go take a tour of the nursing homes you might like. Consider such issues as how long it will take a family member to get there, or how much parking is available. When you've decided on a nursing home, let the discharging facility know your choice. It's best to have a back-up facility in case the first one isn't able to accept the patient.

What to Look For When Touring a Nursing Home

When attempting to choose a nursing home for your family member, it's important to recognize that they're trying to make a sale. Their marketing director will show you the areas of the nursing home that look the nicest and might possibly leave out the area where your family member would actually stay. Many nursing homes have a professionally decorated room set up just for tours, even though there's absolutely no chance your family member will end up in that room. As they walk you through the facility, they are somehow alerting the staff to remain on their best behaviors and keep the "difficult" patients hidden away (this is often accomplished by the person leading the tour holding a brightly colored folder).

Feel free to call ahead and make an appointment with the Admissions Coordinator for a tour of the nursing home. During your tour, peek into patient rooms as you pass by to see if their rooms are comparable to the room you were shown or if that room appears to be well-maintained only for touring purposes. Afterward, go back at different times (such as breakfast or dinner time) to see how patients are treated when members of administration aren't usually around.

An important thing to look for when walking through the nursing home is the staff and patient interactions. If there are smiles all around and the atmosphere is relaxed, that's a good indication of the care provided. Do staff members address patients by their names? Staff and residents who appear stressed and uncomfortable can be an indication of a poorly run facility, although they might just be having a bad day.

When touring the nursing home, it's best to ask whether the patient will be showering in his room or if it will be in a common area. Even if a shower is located in the patient's room, it's possible that he'll be showered in a common shower room. Patients who are showered in their rooms don't have to suffer the indignity of being wheeled half-naked through a public area.

Many nursing homes will tout their non-profit status as an indicator of excellence. A non-profit status doesn't mean that a facility is better; every nursing home is required to follow the exact same state & federal laws. Non-profits are no better or worse than any other facility; nursing homes that don't break-even on expenses won't be in business long. There are many things to look for when choosing a facility:

- Are you able to reach a staff member to set up a facility tour? If they are too busy to give a tour, they might be too busy to provide personalized services to each patient.
- Is there enough parking available? If there aren't enough parking places, family members might not be able to visit as often.

- Are there activities posted in a public place? Do the activities posted look interesting for an elderly person?
- Do they take patients on trips outside the facility? Does the facility have a wheelchair equipped van to transport patients to the doctor's office?
- Do staff members call patients by their names in a respectful manner?
- Do patients have personal items in their rooms, or does that appear to be discouraged by the management?
- How does the facility smell? If it smells strongly of urine, there's a problem. But if it smells strongly of cleaners while you're there, go back at a later time and see if it was an attempt to cover up unpleasant odors during your tour.
- Are the patients lined up in the hallways, looking bored? Although residents tend to congregate around the nursing stations, if this is happening at all hours it's possible the activity program is lacking.
- Does the staff appear to be disorganized, with paperwork everywhere?
- Are there medications sitting out unattended? This is unsafe (at best).
- Are telephones answered in a reasonable amount of time, or are they ringing off the hook?
- Are multiple patient call-light alarms ringing off the hook?
- Are there outside areas available for the patients, with enough shade? Are these areas easily accessible to patients and family members?
- Is the facility well known in the community for having a high staff turnover? If a facility can't keep its staff, that's an indication of problems.
- Look on the Medicare site (www.Medicare.gov) and review the information listed in Compare Nursing Homes under the Facilities & Doctors tab.
  - o If there is a red circle with the letters "*SFF*" next to the nursing home's name, this facility is a *Special Focus Facility.* Special Focus Facilities are those with a history of serious quality issues so egregious that the Medicare program is closely monitoring them. If they don't improve their care, these facilities are in danger of losing their Medicare and Medicaid certification and payment. If that were to happen, it often means that the facility will be closed and the state will help the patients move to other facilities that could meet their needs. It's rare that a facility will remain open if it permanently loses its certification.
  - o How many stars does the nursing home have? There is a five-star rating system that reflects the most recent state inspection. While not the only thing to look for, it should be taken into consideration.
  - o Compare the nursing homes in your area; don't just look at one specific facility. Be open to looking at all the nursing homes in your area.

- Call the state ombudsman and ask about the facility. They might tell you if any problems have been identified, but won't be able to discuss ongoing investigations.
- Read the nursing home's last inspection – the nursing home is required to have it available for your review. If it's over a year old, they probably aren't including the results of the last inspection. Why?
- Request the inspection results from the state board of licensing to compare with the one they have posted; it's possible they've omitted some pages or changed some of the information to give the appearance that the nursing home provides better care than it actually does.
- If the nursing home's admissions are currently being 'held' but they'll put you on a list – why are they being held? CMS holds new admissions only for facilities with severe problems.
- Ask friends, neighbors, or anyone else if they've had any experiences with the nursing home; if one has had a bad experience that's to be expected, but if several people have – consider another facility.
- Use the Internet to help:
  - Search online for information about specific nursing homes.
  - Search information about the parent corporation of the facility if it's a chain of nursing homes.
  - Search the administrator's name. Has that person been fined by his/her board of licensure for misconduct or improper dealings?
  - Search the director of nursing's name. Has that person been fined by his/her board of licensure for misconduct or improper dealings?

l.e. green

Checking the Nursing Home's Performance Ratings

Nursing homes are monitored by different state and federal agencies, and undergo different types of annual inspections that are formally referred to as *state surveys*. These inspections are comprehensive audits of all facets of the nursing home, and while they don't find every problem that exists in the nursing home, there's a pretty good chance that serious problems will be identified. After the survey has been completed and the nursing home has had time to address any problems identified, the results are posted on the Medicare website at www.medicare.gov.

Even though the Medicare site can be difficult to maneuver around for the non-internet savvy person, it's important to review all of the information provided for any facility to which your family member might be sent. To make it easier to understand, Medicare has created a five-star rating system. The overall five-star rating relies upon a confusing, convoluted formula that compares the nursing home to others in the area; only a certain percentage can be rated as below average or above average, so even a poor performing nursing home can be rated "average." In other words, a nursing home that provides poor care can receive the same overall rating as others in the area that provide substantially better care.

There are also many privately owned websites that are more user-friendly; they post the same ratings as Medicare but they are easier to navigate. In addition to the Medicare five-star rating, these websites might include their own customer comments, but basically the information they provide is the same as that which can be found on the Medicare website. Most of these companies charge for the same information that is offered for free on the Medicare website, and in many cases their information is outdated. Unless they update their ratings on a weekly basis it's possible that the information that they've posted might be outdated. Regardless of where the ratings can be found, the information can be somewhat misleading.

In 2012, the Medicare website began posting the actual inspection results, any financial penalties that have been assessed, and complaints that have been filed against each nursing home (prior to 2012, the information provided was non-specific). As with everything provided on the Medicare website, this information can be difficult to find and even harder to understand. It's important to note that the posted results can – and do – change. The initial findings will be posted soon after the survey; however, a nursing home that receives a substandard survey often negotiates a settlement with CMS, and the website will be changed to reflect the watered down (negotiated) overall ratings, not the initial inspection.

Something else to consider when researching a nursing home is that there can be a substantial lapse in time between the inspection and the date that the information is posted on the website. A facility that appears to have no problems might have received a substantial downgrade in its rating without the general public being able to access the information for several months, or even years. As mentioned above, the survey results can change – so it's important to check the website on a regular basis and to consider more than the five-star rating that Medicare assigns. Facilities with deplorable inspection results that were fined to the fullest extent of the law can rate "average" or above. Potential customers who view the website won't ever know there were changes unless they check the website on a regular basis, or if they take the time to review the actual survey findings from the state agency that surveys nursing homes.

One way a nursing home with consistently poor inspection results can be easily identified on the Medicare website is if it is included on the list of *Special Focus Facilities.* To attain the dubious honor of being listed as a Special Focus Facility, the nursing home must meet the following guidelines:

- It must experience substantially more problems than other facilities,
- The problems must be serious in nature, including actual harm or injury to patients; and
- Show a pattern of at least three years of serious problems.

Special Focus Facilities identified on the Medicare website by the letters SFF; they are inspected at least twice each year and are under intense scrutiny by both the state and federal governments. If the nursing home doesn't improve, it faces the very real possibility of being terminated from the Medicare and Medicaid programs, essentially closing the facility's doors. There is limited funding available for the SFF program, meaning that only the worst of the very worst make the list (136 nursing homes out of the approximately 16,000 that are operating in the United States). Obviously, many nursing homes that should be on the list don't make it due to the lack of funding available.

Because the possibility exists that a nursing home could experience severe problems without it being posted on the Medicare website, it's advisable to look at the actual inspection form that was generated during the survey. This form, called the *2567 form*, must be made available to consumers in a common area in the nursing home. Some facilities require you to ask for the form and then will only allow you to read it in the front office while a staff member is present. It's intimidating to read the survey results with someone standing over you, and if this is the case, you might wish to find a nursing home that doesn't have anything to fear. Depending upon the state in which you live, the 2567 might immediately be posted on the state website (often listed under the state Department of Health) or you can request a copy of the form by calling the bureau of licensure or health department. Again, this form – or a watered-down version of it – will eventually be posted on the Medicare website, but when you're looking for a nursing home for your family member you might not be able to wait until CMS updates the website.

The information that is posted on the Medicare site might not tell the whole story. When a nursing home experiences a particularly bad survey, the first thing that they will do is appeal the findings. If the results were bad enough, they will continue to appeal the findings until the federal government finally decides that the amount of the fines they'll receive is less than the cost of prosecuting the nursing home. The ultimate goal is to change the nursing home's behaviors, and an expensive, drawn-out investigation can accomplish this (or not). The information that is posted on the website will reflect the negotiated findings, not the original (awful) survey results.

I've seen substandard results and allegations of abuse changed from *Immediate Jeopardy* (meaning that the facility's patients were in immediate jeopardy of harm) to mediocre results. No one would ever know that there had been serious problems that nearly cost them their business unless they read the actual 2567 form.

Another way for a poor performing facility to make it difficult for the general public to find out about its record is for the corporation to sell the facility – or pretend to sell it by changing the name of the nursing home and/or the corporation that owns it. The survey results that will be available might be those that occurred after the name change, making it more difficult for prospective patients and their families to research a facility's history.

James is looking for a nursing home for his mother. He has heard that the worst facility in town is called "City Rehabilitation Services," and intends to avoid this facility if at all possible. He attempts to look up the facility's most recent inspection results, but the Medicare website reports no facility by that name. James' mother is sent to a facility by the name of "Pine Valley Rehabilitation."

James later finds that Pine Valley Rehabilitation is actually City Rehabilitation Services, having legally changed its name to "Pine Valley Rehabilitation." Each nursing home owned by the parent company is actually its own LLC, and the administrator is the CEO of that corporation. The parent company collects a "management fee" each month, which is essentially the profits that have been generated by the nursing home. This method of operation protects the parent company and every other nursing home it owns from liability from prosecution. If there are substantial problems with the nursing home, they can simply "sell" (transfer) it to another corporation.

Because the Medicare site no longer lists the facility under its former name or ownership, James had no idea his mother was going to the *one place* he feared.

Locating the actual 2567 form – the survey results – on the Medicare website takes six separate steps and can be hard to find if you don't know where to look. To access the inspection results online:

1) On the Medicare.gov website, choose "**Find a Nursing Home**" on the left.

2) Search the nursing home by Zip Code, City or State.

3) Select the nursing home(s) by checking the box and pressing the "**Compare Now**" button at the bottom of the page.

4) Click the "**Inspection Results**" tab.

5) Click over the words "**Health Inspection Details**."

6) Click "**View Full Report**."

The survey results can be somewhat misleading; even the most minor of infractions appears to be serious when written on the 2567 form. The actual form explains the violation, but it's often difficult to interpret. Unless the form assigns actual harm, it's best to ask a professional such as a social worker or nursing home ombudsman to help you interpret the findings. This form should be viewed as a part of the overall picture and is not necessarily the only indicator as to how the nursing home is performing. However, if there is any mention of abuse or what appears to be a serious infraction involving the administrator or director of nursing, it might be best to find another nursing home unless you are aware that the responsible staff member has been replaced.

When researching a nursing home's record, remember that the information on the Medicare website might not be current – it can take months or years for the results to be posted. It is possible to obtain the most current results directly from the agency that gathered it. Each state has a different name for the survey agency (a complete list is provided at the end of this book), and has its own procedures when it comes to providing the information to the general public. The agency contact information can also be found on the *Medicare.gov* website on the page of each specific nursing home. A quick phone call to the agency will let you know if the results are posted online, and where to find them. Sometimes the information is easily found and understood, while other times it's hard to find and even harder to understand.

There are basically two types of inspections: *Annual State Inspection Surveys* and *Complaint Investigations*. Although the annual inspections can occur at any time, they usually occur anywhere from eleven to thirteen months after the last annual inspection. Complaint investigations can occur at any time, either by a team of workers or by one surveyor who reports back to the team.

Annual State Inspections (Surveys)

Every nursing home is audited on an annual basis to ensure that the patients are receiving appropriate care, that all applicable laws and rules are being followed, and that the nursing home has developed and is following a *care plan* that addresses the individualized needs of each patient.

A survey team enters a nursing home for its annual inspection and requests several charts. The administrator and several other staff members quickly review the charts. Any missing documentation can be falsified (recreated), and problem charting can be removed from the chart because it's better to have missing documentation than incriminating notes. Please note that changing the charts in any manner is illegal and considered to be falsification of a legal document, but this doesn't deter unethical administrators.

Although the survey team has asked to be left alone, staff members will be sent in offering water or snacks. In this particular nursing home, the staff will be asked to look at the open charts on the table and report upon which areas the surveyors appear to be focusing.

During the survey process, if a potential problem is suspected, the administrator might attempt to access the charts while the state workers are using them. One method of doing so is to page overhead that the patient's doctor is on the phone; a staff member will enter the room and request a chart in order for the nurse to provide information to the doctor. The documentation in question is either removed or slipped into the chart, and then the chart is returned to the surveyor. Hopefully the surveyors won't notice the discrepancies.

At the end of every day that the surveyors are present in the facility, the administrative team questions every nursing home worker to whom the surveyor has spoken and attempts to address any areas the survey team appears to be focusing. Workers often stay well after their shift to fix any problems that have been identified.

When the state workers enter the facility, they present their identification to the administrator and request a pre-selected sampling of patient charts. The facility is required to immediately surrender the requested charts to the state survey team, although I've seen facilities that forced the state to wait while they pored over the charts in an attempt to change any documentation they believed to be problematic.

This behavior is highly unethical and illegal (this is considered to be falsification of a legal document), but it happens all the time because it's hard to prove that anything was changed unless it's been observed by the surveyor.

Nursing homes can be creative when it comes to *"scrubbing charts."* More than one nursing home administrator has told me it was company policy to scrub any chart prior to providing it to a surveyor, although I wasn't ever able to locate this policy in the employee manual.

In addition to chart reviews, the audit will consist of patient/staff interviews, kitchen inspections, physical plant inspections, business office audits, and medication audits. Even though this is a scheduled annual event, a full-blown survey can occur at any time if an investigating agency has cause to suspect ongoing problems. These audits take 1-4 days on average.

The state survey team will generally review about 10% of the active patient charts and a smaller sampling of closed charts. They will also request the charts of patients who recently filed complaints, or review those of patients who have complained in the past. They will follow staff members as they pass medications, perform treatments and otherwise provide their day-to-day services to patients. Surveyors also review the alarm systems, kitchen and grounds, and meet with patients both 1-1 and in large groups to gain their input about the nursing home's day-to-day operations.

Many nursing homes respond to the state survey by adding extra workers to the medical floor while the surveyors are present. The corporate office will send multiple staff members to oversee the process, and the nursing home will be cleaner than ever. Patients who are used to waiting over an hour for assistance will find that their call lights are answered promptly and that workers are on their best behavior. Overhead pages will be held to a minimum and family members will be treated much better than usual. The activities will be a little more active and the food will be substantially better while the surveyors are present in the building. The state's presence in the facility will be nerve-wracking for staff members, but the patients and families will love it.

During the time that the state is completing the audit, the facility will post notices at the entrances explaining that a survey has begun and how many days the state survey team anticipates it will be present. The notices include instructions as to how family members can arrange to speak with a member of the state team if they wish. Don't feel intimidated; families are welcome to speak freely with the state and the nursing home can't retaliate against the patient if they do. The inspectors also conduct a patient meeting during the survey process, which allows patients the opportunity to discuss any concerns that they have. Nursing home staff members generally aren't allowed to be present for this meeting. Although these meetings are designed to seek out problems, it's also common for patients and families to provide positive feedback as well. A patient who resided in a nursing home where I worked told me that she had been promised extra snacks if she complimented the nursing home during such a meeting.

When a state surveyor interviews staff members, they're often afraid to candidly discuss any problems that might be occurring in the facility. This is because the 2567 form identifies the staff member who discussed the issues for that specific patient. For example, the form will list "*CNA*" (certified nursing assistant) and what she said. If this CNA previously spoke with her supervisor about that patient, it's a sure bet that was the staff member to whom they're referring. If the form lists "social worker" and there's only one social worker on staff, that too is a no-brainer. Even if it's difficult to identify the staff members from the information provided by the state workers, the administrative team might go to great lengths to determine who it was that cooperated with the surveyors and retaliate against him/her. Not all nursing homes operate in this manner, but it happens. If the worker values his job, he'll be extremely cautious with his answers.

Once the survey has been completed, the team will meet with the nursing home administrator, director of nursing, and corporate representatives to conduct an *exit interview*. They will present the findings and discuss their recommended outcome. Much of the time there are no serious findings, but if a problem is identified the administrative team might know about it immediately. It's possible that additional issues will be revealed when the nursing home receives the formal report a couple of weeks later. If the nursing home fails the survey, the team will return for another inspection at least once; depending upon the severity of the problems uncovered it's possible that the state will return several times.

State survey results are revealed in their entirety on the 2567 form, which the facility is required to make available to the general public. The form lists all identified problems (known as deficiencies) and any improvements that the facility must make in order to meet the minimum standards required by all applicable laws and rules.

The 2567 form will remain the same whether or not the deficiencies are successfully appealed later on, although they will probably be accompanied by a letter that states that the severity of the deficiencies and amount of the fines were negotiated down by the facility. The form that is posted on the Medicare website is neatly typed, while the one that is available in the nursing home and the surveying agency will contain both the state's findings and the nursing home's response. Regardless of the original findings, after a successful appeal the survey results (including the level of harm and amount of people affected) will change for the better.

Deficiencies that are egregious in nature and that affect the health, safety and/or well being of the patients will be assigned a higher level of harm. The degree of seriousness is reflected in this number; the higher the number assigned to the violation, the greater the violation (most deficiencies are assigned a "1" or "2," anything greater than that is serious). The categories for number of patients affected are *Few, Some, and Many*. Generally speaking, any violation assigned a "three" or higher which affects at least "some" people is fairly serious. Because the website and its five-star rating is changed to reflect the negotiated findings, it's important to view the actual 2567 form to gain a clear view of the problems that were found during the survey. Otherwise, you might choose a sub-standard nursing home for your family member.

It's possible that the nursing home will be sanctioned for survey results, including monetary fines, admissions being held until certain criteria has been met, or the withholding of payment for Medicare and Medicaid patients until the identified problems can be corrected. In nearly every case, the nursing home will appeal the findings, which can cost tens or hundreds of thousands of dollars in legal fees. Those issues that can't be resolved after multiple surveys can result in nursing homes permanently losing their funding. This doesn't happen very often, but you can be sure that if it does there were some pretty awful things going on in that nursing home.

When a nursing home has experienced a particularly bad survey, they usually hire a law firm that specializes in such appeals and the process will drag on for years at a cost that can easily pass $100,000.00. After a few years, CMS eventually allows a settlement to be negotiated because the fines that the government assesses are substantially less than the costs of continuing to prosecute the matter.

If there are negative findings, it's possible that the administrator will start a witch hunt and urge the staff to report on fellow workers in an attempt to deflect the blame. Intimidation is a powerful tool in the context of ending a person's job or chosen career. Staff members who are suspected of participating in investigations are often fired or might suffer retaliation to the point that they quit. In addition to being fired, the facility might harass those employees suspected of cooperating in an investigation and attempt to have them blacklisted in the local medical community. Complaints may be filed against the professional licenses of these employees in an attempt to discourage them from cooperating with the state, or at least in an attempt to ruin their credibility in the ongoing appeals process. Not every nursing home will act in such a manner, but enough of them do that the message is clearly understood by everyone in the industry. It's a given that the corporation will believe the administrator over the subordinates nearly every time.

Of course, there are laws that are supposed to protect health care workers who report fraud and abuse from suffering retaliation, but it's difficult to prove that a staff member was fired as a result of their cooperation with the surveyors. I've personally experienced the effects of a nursing home removing documentation from patient charts and replacing the forms with manufactured documents that gave the appearance of the employee having a vendetta against the nursing home.

In one particular case, a new administrator brought a nurse along with whom she had a long personal and professional relationship, both of them having been cited for abuse twice in the previous two years. During a complaint investigation, the nurse was found to have shaken patients, withheld medications, verbally abused them, and physically assaulted another employee. The administrator lied to the state investigators, claiming that she didn't know the nurse well (they lived together) and wasn't aware of any previous abuse allegations. This triggered a full inspection wherein the facility was cited for knowingly hiring staff members with a history of abuse.

In that instance, the administrator fired those employees she suspected of cooperating with the state investigation, and attempted to intimidate me by filing a complaint against my professional license. I successfully defended my professional license, but it took over three years for the ordeal to be over and my career will never fully recover. Several of the staff members who wrote letters in support of the administrator (implying that I was a horrible person) later apologized to me and said that they had felt bullied into doing so. The experience was devastating.

Unfortunately, in order to successfully win a lawsuit for such a retaliatory firing, it's up to the staff member to remove proof from the nursing home. It might even be necessary to violate healthcare privacy acts in order to defend oneself from such a firing by removing documents that include patient information. In this particular case, that wasn't necessary; the administrator herself provided overwhelming evidence that she and her staff had lied to the investigators, falsified emails and faxes to make it appear that the employee had received written warnings and participated in a cover-up, all the while, the nursing home corporation stood firmly behind the administrator. The Medicare site was amended to reflect the negotiated findings and, unless they knew where to look, customers weren't aware that there had been any problems at all.

Even though that situation occurred several years ago, the nursing home's current overall rating has continued to be "above average" even though the inspection ratings have remained "below average." My point is that these ratings can be misleading and shouldn't be the only method used to choose a nursing home.

Again, many nursing homes wouldn't respond to a poor survey in this manner and would fully investigate any issue long before things became so serious that the facility would fail a state inspection. In my opinion, most nursing homes are honest and caring in their mission. However, knowing that such a situation can occur makes it harder for workers to be completely forthcoming during investigations.

Complaint Investigations

That a facility is the subject of a complaint investigation isn't necessarily indicative of a problem because anyone is able to file a formal complaint against a nursing home. The complaining party could be a patient or family member, member of the community, staff member, or even the nursing home itself. In fact, the nursing home is required to notify the state if there are allegations of abuse, whether on the part of a patient, staff member, visitor or other person in the facility. Each complaint might not trigger a formal investigation; it depends upon the nature of the complain as to how the incident will be investigated. People can call and complain about anything and it's up to the state agency accepting the complaint to determine whether or not an investigation is warranted.

A complaint investigation usually consists of a single state investigator who arrives on-site, introduces himself to the administrator and begins his investigation. The nursing home is required to cooperate and provide access to the patients, employees, and to all documents such as patient charts and medication administration records. The investigator is able to contact his office and request follow up if he uncovers something that he believes warrants further action. After an investigation has been completed, the worker will meet with the administrator and any other staff members that the administrator chooses to include in the *exit interview,* during which they discuss the findings and recommendations.

A complaint investigation might end that day, or it might trigger a full inspection (survey). It is possible for a facility to have multiple inspections or complaint investigations in a single year. Again, information regarding investigations can be found either on the Medicare site, state website or by requesting a copy of all annual surveys and complaint investigations from the state licensing agency.

When choosing a nursing home for your family member, don't trust that the nursing home representative will be honest when you ask whether there are any ongoing investigations. The admissions representative doesn't hold any kind of professional license and is under no legal obligation to be honest with you during your tour of the facility; in fact, they might not even know that there have been serious allegations of abuse or neglect. Check with the state licensing agency to find out whether or not there is an active investigation about the nursing home. The only way you can be sure to have a complete picture of the facility is to verify the information for yourself.

If you believe that your family member has been mistreated, you have every right to speak with the administrator or to call the nursing home ombudsman. You also have the option of calling the state licensing agency to report your concerns. Any of these actions might trigger a complaint investigation, which isn't necessarily a bad thing. No complaint is too trivial, such as the incident below:

Margaret is a 95 year-old resident of the 200 hall in a nursing home. She tells her daughter Mary that there are never any snacks available after dinner, and when she asks for tea she is told she can't have tea after dinner. Mary speaks with the charge nurse, who tells her that the nursing staff has reported that her mother is becoming increasingly confused. However, the charge nurse assures her that they will offer tea to her mother from that point on. Margaret continues to complain about the lack of snacks, and says that the staff makes fun of her when she asks for tea. Mary chalks it up to her mother's increased confusion.

Mary never speaks with the administrator about this issue, nor does she check to see if any complaints have been filed about the lack of snacks at night. Had she checked with the state, she would have found that the nursing home has been written up multiple times for not providing snacks on the 200 hall.

Mary also would have found that not only is her mother alert & oriented with no confusion, the staff member who Margaret claimed was making fun of her (the charge nurse) had been suspended for the same behaviors while working on other halls Mary's reporting of this seemingly meaningless issue could have saved her mother months of anguish.

When a complaint investigation is underway, the administrator might not be honest with the investigator. It can be difficult for the state to prove that the nursing home was withholding information or that documents were falsified or amended in any way. In most cases, a nursing home would rather remove documentation from the chart and pretend it couldn't be found than to present damning information that will trigger further investigation into the incident. However, if the investigator suspects that the nursing home is hiding something, there will probably be further investigation and it's even possible that the incident will be referred to a law enforcement agency.

Don't trust that the nursing home will inform you about any ongoing investigations that begin after your family member has been admitted. Nursing homes have no legal obligation to advise patients and their families about any recent complaints that have been filed. Even if the nursing home had no problems on the day that the patient was admitted, there could be serious allegations of abuse and families filed since that date. In order to protect your family member, it's best to contact the state agency for updated information several times a year (a few weeks after the annual inspection or a complaint investigation). This ensures that the patient and family will remain informed about all investigations and annual inspections. Even a meaningless complaint can be indicative of abuse (in the previous scenario, this would be considered verbal abuse and also neglect for withholding the snacks; it might also be falsification of a medical record if the nursing home has recorded confusion that doesn't exist).

Although it's quite rare for current employees to volunteer their help during a complaint investigation, sometimes employees will save a copy of the offending documents and sneak them to a state worker. Employees who are willing to cooperate in such an investigation should be commended, although chances are pretty good that they'll be fired if they're caught. The employees are then the subject of retaliation as the administrator freely shares his suspicions of the offending staff members with other administrators, often embellishing the information to make them appear to be vindictive, horrible people. The employees' reputations can easily become the facility's defense against allegations of wrongdoing. Eventually, the workers might be forced to find another line of work or move away in order to find a job. Of course, this is illegal behavior on behalf of the nursing home administration, but it's difficult to prove and the legal fees can easily bankrupt the now ex-employee. The odds are always in the company's favor in these instances.

Again, in most cases nursing homes are operated appropriately and many complaints are found to be without merit. However, if there is a pattern of a specific type of complaints, even if the state doesn't find any problems it might be best to discuss your concerns with the administrator or to move your parent to another facility. There are many things that can happen to a nursing home resident, and they don't necessarily mean that the nursing home is at fault. However, if a nursing home doesn't appear to provide the highest quality of care you have the right to complain, have him transferred, or both. Your concern is your family member, not that the nursing home needs revenue.

If the nursing home doesn't meet the quality requirements of the patient and family for any reason, they have every right to move the patient to another facility *as long as they are able to find one that will accept the patient.* This could be difficult, because the current nursing home will forward information about the patient to the new facility the family has chosen. Since they don't want to lose the patient and might have to explain to the parent corporation why he is leaving, the current facility might do everything possible to block the discharge. It may be necessary to meet with the admissions coordinator or administrator of the preferred nursing home and explain why the last facility wasn't able to meet the patient's needs. Once the patient has been accepted, the discharging facility can't block a transfer by refusing to cooperate with the family or the accepting facility. If you request a transfer and it isn't completed within a few days, call the state ombudsman for assistance.

It's also important to remember that nursing homes with poor inspection results can and do improve. If you like the facility where your family member resides and see positive changes occurring, it might be worth it to leave the patient there but to visit more frequently. It can be traumatic for a patient to move to a different facility and have to get used to a new environment.

For those patients residing in a facility designated to be a ***Special Focus Facility***, the family should definitely visit more often and pay special attention to the 2567 form. However, there are over 16,000 nursing facilities in the United States and only 136 included in the Special Focus program, so not being included on the SFF list doesn't mean that a nursing home provides quality care. If more funding was available, hundreds or possibly thousands more would be placed on the watch list. Any nursing home with a poor track record, multiple deficiencies on the annual survey, or that has experienced a hold on payments or admissions should be visited frequently by family members and monitored to ensure the patient receives appropriate care.

Another reason to visit the nursing home frequently is to monitor the progress of a new administrator or director of nursing. If the nursing home was recently sold to a new corporation, that too would be a reason to visit more often. It wouldn't be unreasonable to move the patient to another nursing home if you believe that the quality of care has significantly declined, even if the patient appears to be happy where he's at. The bottom line is that in every case you should do what you believe is appropriate to ensure the patient's safety and well-being.

A recent trend in state abuse investigations involves placing cameras in patient rooms (with patient/family permission, of course). Nursing homes should have nothing to hide, but recording the goings on can verify that the patient is receiving appropriate care. Staff members have been fired, and even sent to jail for abuse that has been caught on camera. Nursing homes hate when patient care if filmed – not because of the potential violation of privacy, but because of the element of surprise. Some facility staff members don't like having their behaviors monitored, but if they're doing nothing wrong they shouldn't have to worry about being filmed.

I worked in a nursing home where the floor supervisor demanded that a family member immediately surrender his/her camera, insisting that they're not allowed to take photographs. The family solved this issue by calling the police, who escorted the family member from the facility *with their camera*. Although you aren't allowed to take photos of other patients or staff members without their permission, the nursing home isn't a prison. It is legal to take photographs of your family member and his environment. If a nursing home employee attempts to take your camera, you have every right to call your attorney or 911 if you feel threatened. They can't legally force you to turn your private property over to them.

Without the intervention of brave staff members or patients' families, nursing homes would operate however they wanted without being caught. All that the corporate ownership sees is the financial profits, and the nursing home administrator earns huge bonuses as a result. Unless a staff member is willing to risk his career by coming forward, no one will ever know what's going on every day in that particular nursing home.

In a recent case, a nursing home administrator intimidated workers, patients & families while she inserted herself into every facet of the facility operations. She refused to allow the nursing home's patients to discharge before the facility milked every Medicare dime possible, bullied chemotherapy patients into participating in therapy even though they were too sick to do so, demanded that her staff send patients with dementia to a psychiatric ward in order to bill Medicare for rehabilitation upon their return to the nursing home, and refused to allow patients their right to choose their aftercare providers. She forced staff to change documentation in order to substantiate higher billings, and stated in meetings that the patient and/or physical therapist didn't decide when a patient had completed his therapy; she asserted that it was *her* decision.

She also did many things that seemed to have no motive beyond her wish to control people; she had her staff move patients from room-to-room, used an unlicensed social worker along with her favorite LPN to arrange for inappropriate discharges and would only refer to one home health agency and one equipment agency. This resulted in a patient being discharged to an unlicensed facility without any arrangements having been made to provide for his oxygen; he was sent to the hospital soon afterward. Since discharge planning is a huge issue for patients, her policies placed patients in jeopardy of serious harm.

This administrator threatened her employees by insisting that she made the corporation millions of dollars and anyone who crossed her not only wouldn't be believed, but she openly guaranteed they wouldn't have a career by the time that she was done with them. She bragged in open meetings about her ability to manipulate the system, and ran the nursing home in this manner for more than six years before I arrived on the scene. Even though at least five social workers had worked there before me, none were brave enough to report her behaviors to the corporation. I was rewarded for my bravery by not only being suspended, but the company never even paid out my final check.

The administrator was fired, but of course she was paid out her wages and found another job in the industry immediately (although she did suffer a huge pay cut). Her behaviors were never addressed by her licensing board; in fact, her former company seems to have never reported the problems and without the cooperation of the company, there was no proof of her wrongdoing. Her new employer and licensing board will never know the type of manager she was prior to coming to work for them.

Administrators get away with this behavior because companies rarely question the day-to-day operations of a profitable nursing home, even if it's abnormally profitable. There are many redundancies built into the system that can make it difficult for nursing homes to act in a fraudulent manner, but with perseverance it's possible for an administrator to manipulate the system. For example, every discipline's charting must match in order to justify billing at a higher rate (but only if that chart is ever audited). Nursing homes can attempt to mask their actions by reviewing everyone's notes and have them re-written (illegal, but when threatened with their job every employee will have to make hard choices).

When an auditor reviews the chart information, any discrepancies will raise red flags and eventually result in financial penalties – but the odds that the chart will never be reviewed are in the nursing home's favor. The greatest barrier to an honest, well-managed nursing home is the lack of oversight. There simply isn't enough money to provide effective oversight to nursing homes or other providers. The state surveyors might do an excellent job of identifying fraud, but since 2005 many states have cut this program to the bare minimum. The workers have more facilities to audit and less time to perform their job.

The nursing home ombudsman programs have also experienced severe cutbacks; some states rely upon volunteers to advocate for patients in nursing homes. Since volunteers are either retired or otherwise unemployed, they might not possess an adequate knowledge base of the applicable rules and laws regarding care in a nursing home. These are the agencies that are charged with advocating for vulnerable patients, and they should only rely upon licensed, professional workers with years of experience in providing services to seniors. In many areas, these programs have little or no funding and so they take whatever help they can get.

Some states are cutting costs by mailing self-evaluations to smaller group homes, skipping their survey process altogether even though they provide a level of care comparable to that of a nursing home. In a time when oversight is so badly needed, there are less surveyors to go around and those that are hired are paid substantially less than if they if they worked in the private sector. This is why family members and outside agencies such as hospices must ensure that patients are well-cared for and that facilities are following the appropriate laws and rules.

Again, it is important to review a nursing home's history of caregiving before allowing your family member to be admitted. A recent study found that the Medicare program paid 5.1 billion dollars to private facilities to provide substandard services to their patients in 2009 (the most recent year for reporting purposes). The problems that were identified included inappropriate monitoring of psychotropic medications, providing therapies that patients didn't need in order to receive higher payments from Medicare, and inappropriate discharge planning. The study recommended that payment to nursing homes be tied to their inspection results; with those nursing homes with substandard survey results being penalized financially until they raise their scores. Of course, the nursing home industry opposes this idea and has suggested that the Office of the Inspector General change their criteria rather than to admit there are real problems out there that need to be addressed.

If you suspect that a nursing home is mistreating your family member or another resident, you have the right to call and report it to the state regulatory agency. The contact numbers for these agencies are posted on bulletin boards in a common area of the facility, and I have included contact numbers in the chapter entitled _Nursing Home Survey Agencies_ at the back of this book. Each nursing home is required to post the patients' rights and responsibilities and to follow them; patients have the right to be treated with respect and dignity.

Nursing homes are no longer prisons to send old people when they are dying. They are now places that must provide quality care for the elderly where they can live out their final days in an environment where they are free from abuse and neglect. The nursing home is there to meet their needs, and they can't be forced into accepting treatments or therapies simply so that the nursing home can earn more money.

If your family member is in a facility and the annual survey is in process, feel free to discuss any concerns that you might have with the surveyors. It would be helpful to have dates, times, places and the name of the employees involved, if any. Don't allow the nursing home staff to interfere with this discussion, or to deter you from meeting with the surveyors. You have the right to meet with them without fear of retaliation.

Determining the Payment Source

Most people don't understand the many different types of care provided to patients, and that there are multiple sources of payment for care in nursing homes. The general misconception seems to be that all you need to do is walk in the front door and somehow the bill will be paid. Although this once was true, things have changed dramatically. In nearly every instance, patients aren't allowed entry into a nursing home until a payment source can be secured. The reason is simple: once a patient has been admitted, the nursing home has a responsibility to care for him. If a patient has no payment source or safe discharge plan, the nursing home could be stuck caring for the patient for a long, long time.

Nursing homes walk a fine line when considering whether or not to accept a patient; they must take enough time to ensure they'll be paid, but if they take too long the patient will go elsewhere and they'll lose some much-needed revenue. They'll gather the information as quickly as possible in order to make their decision, and hope for the best.

There are many different types of payment possible for nursing home placement; some are designed to be short-term while others, such as Medicaid, pay for placement as long as the patient needs it. It really does matter to the nursing home how the patient will pay for his stay because, the higher the reimbursement, the more desirable the patient will be and the harder the nursing home will work to get the patient in the door.

Traditional Medicare (Original Part A)

Patients receiving therapies or treatments under the Medicare Part A benefit provide the highest amount of reimbursement for nursing homes. Those patients who appear to require the full 100 days worth of treatments and therapies (and who possess a Medicare supplement that pays 100% of the copayments) are greatly desired. The Medicare nursing home payment system is very complicated, but essentially the more therapies (speech, occupational and physical therapies) in which the patient participates, the greater the income to the nursing home will be.

Most people are under the impression that Medicare pays for a full 100 days in every instance, but that's simply not the case. The benefit will pay for up to 100 days worth of skilled nursing services or therapies (physical, occupational and speech therapies), but the patient has to demonstrate a need for it and also be progressing toward a goal. If the patient is walking 20 feet when he arrives, and is walking that same 20 feet a month later, the nursing home isn't able to show that he is progressing toward a goal. The program is set up to help people recover from a hospitalization, not simply to give them a place to go for awhile. Medicare pays thousands of dollars each month to help patients meet their goals, and nursing homes compete for these patients.

The nursing home's marketing efforts will include providing lunches, gift baskets, pens and other trinkets to doctors and hospital discharge planners. Most of the nursing home's marketing is targeted toward these professionals and not toward the family members and patients, even though the families and patients ultimately choose where the patient will go for rehabilitation. Over the years, family members have told me that they felt "railroaded" into sending the patient to a certain facility, which probably was the one with the most aggressive marketing campaign at the time of the patient's admission. Either that, or the nursing home probably has a relationship with the hospital discharge planner or patient's doctor.

Medicare does require that a patient be admitted into the hospital for a 3-day qualifying stay prior to being admitted to the nursing home; there is absolutely no way to get around this requirement (which actually means "over three midnights."). It doesn't matter whether the patient's primary physician believes that the patient requires skilled nursing services and is willing to write an order to that effect, if the patient hasn't been in the hospital for the required three day stay he won't be eligible for Medicare Part A to pay for any part of his stay in a skilled nursing facility (also referred to as a nursing home).

In order to qualify for Part A to pay for rehabilitation in a nursing home, a patient must be a "full admit" to the hospital. It doesn't count toward the 3-day qualifying stay if the patient was held so that the staff could observe him to ensure his symptoms don't return or worsen. It's important to explain to the doctor, social worker or case manager that the plan is for the patient to be discharged to a nursing home when he leaves the hospital; if they are able to justify his being a full admission from the start it will help to ensure that he meets the necessary 3-day requirement. Some doctors are suspicious when they're told that the plan is for the patient to go to a nursing home (a doctor accused one of my patients of being too "lazy" to care for her husband...), but don't let their attitude deter you from getting what you need. If the patient requires hospitalization, it's not an abuse of the system for him to be a "full admit" from the day he arrives.

As recently as twenty years ago, pretty much any patient could be held for three days with the expectation that Medicare would cover the bill. This is no longer the case; these days the hospital will only allow the patient to remain in the hospital for the full three days as long as the patient's *medical necessity* warrants the admission. Medicare will not pay the hospital bill if the patient's only reason for being there is to qualify for nursing home placement. The hospital has agreed to accept the amount that Medicare approves, and if Medicare denies the bill outright, the patient isn't responsible to pay it. Hospitals won't keep patients if they're not going to be paid for the service.

After leaving the hospital or acute rehabilitation facility, the patient isn't required to go straight to the nursing home; he actually has a 30-day window starting from the date of hospital discharge during which he can be admitted to a

SNF under the Medicare benefit. As long as he is admitted to the SNF within those 30 days and presents a medical need, Medicare will pay for him to receive services in a nursing home. There is absolutely no way to extend the 30-day window; if the patient has been out of the hospital and hasn't received care in a facility under the Part A benefit for 30 days he doesn't qualify to receive skilled services under the Medicare benefit until he has returned to the hospital for another 3-day stay.

Patients don't always meet the criteria for Medicare to foot the bill on the day that they arrive at the nursing home. Sometimes they need time to recuperate before they are able to participate in therapies, and have no other skilled need when they leave the hospital. An example would be a patient who had surgery such as a hip replacement, and isn't able to bear weight for six weeks while his bones heal. It's possible that Medicare will pay for a few weeks of therapy in order to strengthen his upper body and to help him with transferring from bed to wheelchair, but the Medicare benefit pays only as long as the patient is able to progress with these tasks. Once the patient has met these goals, he'll need to have another source of payment for his room & board while he waits to start physical therapy.

If the patient isn't able to pay an average $200 per day and isn't eligible for Medicaid or another type of payment for his room & board, it's possible that he will have to go home until he is ready to start a comprehensive therapy program. Unfortunately, Medicare does not consider a patient's lack of ability to care for himself to be a medical necessity to remain in a nursing home.

Some nursing homes are willing to risk their future with the Medicare program by lying about the amounts and types of therapy the patient is receiving during this time period. Even though it's becoming increasingly harder to fraudulently bill Medicare, it's still possible for nursing homes to falsify their documentation and continue to bill Medicare during the time that the patient is waiting to begin comprehensive therapy services. Not only is this illegal, it also means that the patient will have less time available for rehabilitation later on when he really needs it. If the nursing home is caught fraudulently billing Medicare, it will be forced to return thousands of dollars and can also lose its ability to bill Medicare and Medicaid in the future. Most nursing homes aren't willing to take such a risk, although there are always a few who believe themselves to be above the law.

If the patient is able to participate in therapy but the 30-day window has passed, he will have to return to the hospital for another 3-day stay in order for Medicare to pay for the services. However, the patient will have to *present a medical need for hospitalization* at that time – meaning that he will need to be sick enough to require hospitalization. If the patient isn't admitted into the hospital, he won't be able to use Medicare to pay for his stay in the nursing home and will either have to pay privately for his room & board and use the extremely limited Medicare Part B benefit for therapy, or go home with home health care or outpatient rehabilitation.

All of this can be confusing to the customer. The patient who was receiving therapy – but stopped for a short while – will pick up the therapy days at the point that he stopped; if he used 30 days, he will have 70 left when he is ready to start again. The Medicare benefit will only regenerate to the full 100 days once the patient hasn't used the Medicare Skilled Nursing Benefit for sixty consecutive days. At that point, the patient will have to be admitted to the hospital for another three days. Following the Medicare rules can be frustrating, as well as stressful for the patient who doesn't qualify for Medicare but isn't ready to return home.

Nursing homes that previously refused to accept a patient for long-term care under the Medicaid benefit because there were "no beds available" are often willing to accept him for skilled services with the plan of his staying long-term. After the nursing home has reaped the benefits of the higher Medicare payment source, the patient's payment source will "roll over" to whatever payment source he has for his long-term care. For example, if the patient's payment for long-term care is Medicaid, he will be admitted under the Medicare benefit and stay on a long-term basis with Medicaid paying his room and board. The nursing home can't make the patient leave unless there is a safe discharge plan that is agreeable to the patient and his family. I've seen many nursing homes discharge patients and tell them they'll place them on a list for readmission as soon as they have a bed available; in reality, the patient could have refused to leave and the nursing home would have been forced to keep him on a long-term basis.

The billing model that Medicare uses to pay for skilled services is confusing; the program uses a complicated formula called **RUG (Resource Utilization Group)** rates that take into account the patient's capabilities, the amount of skilled nursing care provided, and the number of therapy minutes the patient requires. Facilities provide the maximum amount of services possible in order to have a higher **RUG** score, but the Medicare system doesn't make it easy to bill at the higher levels. It's nearly impossible for nursing homes to falsify all of the chart documentation necessary in order to justify billing at a higher rate than the patient's physical status allows. Remember, though, that in most cases a very small number of charts are audited and nursing homes are rarely caught overbilling.

Nursing homes can be caught committing fraud in several different ways, the most common of which is a Medicare audit of all of the therapy charts for a given period of time. Medicare employs companies called **Medicare Administrative Contractors (MACs)** that audit patient bills looking for trends that appear to be out of the norm; those nursing homes that trigger an investigation will be directed to send certain patient charts to the designated Medicare Administrative Contractor for further investigation.

Another way that fraud can be discovered is when an investigator discovers evidence of wrongdoing during a complaint investigation or state inspection. The surveyors are instructed to look for indicators of fraud and to report their suspicions to the MAC for their region. In order to get away with fraudulent billings, all of the staff members that interact with the patient would have to falsify their documentation, along with the physician's office and any consultants who have seen the patient. It's nearly impossible for every entry in the chart to match exactly, and those that do raise suspicions of fraud.

Facilities are penalized financially if they're caught billing for services at rates that can't be justified, and can even lose their license to operate. Nursing home administrators can also lose their ability to participate in the Medicare/Medicaid programs, meaning that they will be forever prohibited from working for a company that participates in billing these federal programs. This will eventually result in ending their careers in the medical field, although it takes years to formally lose a professional license. Most companies look at an administrator's past survey results when hiring, as this is an indication of his/her professional performance.

Patients, families and even nursing home employees can call the Medicare Fraud Hotline at (800) HHS-TIPS or (800) 447-8477 to report suspected fraud. Employees who work for publicly traded companies are able to file a lawsuit on behalf of the government, called Qui Tam lawsuits, and can be awarded a portion of the monies recovered. However, these workers have to provide actual proof of the fraud, meaning that they will have to smuggle items out of the office that could possibly result in their being arrested for corporate espionage and violation of HIPAA laws. At the very least, they will probably lose their jobs and remain unemployable in their chosen field for many years. These lawsuits can actually be filed against any company, public or private; but in the years that it takes to successfully prosecute such a lawsuit, a privately held company can easily hide assets and become judgment proof. It's not easy to get away with fraud, but unfortunately it does happen. As I mentioned before, nursing home corporations often fail to ask questions about the methods that their administrators use to make money as long as the facility is reaping huge profits.

Many nursing home companies are adept at structuring their business to render them judgment proof; each individual nursing home is its own corporate entity and the nursing home pays a "consulting fee" to the parent corporation each month. This "consulting fee" is basically the profits that the nursing home makes, so if a specific facility is sued, the parent corporation is safe. As a worker in a facility that was structured in this manner, I was instructed to report any wrong-doing to the administrator. However, since she was the person who was responsible for the problems, I was actually let go when I reported her actions to the parent corporation. I had no recourse, even though she was later fired as a result of my reporting. The odds are rarely in the favor of the little guy.

The Medicare Part A Skilled Nursing benefit pays nursing homes a daily rate depending upon the RUG rate that they've been assigned. Nursing homes are required to provide their patients with all of their medications and therapies out of the amount that Medicare pays, regardless of the actual cost to the nursing home. An error in judgment could cost the nursing home hundreds or even thousands of dollars every day, which is the reason that nursing homes prescreen patients and do their best to closely manage the care they will provide.

Patients who require expensive treatments such as certain IV antibiotics or chemotherapies that cost more than the facility will be reimbursed probably won't be admitted to begin with. If such a patient is admitted with a treatment plan that costs the facility thousands of dollars each day, nursing home administrators will often attempt to get the patient's doctor to change the medications or treatments to a cheaper regimen, or to delay the treatments until after the patient has been discharged from the facility. This could be life-threatening; the patient might not be able to wait several months to start chemotherapy. Patients can speak with their doctors and refuse to allow the change in medication regimen; nursing homes will have a difficult time forcing the patients to follow a treatment plan *if they know about it*. The nursing home won't want you to know they're struggling with the cost of a patient's treatments; much of the time all of this negotiating goes on behind closed doors and the patient might never find out his treatment is being delayed. It's important to ask questions about treatments and medications while a family member is in a nursing home.

Nursing homes often negotiate contracts with providers who can administer radiation treatments at a lesser cost than if they were conducted in the physician's office. As long as the treatments are the same, it shouldn't be a problem as to where they're provided. Radiation treatments are the source of huge profits to the providers; many physicians offer this service in their office or invest in clinics in order to keep the profits in-house. If your family member will be receiving radiation at a different provider than the one your physician orders, ask the doctor to verify that the treatments will be the same. If the nursing home attempts to decrease the frequency, make sure that this won't affect the patient's care. Call the state if you must, but don't allow the patient's health to be compromised because the nursing home is attempting to save money.

Regardless as to whether the nursing home administrator is willing to authorize these very expensive treatments, the staff might be instructed to do their best to encourage or possibly even force the patient to participate in physical or occupational therapy at the very highest level in order to make enough money to help offset the cost of the treatment. The nursing home staff can come up with all sorts of reasons that the patient would benefit from intense therapy, but if the patient feels awful and doesn't feel like participating in intense therapy he doesn't have to do so. The nursing home's bottom line isn't a reason for a patient to push himself beyond his limits.

If the administrator can't get the patient to participate in the maximum amount of therapy, it's possible that the patient's chart will be falsified to reflect him having received therapies that he never actually received in order to offset their losses. One administrator I knew of yelled at a patient in order to force her to participate in therapy; when that didn't work she was heard openly stating that the facility would "just have to bill as if she did it." While illegal behaviors such as this aren't common, they do exist.

If the nursing home staff makes a mistake and admits a patient with expensive treatments that the doctor refuses to change, the facility is required to follow the treatment plan as ordered unless his care can be provided in another setting and the patient and/or family is agreeable to a transfer. For example, if the patient is able to receive the treatment at home or on an outpatient basis, the nursing home can discharge the patient after making the arrangements for him to receive the care he requires. It's not enough to ensure that the patient can access the care; he must be able to pay for it (arrangements that must be made in advance) and he must have reasonable access to transportation. A treatment that is too expensive for the nursing home might possibly be expensive for the patient after he's discharged; if he can't reasonably afford the care, the nursing home isn't able to discharge him. This information might be something that the nursing home "forgets" to mention to the patient and family, because they are hoping to get rid of him as soon as possible.

It can be intimidating when the administrator and director of nursing meets with the patient and family, insisting upon a change to a less expensive course of treatment. The nursing home can't arbitrarily change a patient's treatment plan due to the cost; even if the doctor bows to the pressure and agrees to delay treatment, the patient doesn't have to accept this decision. A quick call to the ombudsman or an attorney will change the nursing home's mind. After all, they intend to remain in business and this issue could ultimately cause them to lose their license to provide patient care. Don't allow a nursing home to intimidate you or your family member into changing the treatment plan to something more convenient for them.

I've been present when an administrator claimed that they weren't able to provide transportation to necessary treatments; she told the family that the facility van was there as a courtesy but that it was the patient's responsibility to access his own transportation. The nursing home is responsible for providing transportation to and from appointments, either via the facility van or by paying another provider for the service. Something isn't true simply because the nursing home administrator says so.

Another way that the nursing home might be able to avoid treating an expensive patient is to encourage him to leave AMA (against medical advice). Nursing homes can encourage patients to leave AMA by threatening them with huge bills, when in actuality the nursing home can't legally bill beyond the copayments and deductibles that Medicare allows. Once the patient has physically left the building, the nursing home is no longer responsible for his care and isn't obligated to readmit him if he wants to return. The nursing home also isn't responsible for setting up aftercare treatments and services for patients who leave AMA because the recommended plan of care was for him to remain in the nursing home, and he chose not to follow the plan of care.

It's important to understand that Medicare will only pay **room & board** in a nursing home, also referred to as **custodial care**, as long as the skilled treatments the patient requires can't reasonably be provided at home. It's reasonable to pay for a patient to stay in a nursing home if it would cost substantially more for the Medicare program to send therapists and nurses to his home for several hours each day. Medicare pays for specialty nursing services such as IV treatments or wound care, physical therapy, occupational therapy, or speech therapy for *up to* 100 days as long as the patient continues to require skilled services that can't be provided in another setting.

The original Medicare Part A Benefit has the following out-of-pocket costs to the patient for skilled nursing services in a facility:

> **The first 20 days** in a benefit period are covered at 100%, and are essentially free to the patient.
>
> **Days 20-100** require a copayment from the patient in the amount of $152.00 per day (2014 amounts). This amount is often covered at least in part by a Medicare supplemental policy or might possibly be covered by Medicaid, if the patient is eligible.

If a patient is discharged from the Medicare benefit before he's used the full 100 days, he can be readmitted onto Medicare services within 30 days without having to go back to the hospital as long as the nursing home is able to justify the need for treatment. His Medicare benefit will pick up where he left off – for example, if a patient with a broken hip previously used 40 days but stopped receiving therapy due to not being able to bear weight, he'll start at day 41 as long as he is able to bear weight and resume therapy within the 30-day time frame.

If the patient requires custodial care without presenting the need for skilled services, Medicare will not pay the patient's room & board regardless of whether he was recently discharged from the hospital. Most nursing homes can justify at least a week's worth of therapy, as long as they're creative. Those patients who simply don't need therapy or other skilled nursing services will have to be discharged from the nursing home, or must remain there under another type of payment.

It's important to understand that the patient doesn't actually have to be discharged from the nursing home when Medicare will no longer cover the cost of rehabilitation, but that Medicare will no longer pay for him to remain in the facility. If a patient doesn't have a payment source available for custodial care, he will probably be discharged to his home. He can be readmitted under the Medicare benefit within 30 days as long as the nursing home as a bed available and is willing to accept him. Patients who leave the nursing home are able to return within those 30 days and pick up where they left off in the 100 day Medicare benefit as long as the nursing home has a bed available and is willing to accept them.

Once the patient has passed the 30-day mark without having been provided with Medicare services, the only way that the program will pay for the unused portion of the 100-day benefit is for the patient to be admitted to the hospital for another 3-day qualifying stay (as long as the hospital is able to justify the patient's need for hospitalization). If there is no medical reason for the patient to be admitted to the hospital, he probably won't be able to return to the nursing home. Nursing homes might be able to circumvent this rule by sending patients to acute rehabilitation facilities (ARF) for three days in order for the patient to resume his treatment at the nursing home (as long as the ARF is willing to go along with the plan and the patient meets the requirements for admission to an ARF).

After the patient has utilized all 100 of his Medicare SNF days, he will have to wait until he hasn't used the Medicare Part A skilled nursing benefit for a full 60 days in order to "recharge" the 100-days all over again. This is the case even if the patient continued to require the level of care that was previously provided under the Medicare benefit. After those 60 days are up, he must be readmitted to the hospital for another 3-day stay for a new benefit period to start before receiving services under the Medicare Part A skilled nursing benefit, and the hospital admission must be for a reason unrelated to the previous admission.

For example, once a patient has received 100 days of skilled services related to a feeding tube, Medicare will no longer pay for his room & board, whether or not he is readmitted for a 3-day qualifying stay, unless 1) he hasn't used Medicare Part A benefit for 60 days, and 2) his medical need isn't related to the feeding tube. to remain in the nursing home. Even if Medicare isn't billed for his care for 60 consecutive days, it won't pay for him to receive skilled nursing related to his feeding tube if he is readmitted to the hospital for a 3-day qualifying stay. The nursing home will only be able to bill Part A for therapies or other services that are unrelated to the feeding tube. However, when it comes to billing Medicare a nursing home can become real creative. If a nursing home is willing to jeopardize its ability to participate in the Medicare and Medicaid programs, it's possible to come up with all sorts of billing codes.

The nursing home is required to report to the Medicare program constantly during the patient's stay via a formal assessment system called the *MDS* (**M**inimum **D**ata **S**et). Over the first few days of admission to the nursing home, the staff evaluates the patient's needs and sets his treatment goals. This is part of the process in developing a *plan of care* (also called the *care plan*). Each nursing home department contributes to the care plan, which is completed under the direction of the patient's primary physician. Any change to the patient's treatment plan requires an addition to the plan of care.

There is at least one nursing home employee, usually an RN, who is responsible for completing and transmitting the MDS. With the input of many other staff members, the MDS coordinator ensures that the assessment is electronically transmitted to the provider contracted with CMS to accept and review the assessment forms. The information contained on the assessment determines the amount that the nursing home will be paid, called the **RUG** rate (***Resource Utilization Group*** rate).

As I mentioned before, Medicare will only pay for room & board in a facility as long as the patient is progressing toward a goal or requires specialty medical care. In the case of those patients who are receiving therapy, their ability to continue isn't based on how many of the 100 days they have used. Once a patient has attained his highest level of functioning (plateaus), he won't be able to remain in the facility with Medicare as his payment for his room & board. This is because Medicare doesn't pay for custodial care in a nursing home. Regardless of whether the patient is able to go home and care for himself independently, lack of a caregiver at home is not a legitimate reason for Medicare to continue paying for his room & board. The only way that Medicare will pay for a patient's room & board is if he is receiving skilled nursing or therapies under the Part A benefit.

Admission to Nursing Home via Medicare Part A Benefit

To qualify to use Medicare Part A Skilled Services 100-day Benefit

1 Patient must have Medicare Part A; and

2 He must have stayed in hospital over 3 midnights (aka "qualifying stay;" and

3 He must have "skilled need" requiring the services of a Registered Nurse or Physical, Occupational or Speech Therapist on a daily basis (need must be documented by a physician); and

4 He must begin the skilled services within 30 days of leaving the hospital; and

5 If part of the 100-day benefit has already been used, he may utilize the rest of the days left in the benefit period if the services start up within 30 days of the date the patient was discharged from the Medicare level of care. Otherwise, the patient will require another 3-day stay in the hospital; and

6 The Benefit Period ends when the patient hasn't received skilled care under the Medicare benefit for 60 days in a row.

Medicare Part A doesn't pay 100% of the charges for the entire rehabilitation stay. The copayment amount is adjusted every year – the 2014 amount is $152.00 per day for days 21-100 – and a patient's ability to pay for the co-payment is usually a factor in the nursing home's decision to accept or reject a patient. The patient might pay for this amount out of his pocket, or he might have a secondary insurance policy that will cover the co-payment. There are many different secondary insurance policies available, for more information please refer to the chapter *Medicare Supplemental Insurance Policies* in the **_Medicare_** section of this book.

As I mentioned above, a patient's secondary insurance might – or might not – cover the cost of the SNF co-payments. Each supplemental plan has different coverage. Secondary insurance plans will usually pay any provider that meets Medicare criteria, with the only exception being if the patient has chosen a Medicare Select Plan. Select plans contract with specific facilities and limit the patient's choices in the process. In most cases, as long as Medicare is the primary payment source the patient will have the opportunity to choose which nursing home will provide his care.

Don't assume that a federal insurance plan (one that is provided to retired federal workers) provides excellent coverage, or that a union insurance policy is the best one available. It's important to check the coverage provided under the secondary insurance, also known as *Medigap Insurance*. It can be devastating for a patient to find that he doesn't have the fantastic coverage that he thought he did, and that the thousands of dollars in premiums he paid over the years were wasted. It is possible to change secondary insurance providers to ensure the patient has the best coverage possible. For more information about changing plans, visit the Medicare website or call a secondary insurance provider directly.

Medicare Advantage Plans – Medicare Part C

Medicare Advantage plans are *HMO's* (**H**ealth **M**aintenance **O**rganizations) and *PPO's* (**P**referred **P**rovider **O**rganizations) specifically designed for Medicare recipients. These plans are discussed in detail later in this book. Like traditional Medicare under Part A, Medicare Advantage plans aren't actually a payment source for custodial care in a nursing home, although they do pay for room & board while patients receive skilled services such as specialty nursing and physical therapies.

Advantage plan providers develop contracts with specific nursing homes to provide skilled services to their patients, so customers might not have a choice as to which facility they'll be sent for rehabilitation services. It's possible for patients to be sent to nursing homes 50 or more miles away because there's no contracted facility closer to their home. Part C Plan providers must ensure that the service is provided, but they're not required to consider how convenient the facility may be for the patient and family. Depending upon the size of the city and how many SNF's are available, it's possible that the contracted provider doesn't provide long-term care at all. The facility's focus might be on short-term rehabilitation services only. If it appears that a patient will require long-term care afterward, the plan will probably need to find another facility for his rehabilitation. Any delay obtaining a long-term payment source can cost a nursing home that only serves patients on a short-term basis thousands of dollars in lost revenue. The need for long-term care tends to limit the choices of a patient who is enrolled in an Advantage plan even further, and the patient/family may be given little (if any) choice of facility.

Part C Advantage plans might have a local back-up facility for such a scenario; if not, the plan will need to develop a one-time contract to serve that patient and ensure that the nursing home is working toward a long-term plan. Since the goal of Part C Advantage plan provider is to hold down costs, the amounts that they pay for skilled services might not be attractive to another nursing home. The insurance provider will either have to increase its rate, or the patient might be sent to a nursing home that is less-than-desirable to the patient and his family.

If the nursing home that the patient prefers isn't a contracted provider for that insurance plan, it might be possible for the insurance to negotiate a one-time contract so the patient can go there (although this is a rare occurrence). The patient's preferred nursing home is under no obligation to accept the amount that the insurance will pay; these plans often pay substantially less than the Medicare Part A rate. Simply stated, a nursing home might not be willing to take a patient at a loss when they can easily fill the bed with a higher-paying patient. They can't charge the patient the difference; it's illegal for any nursing home to charge the patient any amount beyond the regular copayments authorized by the insurance plan in order to be accepted. Generally speaking, Medicare Advantage plans will send a patient to a non-contracted nursing home only if there is no other available option.

Once he's been admitted to a nursing home, a Medicare Advantage plan patient will be monitored closely by an insurance *case manager* whose job it is to ensure that the patient's needs are met while holding down costs. It's common for the insurance provider to require weekly updates in order to issue authorization for the next seven days. As soon as the case manager believes that the patient is no longer appropriate to receive skilled services, the nursing home will be instructed to issue a *NOMNC* notice to the patient and/or family that the services will end. The notice will include information as to the appeal process and the nursing home social worker will assist with the appeal if necessary. Patients can – and do – successfully appeal these notices. For additional information about NOMNC's, refer to the chapter **Understanding How a Nursing Home Operates**.

The 20/80 day rules of traditional Medicare don't apply to Advantage plan participants; the amount of skilled nursing services provided depends on the rules of the specific Advantage plan the patient has chosen. Some plans don't require the 3-day qualifying stay and the copayments are often different than traditional Medicare. Some Medicare Advantage plans (PPO's) also allow patients to use non-contracted providers, although the patient will be left with a much higher out of pocket cost. Because the skilled nursing benefit can vary from plan-to-plan, it's worth checking into the coverage provided before choosing a Medicare Part C Advantage plan.

Private Insurance Policies

Patients who aren't yet 65 or who don't have Medicare as their primary insurance might have benefits through a current or former employer, or might possibly be paying privately for their health insurance. Most insurance companies develop contracts with specific nursing homes, and generally use the same criteria for a patient to qualify for skilled services as Medicare. In order for the insurance company to authorize the care, the services can't be reasonably provided in the patient's home and there are limitations, copayments and deductibles. Like Medicare Advantage plans, most insurance plans employ case managers whose sole purpose is to monitor patient services and hold down costs.

Each insurance company privately negotiates its own contracted rates for the services the nursing home will provide, and it's possible that the patient will be able to choose between several different facilities in the area. There is no requirement for insurance companies to develop a contract with a facility in every town, nor is every nursing home required to negotiate a contract with every insurance plan. In rural areas, it's possible for plan members to travel several hundred miles in order to receive care from an in-plan provider. Just like Medicare, private insurance companies provide skilled services for a limited amount of time and if the patient will need to stay in the facility on a long-term basis, it will be necessary for the patient to have another payment source in place when the insurance company stops paying.

Private Pay

Patients who have the ability to pay out-of-pocket for their long-term care (custodial care) are considered to be *Private Pay* patients. According to a MetLife survey in 2004, the average cost of nursing home care in the United States tops $70,000 per year. Unless a person has substantial assets, he might not be able to pay privately for very long. Private pay patients generally are paying for room & board; they may still be able to receive therapy via the Medicare Part B benefit or via their private insurance if they don't have Medicare. If for some reason they don't have private insurance, they can also pay privately for therapy (although this is prohibitively expensive).

Every patient who is paying privately for his room & board should meet with an *elder law attorney* who specializes in Medicaid planning to see if the patient might possibly become eligible for Medicaid, whether now or in the future. This type of law is different than estate law; an elder law attorney is knowledgeable about the eligibility criteria for Medicaid and might be able to use the legal loopholes in the program to pay for the patient's care. I've seen many people who don't believe that they're eligible later find that, with a little planning, they would have been able to preserve some or all of their assets. Even if the patient isn't eligible when he is first admitted, an elder law attorney might be able to reduce the amount of money the patient must pay out of pocket before he qualifies for Medicaid. A patient doesn't necessarily need to be elderly in order for an elder law attorney to be helpful.

Patients who pay privately for their room & board are usually charged extra for such items as oxygen, briefs/pads, and miscellaneous supplies such as shampoo, lotions, etc. These same items are included in the daily rate for patients whose payment source is Medicare and Medicaid, but because the patient is paying privately the nursing home is able to charge for everything beyond the basic room & board. It's possible to bring your own supplies into the nursing home to cut back on the out-of-pocket expenses, but if you choose to do so it's important to monitor the supplies you bring in to ensure they aren't being used for other patients.

Items such as specialty mattresses, wound care supplies and feeding tube supplies can cost hundreds – or thousands – of dollars each month in addition to the cost of room & board; again, these same items are provided at no extra cost if the payment source is Medicare and Medicaid. Even though these supplies are necessary medical items, Medicare and most private insurances do not pay for these items on an ongoing basis for patients who are located in nursing homes. Nursing homes charge exorbitant amounts to rent specialty items *because they can*, but patients have the right to purchase them outright from equipment providers or even private parties.

Nursing homes don't always pay full price when they purchase or rent these items, but will charge full price (and more) to the patient. I worked for profit-driven nursing home that attempted to cajole a grieving family member into donating a $6,000 specialty mattress to the facility because they would be able to charge another patient over $100 per day to use it. The family instead chose to donate the mattress to a non-profit agency – not only were they able to take a tax write-off, they also provided comfort to patients in need. The nursing home administrator was angry about the loss of revenue.

Traditional Medicaid

Traditional Medicaid is a health insurance program provided to people who are low-income and who don't reside in nursing homes; they might live at home or in an assisted living facility. There are many different types of Medicaid programs that vary according to the recipient's age, income and location of residence; the eligibility for these programs is changing due to the Affordable Care Act. It's safe to say that a person is eligible for traditional Medicaid if he has Supplemental Security Income but any other questions about eligibility should be directed to the Medicaid program in the state where the patient resides.

Regarding nursing home placement, it is possible for traditional Medicaid to pay for a few days in a nursing home; however, if the patient remains in the nursing home longer than 30 days (whether or not Medicaid is paying the bill), the Medicaid program rules will probably require that his case be transitioned to the institutional program. Once he is discharged from the nursing home, his Medicaid will probably be changed back to the type of services (traditional Medicaid) that he had before he was admitted to the nursing home. The only exception would be if he were approved to receive services via a Medicaid waiver program when he is discharged from the nursing home.

Institutional Medicaid is the name of the program that pays for long-term care. There is a difference in the eligibility criteria between traditional and institutional Medicaid, and there's no guarantee a person who qualifies for one program will qualify for the other. A patient could have gifted away tens of thousands of dollars to family members a few months before he lands in the nursing home and still qualify for traditional Medicaid, but he won't be eligible for the institutional program. The application to transition a patient from traditional to institutional Medicaid is often completed by the nursing home business office without the family's knowledge.

Many nursing home admissions and office staff aren't aware of the differences in eligibility criteria between the different Medicaid programs. There is no specific educational requirement to work in either of these jobs, and they might possess no practical knowledge of the Medicaid program. This can be beneficial to families, who can use the facility's lack of knowledge about Medicaid in order to have the patient admitted. As long as the family doesn't accept personal responsibility for the patient's medical bills, in most cases the only money that the nursing home can ask for is the patient's share of cost. Refer to the chapter on **Medicaid** for more information about Medicaid eligibility.

A nursing home for which I once worked hired a new office manager, who approved a patient's based on the fact that her payment source appeared to be Medicaid. After the patient was admitted into the facility, it was found that she wasn't eligible for the institutional program because she had sold a home and gave the money to her children. This lack of knowledge cost the nursing home thousands of dollars in unreimbursed care that they provided. Had the office manager asked me or any number of other staff members to review the application, the patient never would have been approved.

"Pending" Medicaid
When a patient is attempting to gain entry into a nursing home, he will need to have a payment in place. If the payment source will be Medicaid, it will be necessary for the patient to apply for *institutional Medicaid* to pay for his room & board. Even if a patient has been approved for traditional Medicaid in a home-

based setting, an application will need to be placed for the institutional Medicaid program.

Eligibility for the institutional Medicaid program is confusing; a patient isn't eligible for Medicaid until he's been admitted into a medical facility, yet he generally won't be admitted into a nursing home until he has a payment source (Medicaid) in place. The application can be submitted while the patient is in the hospital or other facility, but since most hospitalizations last less than a week it's highly doubtful that the Medicaid will be submitted, much less approved, in time for the patient to be sent to a nursing home. An uncomplicated Medicaid application can take up to 90 days for approval, while an application with multiple issues to address can take six or more months to become approved. The application can't be submitted while the patient is at home; any application submitted before the patient arrives at a medical facility will be denied *because he must be physically located in an inpatient setting in order to be eligible for institutional Medicaid.*

Patients who have applied for institutional Medicaid and are awaiting a decision are considered to be "*pending Medicaid*" and are often referred to as "*penders*." The Medicaid application can be approved retroactively up to three months prior to the date the application was placed as long as the patient was otherwise eligible for that time period (this helps to cover hospital bills). Anyone is able to place an application for Medicaid, but there is no assurance that a patient is eligible for the program until the application has actually been approved. Because of this, many nursing homes won't accept a patient without the Medicaid in place, or will require some type of guarantee that they'll be paid in the event that the Medicaid is denied.

A guarantee is exactly what it sounds like; a person or agency is guaranteeing that they will pay for the patient's room & board if for any reason the Medicaid is not approved. There could be any number of reasons that that Medicaid might not be approved, and without a backup payment source the nursing home will be stuck with a non-paying patient. If the patient can be admitted via another payment source (such as under the Medicare Part A benefit or via a hospice respite admission), it's possible that a guarantee won't be required. Each facility is different.

The best way to get a patient accepted for long-term care is to be admitted directly from the hospital via the Medicare Part A benefit and immediately placing an application for Medicaid. Depending upon the area in which the patient lives, a Medicaid application can take anywhere from a couple of weeks to several months to be approved. There's a good chance that an application that has been submitted when the patient first arrived in the facility will be approved before the Medicare services have been completed. If the Medicaid application hasn't been approved by then, the nursing home might ask the family to pay for his room & board, but as long as the family didn't issue a personal guarantee when the patient was admitted it's not their responsibility to pay for the patient's room & board. The nursing home can't discharge the patient if he doesn't have a safe discharge plan, yet doesn't have a payment source in place.

Another way for a patient to be admitted would be for him to pay privately for a few months, and then apply for Medicaid when he runs out of money. This works as long as the patient has enough money to pay out of pocket for awhile, but if he runs out of money before the Medicaid is approved, the nursing home will probably look to the family for payment. It's important that the family not sign any forms accepting financial responsibility for the patient, otherwise they'll be responsible for paying the patient's bill until the Medicaid is approved. Many nursing homes bury the payment guarantee deep within the admissions agreement and hope that the family members will inadvertently sign it. Please refer to the section *Signing The Intake Packet* for additional information.

If the patient doesn't have the ability to pay privately for awhile, it's possible to find a nursing home that will accept him and help place his Medicaid application after he's been admitted. Sometimes these nursing homes might be less desirable than other nursing homes in the area, and they can't be as choosy when it comes to accepting patients, but it's also possible that the nursing home provides excellent care and that they reason they accepted the patient is because the Medicaid appears to be a sure thing. If the patient doesn't like that particular nursing home he can transfer to another facility once his Medicaid has been approved. The facility is betting that the patient will have become accustomed to live in that facility and won't want to move (people dislike change). The family might be hesitant to send the patient to a nursing home where he doesn't intend to stay long-term, but sometimes they have no other choices available to them at the time. It's frustrating for families who aren't able to care for a patient when they realize that the nursing home they've chosen isn't obligated to accept him.

Nursing homes often look to a patient's family members as another potential source for a payment guarantee. Some nursing homes will allow the family to pay a deposit of several thousand dollars to the nursing home; if and when the Medicaid is approved the nursing home might refund the family's money. Other nursing homes require that the patient's bill be paid in full every month, with the promise of a refund for the months that are covered when the Medicaid is finally approved. This seems extreme, but unfortunately (sometimes) it's the only way to get a patient admitted into a nursing home. It's important to get the nursing home's promise in writing, because if it's your word against theirs you will have no legal recourse if the money isn't refunded as agreed.

The nursing home can't legally charge the patient/family for the same period of time that Medicaid pays (this would be double billing). I have seen some nursing homes refuse to refund the money the family paid out of their own pocket, and start billing Medicaid from the date of approval forward (even though Medicaid was approved retroactive to the day he was admitted into the nursing home). The only reason that the nursing home would keep the private-pay monies would be due to the private-pay rate being higher than the Medicaid daily rate. It depends upon the state as to whether there is a difference in the Medicaid versus private-pay rate. The payment issues are buried deep within the admissions agreement, so be careful what you sign when you admit a family member.

If a patient has Medicaid in one state, it doesn't just transfer when he chooses to move to a nursing home in another state. Even though the eligibility process and rules are basically the same, a new Medicaid application will have to be submitted and the patient will have to undergo the application process all over again. This is frustrating for people who live in an area where the hospital is just across the state line; he might be approved for Medicaid in the state where the hospital is located but will have to reapply in order to be placed in a nursing home near his home. If your family member is admitted to a hospital in another state and will require skilled nursing services when he's discharged, discuss this issue with the hospital social worker or discharge planner in order to ensure that his needs are met.

Nursing homes aren't always forthcoming when it comes to accepting a patient; a former patient of mine whose payment source was Medicaid was accepted into a nursing home in another state when his wife moved there. I was coordinating the discharge, and the admissions representative of the new facility assured me that there was no problem with the transfer. There was no mention of a deposit being necessary; in fact, the nursing home called and said they would accept the patient that weekend. I was assured that the new nursing home had everything that they needed to accept the patient, and it was reasonable to expect that the nursing home wouldn't require a deposit because Medicaid eligibility is pretty much the same from state-to-state.

A close family friend provided the patient's transportation, driving nearly 300 miles round-trip to bring him to the new facility. When he arrived, a worker rushed out to the car and demanded a check for over $6,000 from the friend (who wasn't legally responsible for the patient). They simply would not allow the patient entry without it. Feeling pressured (he had an elderly man who required a diaper change sitting in the front seat of his car), the friend wrote the check. Every month, the nursing home billed this gentleman who had merely provided transportation and threatened to sue him if he didn't pay. The nursing home never assisted with the Medicaid application, and the friend paid the patient's room & board until his death six months later – even though he was under no legal obligation to do so. Had the friend and patient's wife spoken with an elder law attorney, they could have saved months of heartache and thousands of dollars they couldn't afford.

Some states, counties, hospitals or social service agencies will assess a patient's ability to pay and have a process in place to guarantee payment if the patient is denied Medicaid. They generally have their own application process and require the same *verifications* that Medicaid requires, because they are promising to pay for the patient's room and board *forever* if the Medicaid application is denied. The guarantee is provided based on the information that was provided to them and if any eligibility problems are later identified, the guarantee will probably be rescinded. A guarantee can be a useful tool to get a patient into a nursing home, but they're not offered in every area. Agencies that offer guarantees are rare, but they do exist.

Some hospitals will immediately place an application for Medicaid in order to make the patient easier to discharge (and also to help cover the patient's copayments and deductibles in the hospital); this might help to expedite the discharge process. The hospital itself might guarantee the nursing home's payment, or an insurance plan such as an HMO might pay the nursing home for a month or two in order to get hard-to-place patients out of the hospital. For the most part, though, hospitals and insurance companies rarely guarantee the patient's nursing home placement for long-term care.

Placing A Patient "Pending Medicaid."

- Ensure that you have gathered all of the necessary verifications.

- Meet with Elder Law Attorney or other Medicaid Professional to help with the application, if needed.

- Offer ongoing assistance in obtaining any further verifications if at all possible.

- Ask the nursing home if any deposit will be necessary *before* the patient is admitted.

- Don't sign anything personally guaranteeing the patient's payment in the nursing home; have the patient sign his/her own paperwork if at all possible.

- Call the Long-Term Care Ombudsman to help mediate once the patient has been admitted if there are any problems.

It's also possible that the Veteran's Administration will pay for a couple of month's placement while the Medicaid application is in process; this usually occurs when the patient is physically located in a VA hospital and no nursing home is willing to accept him. While this isn't actually a payment guarantee, it does help get the patient placed in a nursing home. The patient has to meet the VA criteria in order for this to be a possibility.

Accepting patients who are pending Medicaid with no guarantee of payment poses a financial risk to nursing homes, and nursing homes do have the right to refuse any patient if they don't believe they can meet the patient's needs. Without some form of guarantee, the nursing home risks the very real possibility that they'll be stuck with a non-paying patient they aren't able to discharge. This is why nursing homes carefully screen patients for potential payment problems before they're admitted. The nursing home can attempt to intimidate the patient and/or family into paying out-of-pocket, but if they can't collect the money they might be providing free services to a patient for a long, long time.

Institutional Medicaid

Institutional Medicaid (also known as *long-term Medicaid* or *nursing home Medicaid*) is a federally funded program that is administered by each state with matching federal dollars which pays for room & board in a nursing home on a long-term basis. This is the type of Medicaid for which a "pender" (above) has applied. Institutional Medicaid pays the room & board for patients who can't afford to pay out-of-pocket for their nursing home placement. The payment system is simple: the unmarried patient pays his income to the nursing home and the Medicaid program pays the difference between the patient's income and the actual billed charges. Married patients might be able to pay less toward their care in order for their spouse to maintain the household expenses out in the community.

Institutional Medicaid might also pay for in-home care under special waiver programs in which the client meets all of the eligibility guidelines for Medicaid (except the part about being a patient in a medical facility). Medicaid waiver programs vary from state to state and often have a long waiting list. These programs do not pay for 24-hour care in the home and aren't the answer for every patient. There are many different types of waiver programs - for additional information about waiver programs contact your local Medicaid office or *AAA* (Area Agency on Aging).

In order to qualify for institutional Medicaid, patients must have less than $2,000 in assets (this amount varies according to state), may own one home, one car, and a burial plan that holds no cash value to them; additionally, each state sets its own income limit. If the patient is even one penny over the asset or income limit, Medicaid won't pay for a patient to remain in a nursing home. The patient can't have given away or transferred assets in the past 60 months (5 years). Please refer to the chapters on institutional Medicaid for additional eligibility information.

Medicaid eligibility is a dirty little secret about which many nursing homes don't like to discuss. This is because they often are able to charge more for private-pay patients and therefore have little incentive to offer information about Medicaid. Even if the Medicaid and private-pay rates are close to the same amount, nursing homes are able to charge for the same ancillary supplies and equipment that they're required to provide to Medicaid recipients for free. Medicaid programs often pay

60 days or more in arrears, while private-pay patients pay in advance. It's easy to see why private-pay patients are more desirable than those who are on Medicaid.

Nursing homes are required to provide information about federal and state programs to help pay for the placement *if the patient or family asks*; if the family doesn't specifically ask, the facility is under no obligation to offer the information. Even if the family mentions to the nursing staff that they're struggling to pay for the patient's room & board, this information probably won't make its way back to the business office. Unless the family discusses this problem with the billing office, the nursing home probably won't know if a patient's family is struggling financially or if the patient is running out of money.

Sometimes it's not enough to speak with the business office manager; she might not have a working knowledge of Medicaid eligibility and therefore won't be able to properly advise patients and their families. Because of the complexity of Medicaid applications, some nursing homes do employ benefits specialists that assist patients with applications – but their services probably won't be offered unless the family asks to meet with them. The end result is that many people aren't aware they are able to qualify the patient for Medicaid, and might pay thousands of dollars out of their own pocket for which they will never be reimbursed.

> Tony's mother transferred her home into his name in 1996; she was placed in a nursing home in 2005 for rehabilitation and wasn't able to return home afterward. A friend whose parents were in a nursing home told Tony that his mother probably didn't qualify for Medicaid, and he believed them because it "sounded about right." He paid for her $6,000 room & board each month out of his own savings account, nearly wiping him out financially. Tony finally applied for Medicaid a couple of years later, and the Medicaid eligibility worker told him that his mother had been eligible the entire time that she had been in the nursing home. This was after he had paid over $125,000 out of his own pocket! When he complained to the nursing home administrator, she told him that he should have asked for assistance because they aren't clairvoyant and had no idea as to whether or not his mother might be eligible for Medicaid. He was never able to recover any of the money he'd paid.

Unmarried patients who utilize Medicaid as the payment of room & board in a nursing home are allowed to keep a minimum of $30.00 per month for a ***personal needs allowance*** (this amount varies from state to state and in most cases hasn't been adjusted for many years). The rest of the patient's income is paid to the nursing home as the patient's ***share of cost***, or ***patient liability***. If the patient is a veteran or the spouse of a deceased veteran, it's possible he'll qualify for a program that will pay him another $90.00 per month that doesn't count toward his share of cost). Even though these programs have nothing to do with each other, the

Medicaid program requires that an application for this VA program (*Aid & Attendance*) be submitted if the patient appears to be eligible. The applications can easily be found online.

Patients who are married don't follow the same rule regarding their share of cost; the *community spouse* (the spouse who remains in the community) is allowed to keep an amount that is determined by Medicaid to be sufficient to sustain the household, usually *up to* $2,500 or so depending upon the amount of household bills (this amount varies from state to state). The community spouse is also allowed to keep some of the joint assets. The program that determines the amount of income and assets that the community spouse will be allowed to keep is called *spousal impoverishment*. This program is part of the application process and automatically calculated into the amount of his income that the married patient has to pay. Although this program is able to preserve some of the spouse's assets, a good *elder law attorney* might be better able to help preserve the spouse's financial position and save the spouse tens of thousands of dollars (or more). Spousal impoverishment does not apply to unmarried patients who cohabitate; it's best to seek the advice of an elder law attorney for situations such as this.

If a patient has a Medigap insurance policy that pays secondary to Medicare, the Medicaid program will probably absorb the cost of the premiums; the patient will continue to pay for the secondary insurance and the Medicaid program will pay that much more to the nursing home. If the patient has no secondary insurance, it is possible that institutional Medicaid will act as a secondary insurance to Medicare for days 21-100 in the nursing home as well as to pick up the co-payments and deductibles that a private insurance policy would normally cover. Since the recession began, many states no longer pay as a secondary and instead allow nursing homes a special write-off at the end of the year to offset their costs. Most states encourage patients to have a secondary insurance plan if at all possible.

Medicaid is a complicated program; unless the patient's finances are simple it's worth the cost of an elder law attorney or other Medicaid professional to help with the application. There are private companies that assist with applications, often staffed by former Medicaid eligibility workers. They generally cost less than hiring an attorney, and if they identify an issue that requires legal intervention they'll refer to an elder law attorney. It *is* possible for the average person to complete a Medicaid application; if you choose to do so, it's important to pay attention to detail. Incorrect information or lack of verifications can delay an application for months, or will result in a denial of payment. I can't stress enough how valuable an elder law attorney can be when it comes to Medicaid eligibility; I've seen people preserve $100,000 in assets while their spouse was approved for Medicaid to pay the cost of the nursing home placement.

Another important aspect of institutional Medicaid is that it is only available to patients who are residents of nursing homes or other facilities (such as hospitals) that meet certain CMS eligibility criteria. Institutional Medicaid recipients who are discharged from approved medical facilities and admitted into non-approved facilities such as hospice inpatient units (facilities that provide *end-of-life care* to patients) or ALF's *are not eligible for institutional Medicaid.* The reason the patient might be moved to a hospice inpatient unit is to provide 24-hour nursing with a physician available at all hours; for patients who are in excruciating pain or who have symptoms that need to be managed closely an inpatient unit is an excellent place to have this care provided. However, by moving the patient out of a nursing home the hospice is jeopardizing his payment source not only for long-term care, but possibly for his hospice care as well.

Many medical providers don't understand the differences in Medicaid and Medicare, and it ends up creating a huge problem for them. This is especially true if the patient's payment for that program (such as hospice) was Medicaid, and the patient is only eligible for Medicaid if he resides in a nursing home. Moving a patient to a hospice inpatient facility is a perfect way for a nursing home to get rid of a problem patient; they can simply refuse to accept him back. The hospice will have a difficult time discharging the patient because his Medicaid is no longer in effect, and he'll have to reapply for Medicaid all over again.

Regardless of whether institutional Medicaid was the payment source in the last setting; the patient loses his eligibility once he is discharged from the nursing home. The Medicaid program will usually terminate the patient from the program at the end of the calendar month. In order to requalify for Medicaid, it's possible that the patient will have to be readmitted to a nursing home on a Medicaid pending basis and endure the application process all over again. The nursing home might have to wait 3-4 months before they receive any payment (including for medications and specialty treatments); this can be a contributing factor to why a nursing home might refuse to take the patient.

If for some reason the former Medicaid patient who was admitted into a non-CMS approved facility is difficult to place, such as displaying behavioral problems, having a high acuity (greater medical needs), or the family is difficult to deal with, the patient probably won't be going anywhere for awhile. It's possible that the facility will be providing free room & board until a safe discharge plan can be developed, because they are required to follow the same rules as other types of caregiving facilities. This is true even if the patient no longer meets the criteria to remain on that program (for example, a patient in a hospice inpatient facility who no longer meets the criteria for hospice care). In these cases, it's possible for the discharging facility to pay for a few months room & board in an ALF until a long-term payment source can be secured.

State or County Placement

It was mentioned in the section on institutional Medicaid that a state or county agency might guarantee payment for a patient who is pending Medicaid. If for some reason the patient is denied Medicaid, the guaranteeing agency might continue paying the patient's room & board indefinitely. These agencies usually put patients through a rigorous application process and are reasonably assured that the Medicaid will be approved. However, they issue their guarantee based on all of the information in the application, and if the Medicaid is denied based on something that was omitted it's possible that they will withdraw their guarantee and the facility won't be paid. This can be confusing, to say the least.

In addition to acting as a guarantor, sometimes state or local programs will pay the room & board in a nursing home for patients who don't qualify for institutional Medicaid. A patient might not qualify for Medicaid for any number of reasons, such as income that exceeds the limit for that particular state. For additional information about the various types of alternative payment for nursing home placement available in your area, speak with a nursing home admissions coordinator, social worker or Medicaid professional. You can also obtain information about available payment sources from your local Area Agency on Aging. This type of payment is fairly rare, because most local government budgets can't afford to pay for long-term care; they exist simply to fill in the gaps where patients aren't eligible for Medicaid and yet can't afford to pay the full cost of placement.

Respite Programs

There are programs, such as Medicaid-based aging waiver programs, that are set up to provide assistance to patients who don't reside in nursing homes yet meet all of the other criteria for institutional Medicaid. These patients are able to maintain in a homelike environment with the assistance of caregivers paid for by the Medicaid program, rather than forced to reside in a nursing home. The criteria for these programs is that patients must require assistance with their activities of daily living, but can't require 24-hour care. If they require too much assistance, they're not eligible – but if they don't require enough care, they're also not eligible for the program. It's a fine line.

Many of these programs offer a respite component, where patients can be admitted to a nursing home for a few days or weeks in order to give their caregivers a break. This is called *respite care.* The patient's program case manager can help to make all of the arrangements for respite admissions, which are provided at no cost to the patient or family. The patient might not have a choice as to where he may go for respite, as the program that is funding the respite will be making the arrangements and will develop a contract with that facility. This is not a long-term solution for the patient, but it does help out. Hospice programs also offer respite to their patients (sometimes they provide respite in their inpatient unit, while other times they utilize nursing homes for this service).

Some local agencies such as the Alzheimer's Association or other public or private agencies might also offer a program that specifically pays for respite care and nothing else; these programs are usually grant funded and the coverage is for a very short period of time. It's worth calling around to ask if this type of assistance is available in your community and how it can be accessed. Respite might also be provided on a daily basis in an adult daycare facility.

Patients or their family members can also pay privately for respite. Because the placement isn't limited due to funding sources, patients can use an assisted living facility, group facility or any setting that will can meet the patient's needs. Many nursing homes don't like to provide respite; these admissions are time-consuming and provide very little profit.

Veteran's Administration (VA)

The VA is limited as to how it pays for nursing home placement; in most cases the VA will only pay for a patient's room & board in a privately owned nursing home on a long-term basis if the patient has a service-connected disability of 70% or greater. The VA develops contracts with specific nursing homes, and has a nursing home geriatric case management unit that works closely to manage the care provided to their patients in each facility. The Veteran's Administration might also provide long-term care in a facility that is owned and operated by the VA, if there is one in the area.

The VA might also pay for a couple of month's placement in a facility if the Veterans Administration is the payment source for a patient in the hospital and there's no obvious discharge plan in place. The only reason that the VA would do so is to give a nursing home enough time to secure a long-term payment source like Medicaid. This doesn't happen very often and is only done on a case-by-case basis.

The VA also pays nursing home room & board in certain circumstances for patients who are currently receiving hospice care and have no other caregiving options. This option is available whether or not the patient's hospice care is paid by the Veteran's Administration or by Medicare; however, the patient may only remain in the nursing home as long as he is receiving hospice care. If he is discharged from hospice (for example, if the patient is sent to the hospital for treatment or if the patient doesn't appear to be declining), the VA will no longer pay for his room & board. This can be frustrating for the patient who chooses hospice and is placed in a nursing home, only to find that the hospice can no longer justify serving him. He will either be discharged to another setting or will have to qualify for another type of payment in order to remain in the nursing home. Hospice programs must work closely with the nursing home to ensure that the patient's needs will be met after he is discharged from their program.

Regardless of the manner in which the patient qualifies for nursing home placement, his care will be closely monitored by the Veteran's Administration. This is to ensure that he receives the services that he requires and that he remains eligible for the VA to continue paying for his room & board. Contact your local

Veteran's Administration office for additional information about nursing home placement.

Other Veteran's Programs

Veterans with a higher pension amount might be able to pay for their room & board in a nursing home out of their pocket; this is considered to be private-pay monies and isn't considered to be a Veteran's payment at all. There is no case manager assigned and the VA will have no interaction with the nursing home at all. Patients who have a VA pension or annuity might continue to receive the same income, as long as the amount they receive each month is enough to cover the nursing home room & board.

If the patient's ongoing income isn't sufficient to pay the full cost of placement, it will be necessary to apply for Medicaid to supplement his income to pay for the cost of the care. At that point, his VA income might possibly convert to a different program called Aid & Attendance and be decreased to $90.00 per month. This might not seem fair, but the $90.00 won't count toward the patient's share of cost and he can use it for whatever he would like (as long as it doesn't exceed the $2,000 maximum assets allowable under Medicaid).

One doesn't have to be receiving a full veteran's pension prior to admission in order to be eligible for Aid & Attendance benefits. A&A is available to those veterans or their widowed spouses as long as the veteran was honorably discharged after serving at least 90 days, one day of which must have been during active wartime. To qualify for the care, the veteran or widowed spouse must require assistance with their activities of daily living. This program is designed to assist lower-income veterans; there is financial criteria that must be met and this program isn't available to every veteran.

Aid & Attendance might available to patients who are residing in a nursing home, regardless of their eligibility for Medicaid. It can also be used to offset the cost of care in an ALF, small group facility, or at home as long as they require assistance to remain independent. The A&A program offers up to $1,758 per month to a veteran, $1,130 for the spouse of a deceased veteran, $1,380 for a veteran with a sick spouse, or $2,085 for a couple who both require assistance. For additional information about the A&A program you can access the VA website at www.va.gov or speak with someone by calling (800) 827-1000. There is also a wealth of information available at www.veteranaid.org.

Applying for Aid & Attendance isn't difficult, although the application itself appears quite daunting. There are companies that offer assistance with the application process, and their brochures or solicitations can be found in nearly every senior center. Using one of these companies doesn't expedite the process, and it's actually illegal for them to charge for assisting with Aid & Attendance benefits. Companies circumvent this rule by charging for "lifetime benefit assistance," essentially offering to apply for any benefits for which the senior might qualify, and it's certainly not cheap. Lifetime benefit assistance" can cost as much as $1,000.00 for the same assistance that can be accessed for free. The Veteran's Administration does certify some agencies or attorneys to assist with the application process, but they aren't allowed to charge for the service either. Many elder law attorneys are certified by the VA and assist with benefits as part of the legal package they offer.

It's important to note that Aid & Attendance isn't an immediate solution; it can take a year or longer to become approved and even longer to start receiving Aid & Attendance monies from the VA. The program pays retroactive to the date of application, which means that first check will include several months of retroactive payments. For Medicaid recipients, this money will count toward the $2,000 allowable asset limit so it's important to use the money to buy items (or to present receipts for items that have already been purchased and reimburse the person who paid for them immediately) for the patient as soon as possible. Many people use this money to help pay for a burial plan, or to pay for caregivers to provide socialization for the patient in the nursing home.

State or Private Veteran's Homes (non-VA)

There are Veteran's nursing homes in many different areas of the country that only accept veterans and charge a lesser amount out of pocket than if the patient had to pay privately - often around 30% of his income. The remainder is made up either by state funding, Medicaid or private pay. These state or private veteran's homes aren't always easy to find and there's usually a long waiting list for the beds. Some families will move a patient hundreds or thousands of miles away in order to secure a bed in a facility dedicated to veterans. This will save him from having to deplete his entire life savings by paying privately for his care, and allow his family members to save their inheritance.

State Veteran's homes are funded with a combination of VA monies and state or private financing, and aren't staffed by VA employees. They are considered to be separate from the Veteran's Administration altogether. Many of them do not have contracts with the VA and won't accept VA funding as a payment source for their patients.

Hospice Benefit

Hospice care is a health insurance-funded program that offers *terminal care* to patients. This type of care is also known as *palliative care,* or *end-of-life care.* Hospice isn't a place; it's an actual type of care that can be provided in just about any setting. Hospice doesn't pay for long-term nursing home placement, although there are two separate levels of care that pay for short-term care in skilled nursing facilities or hospice inpatient units.

One of the benefits offered by the Medicare hospice benefit is ***respite care***, generally a five-day stay in a skilled nursing facility. The respite benefit is provided according to the patient's & family's need; many hospices will limit the respite to once every 60-90 days rather than per event (such as out-of-town weddings, funerals, vacations, etc). Respite care is usually a planned admission, although sometimes ***caregiver breakdown*** occurs wherein the caregiver desperately needs a rest. The hospice will make all of the arrangements for the patient to be admitted to a nursing home for a short period of time. Patients whose hospice payment is Medicare or Medicaid will have these options, but hospice patients with private insurance or even the Veteran's Administration might not have the option of placing the patient in a nursing home for a respite admission. Each case is different; to find out if your family member would be eligible for a respite admission speak with your hospice social worker or case manager.

Hospices and nursing homes must have a contract detailing the services each facility will provide for their patients, and hospices can only serve patients in nursing homes with which they have a contract. This is the case whether the patient has been admitted on a short-term basis or the patient is a full time resident of the nursing home. If the patient's preferred nursing home doesn't have a contract with the hospice serving that patient, it might be possible for them to negotiate a one-time contract. It's up to the nursing home and the hospice as to whether they can come to an agreement on the terms of the contract.

During the time that the hospice patient is receiving respite care in the nursing home, it's possible that the caregiver will realize that it's time to place the patient in a nursing home on a long-term basis. This allows the hospice a short period of time to help the family develop a plan to pay for long-term placement, or to find an assisted living facility or group home that can provide for the patient's needs within his ability to pay. If a long-term placement can't be found in such a short period of time, the patient will probably have to return home until a long-term placement can be secured. If the patient refuses to leave the nursing home, the nursing home will be forced to evict the patient in order to get him to leave. Hospices do their very best to ensure that this doesn't happen, but occasionally a patient or family member with knowledge of the system will refuse to take the patient home once he's got his foot in the door. The nursing home will probably blame the hospice, and this will cause a lot of drama until a discharge can be arranged.

The Medicare hospice benefit also provides for ***inpatient care***, which is a short-term admission to a nursing home in order for the terminal patient to receive 24-hour nursing care for symptom management. Inpatient level of care is provided when a patient would probably have been sent to the hospital, but due to his receiving hospice care such a hospital stay isn't warranted. A patient can be admitted to a nursing home on an inpatient level of care for reasons such as pain management, a change of medications that requires a nurse's assessment every hour, or other symptoms that are out of control. There is no limit as to the length of an inpatient admission; the patient's physical condition dictates how long the patient will need to stay there.

Both the hospice inpatient and respite levels of care can also be provided in a stand-alone *inpatient unit (IPU)* – but many hospices don't own their own inpatient unit. A hospice inpatient unit is essentially a miniature hospital for hospice patients, and due to cost and the staffing difficulties most hospices instead choose to contract with area nursing homes to provide the higher level of care that the patient requires. While Medicare pays the hospice a higher rate as a patient receives comprehensive care under the inpatient benefit, the payment isn't increased while patients receive care under the respite benefit. Respite is a benefit that provides a much-needed rest to the caregivers; Medicare pays the regular daily rate to the hospice and the payment is essentially passed through to the nursing home.

Other than providing payment for short-term services such as respite and general inpatient level of care, hospices don't pay for any type of nursing home placement. The patient will have to use whatever payment source for nursing home placement that he would have used if the hospice wasn't involved. The hospice social worker can assist the patient with information when it comes to placement issues.

The room & board for hospice patients whose long-term payment source is Medicaid is paid differently than the regular nursing home patient. Instead of paying the nursing home directly, the Medicaid program pays the hospice for the patient's room & board at 95% of the nursing home's contracted Medicaid rate. The reason that the program reduces the amount paid to the nursing home is because the hospice provides duplicate services (bathing, medication management, nursing and other services) that the nursing home would have otherwise provided. In other words, the Medicaid program saves money on hospice patients who reside in nursing homes. The nursing homes don't necessarily lose money on hospice patients; CMS allows for hospices to pay the 5% to the nursing homes without considering it to be an illegal kickback. If hospices weren't allowed to make up the difference, nursing homes would have less of an incentive to allow patients to elect to use hospice services (other than the pain and suffering of their residents, which rarely matters to the corporate accounting department). Some hospice companies choose not to pay the difference; these companies might have a difficult time finding a nursing home willing to work with them regarding nursing home placement and respite. Remember that nursing homes are under no obligation to allow every local hospice to provide services to their patients.

Hospice patients whose room & board are paid by Medicaid can be served at one of two levels of care; routine or the higher inpatient rate if the patient requires additional care from the nursing home and hospice as described above. Inpatient care is a very short-term service, and as soon as the patient's symptoms are under control his payment will be dropped back to the routine level of care.

Many nursing homes try to discourage their patients from signing onto hospice programs because the hospice essentially takes over the medical care for the patient and provides the medical oversight to the nursing home. This can create a power struggle between the hospice and the nursing home over who "controls" the patient's care. Hospice is most beneficial to a nursing home patient when he has pain or symptom management issues that the nursing home can't manage, or if the physician won't prescribe the medications the patient needs unless he is receiving hospice care.

Some medical professionals (doctors, nurses, administrators) consider hospice to be unnecessary in nursing homes, and obviously hospices disagree. Hospice intervention can be beneficial because it allows the patient to decline without the nursing home having to continue to attempt to help the patient's condition improve. It can also save the nursing home and/or the patient hundreds of dollars each month by providing equipment and supplies for the patient. Sometimes, however, the patient and family don't notice the difference.

Hospices send their marketers into nursing homes to gain as many referrals as possible, because nursing homes are full of terminal patients. Some nursing homes limit their hospice contracts to only a few companies (which is legal), and strongly encourage their patients to utilize the services of a hospice that is affiliated with the nursing home (which is illegal). I worked for a nursing home that attempted to steer every hospice patient to the company that was owned by the CEO's wife; staff was instructed to document that they offered the patient several options but that the patient chose the affiliated hospice. Staff members who desperately need their jobs probably won't report such abuse to the state regulatory agency.

Long-Term Care Insurance

Long-term care insurance is a type of private insurance policy that pays for some or all of a patient's care when he can no longer remain at home without assistance. These policies aren't always limited to paying for nursing home placement; sometimes they provide for a health-care professional or even a family member to provide assistance in the home rather than to require that the patient be admitted to a nursing home. Each policy is different, and it's the responsibility of the patient/family to ensure that the policy they're buying will meet their needs. Most long-term care insurance policies have a maximum amount of money that they will pay out, or are time-limited (often 3-5 years). The coverage period usually allows enough time for the patient and family to set aside assets in order to become eligible for Medicaid if at all possible.

So far as the nursing home is concerned, patients who pay their room & board with a long-term care insurance policy are considered to be private-pay. Even if the patient assigns the policy to the nursing home, this is a private contract between the patient and the insurance company. In most cases, the nursing home bills the patient the private-pay rate regardless of the amount that the long-term care insurance policy will pay. Hopefully the patient's policy will cover the total cost for room & board, but if not the unreimbursed amounts will be the patient's responsibility.

There are many long-term care insurance providers and they all offer different products. These policies work best for people who aren't wealthy enough to pay outright for the cost of placement, but who don't qualify for Medicaid to pay for the room & board in a nursing home. The cost of the policy is calculated according to the age of the patient, so it only stands to reason that the monthly premium for a person in his twenties will be substantially less than the cost of a premium for a person in his fifties. The longer that a person makes payments, the more money the insurance company will receive to help offset the cost of the patient's care. I've seen policies that cost in excess of $1,000 per month because the insured was in her seventies when she bought the policy. When you take into consideration that the cost of private pay in a nursing home is easily over $6,000 per month, a premium of $1,000 might not seem so bad. In nearly every case, long-term care policies will stop charging the monthly premium when the patient is placed in the nursing home.

Each long-term policy has its own rules and requirements. Some require that a patient use Medicare days before the policy starts paying, meaning that a patient who has been admitted directly from his home might not be eligible to receive any benefits at all. Nearly all long-term policies have a waiting period of some type, and it might not pay for all of the nursing home charges. Some policies don't adjust for inflation, so a policy that would have covered all of the current costs of placement at the time that it was purchased might cover less than half of the charges at today's costs. When shopping for long-term care insurance, it's a good idea to make sure the policy will adjust annually for inflation, although it's still possible for actual costs to be greater than the insurance amount payable.

Long-term care policies usually pay the patient (or his designated family member), who in turn pays the nursing home. However, some policies might negotiate a rate with the nursing home and pay the facility directly. Every policy requires physician certifications to ensure that the patient requires the ongoing care. It's important to read the fine print, because there could be a clause that creates problems later on.

Years ago I knew of a patient whose insurance paid for a maximum of five years; however, after three years the policy required an admission to the hospital and readmission to the nursing home under the Medicare Part A skilled nursing benefit. The patient didn't present a medical need to be in the hospital so the policy stopped paying; his wife spent well over half of their savings to pay for his placement until his death a few years later. Had his wife met with an elder law attorney when he was first placed, he would have been eligible for placement by the time that the three years were up, but no one had advised her to do so.

When considering buying a long-term care insurance policy it's always best to find out what the placement costs are in the community, and then to get quotes from several different insurance providers. Nursing home costs vary throughout the country, and a policy that would easily cover charges in rural Iowa might not even begin to cover the costs in a New York City nursing home. It's always best to meet with an elder law attorney as part of the planning process, as it's possible that the patient can work toward Medicaid eligibility while the policy is paying for the patient's room & board. This can help to alleviate stress when the long-term policy stops paying.

If you are considering buying a long-term care insurance policy, it's important to buy the policy from a stable company with a long history of providing insurance products. Many companies have stopped selling long-term care insurance policies because the rate of return on their investments is much lower than the cost of inflation, and with patients living longer companies are paying out more than they anticipated. Some companies have gone out of business altogether. Instead of buying a long term insurance policy, it's possible that the money would be better invested into a private interest-bearing account rather than buying long-term care insurance. This issue is worth researching rather than blindly following the advice of an insurance agent whose income depends upon you buying his product.

"Free" Nursing Home Placement

Nursing homes do their best to screen patients to ensure that they have the ability to pay, because once the patient has been admitted into the facility it's nearly impossible to discharge him without going through a formal eviction process. There's a saying, "once the head is in the bed..." which means that the nursing home is responsible for the patient once he's been admitted. Even if the nursing home locates a facility that will accept him, the patient can refuse to move and there's little that the nursing home can do. The nursing home can serve the patient (and family) with multiple 30-day eviction notices, but they'll have a damn hard time forcing him to leave. It's the facility's responsibility to make sure the patient has an appropriate discharge plan, which can be a problem if the patient is being discharged for non-payment. After all, if he isn't paying the nursing home, he probably won't pay anywhere else. Even if the patient or family has the ability to pay but simply refuses to part with the money, it's doubtful that the patient will be discharged against his will.

Whether or not he has the ability to pay for his care, once the patient has been admitted the nursing home must ensure that he receives all of the medical care he needs, including medications, lab draws, and specialty equipment, even if the nursing home has to pay these costs out of pocket. This can become very expensive for the nursing home. Most patients have health insurance such as Medicare, but there are still out-of-pocket costs and non-covered medications that can be very expensive.

A patient might not be eligible for assistance to pay for his placement – usually Medicaid – for any number of reasons. If the patient gave away money in the past 3-5 years, or if he owns property with other family members and they're not willing to buy him out or sell the property, he's not eligible. I've seen patients who were denied assistance after they signed their property over to their children and the children refused to return it.

Jane became ill and lived with a family member in deplorable conditions. Adult Protective Services removed her from the home for neglect and she was sent to the hospital. A few days later, she was admitted to a nursing home for rehabilitation services via the Medicare benefit. After the services were completed, the state refused to allow her to return to her home and the family refused to pay the nursing home for her continued stay. A public guardian was appointed for her *person*, but her family refused to provide access to her money and a conservator was never appointed over her finances. The patient remained in the nursing home for over a year without paying a dime, during which time her family freely spent her money. The facility was free to sue the family member for the placement or refer the account to a collection agency, but since the family member didn't sign the admission paperwork he wasn't legally obligated to pay for the patient's room & board.

Sometimes family members bring a patient to the emergency room and then refuse to take him back home; if the hospital is able to keep him long enough it's possible that he'll be discharged to a nursing home via the Medicare Part A skilled benefit. All of the area nursing homes are competing for patients, and they have a short period of time to decide whether or not to accept him. If the hospital discharge planners haven't documented the family's lack of cooperation, an unsuspecting nursing home might accept the patient only to later find that the family isn't willing to assist with a discharge plan. When the patient has completed his therapy, the nursing home won't be able to discharge him. All the while, the family member continues to live in the home and freely spends the patient's money. If taken to court, much of the time a judge won't rule in favor of the nursing home because it's difficult to prove that the transfer of assets (spending of the patient's money) was done maliciously; it's also difficult to prove that the patient was exploited and wasn't a willing participant in the scheme.

There have been a few exceptions; in some instances family members have been found to be responsible to pay for a patient's medical bills. 29 states have some type of *Filial Responsibility* laws on their books that allow nursing homes and other medical providers to recover the cost of an elderly parents medical bills from their adult children. Two states – South Dakota and Pennsylvania – have enforced these laws, but in most other instances they are rarely enforced and the nursing home is stuck with the bills. Filial responsibility laws vary from state-to-state: Arkansas limits the type of care for which a family member is responsible to mental health services, and Nevada only allows a provider to sue if the child made a written promise to pay his parents' bills. It's important to seek the assistance of an experienced elder law attorney if you receive bills from your parent's nursing home. In 2012, the Pennsylvania superior court upheld an earlier verdict holding a patient's son responsible for $93,000 in nursing home related charges even though he had not signed her admission paperwork accepting financial responsibility for her care. Had they been raised from the start, there were several issues that could have changed the verdict in the defendant's favor; an elder law attorney surely would have made a difference in this instance (HCR v. Pittas 2012).

The only way that the "free" patient can be discharged is if he leaves the facility for a time period that exceeds the length of the facility's "bed hold" policy. Usually this is done by sending the patient to the hospital for an acute condition that requires hospitalization; the nursing home isn't legally required to take him back afterward. Whether the patient will be accepted back depends on a number of factors, but sometimes the nursing home will allow him reentry because it might affect future referrals from that specific hospital. Hospital discharge planners often operate under the mistaken belief that the nursing home "owns" the patient if he came to the hospital from that facility, whether he was a patient there for a day or a year. Of course, nursing homes disagree with this attitude and will resist accepting certain patients back.

It's not common for a patient to remain in a nursing home for free, although with the economic downturn I'm sure that it's happening more often. Most patients have some type of payment source available to them, but if not, the nursing home is responsible for patients until they are able to safely return home. It doesn't matter whether the patient remains in the facility for years; once the head is in the bed… the nursing home is stuck with a "free" patient.

The belief that a patient's power of attorney isn't personally responsible for her nursing home payment was challenged a few years ago in Connecticut; the courts found a patient's nephew, her power of attorney, responsible for her payment because he signed his aunt into the facility and didn't write, "*I am not personally responsible for my aunt's bills*" on the admission agreement. He hadn't stolen from her or anything; he simply had not assisted with her Medicaid eligibility by spending her savings to keep her below the $2,000 limit. Because of this, she wasn't eligible for Medicaid and the courts found him personally liable for over $100,000. According to news reports, the family member filed bankruptcy and the nursing home never even recouped legal fees. However, this should be viewed as cautionary story: when signing the documents for a patient to be admitted to a nursing home, clearly write across it, "*I am not personally responsible for my family member's bills.*"

One way to ensure the family isn't on the hook for paying the bill is to have the patient sign his own admission agreement. If he isn't able to do so, the family can refuse to refuse to accept financial responsibility, The nursing home might try to intimidate the family into signing on the patient's behalf, but the only document that truly must be signed is the "permission to treat" form that allows the patient to receive medical treatment (if there is no family available, the physician is able to make the decision to treat the patient without a signature).

If the family member chooses to sign the admission paperwork, he should sign "for" the patient. Examples are *John Doe* by *Mary Doe*, or *Mary Doe* for *John Doe*. The family's obligation is to ensure payment from the patient's finances, not to pay for him out of their personal funds. If a nursing home attempts to force a family member to pay for the patient's placement, it's best to meet with an attorney to ensure that the patient's & family's legal rights are protected. Again, in light of the recent ruling in Connecticut, it's probably best to write the statement, "*I am not personally responsible for the patient's bills*" on the financial responsibility agreement and to obtain a photocopy of the paperwork at the time of signing. That way, the nursing home can't change it after the fact.

As long as the patient's family provided all of his financial information in good faith and has cooperated fully in the Medicaid application process, the facility can't force the family to pay for the placement *unless they personally guaranteed the placement themselves*. If the relative doesn't sign the patient into the facility, it appears doubtful that he can be held legally responsible for a nursing home patient's bills. In most cases, the facility will have to prove negligence – and taking a person to court is expensive; unless the nursing home has in-house counsel, it's doubtful that the issue will ever see the inside of a courtroom. This is especially true, considering the length of time that it takes such a case to wind through the court systems; family members will have sufficient time to hide their assets and file for bankruptcy, leaving the nursing home with a non-paying patient and tens of thousands of dollars in unpaid legal fees. They also will be subject to negative publicity in local (and possibly national) newspapers and over the internet. Even if the nursing home is acting in what they believe to be an appropriate manner, the court of public opinion might think otherwise.

The nursing home administrator will meet with the family and attempt to force them into taking him home or paying out of their own finances; it's one of his job responsibilities to ensure the nursing home is paid. It can be intimidating when the administrator is threatening the family with a lawsuit and ruined credit, but hang tough. Don't sign anything or accept responsibility for the patient's bills, and if at all possible do not meet with the administrator or billing office alone.

I've known some administrators with nasty collection techniques; their job depends upon generating revenue for the nursing home corporation. However, their lack of revenue is not your problem unless you are withholding the patient's money.

If you find yourself in the position of being harassed by the nursing home for payment of a family member's nursing home placement, it's best to contact an attorney to ensure that your interests are represented. In most cases, the nursing home will back down and stop harassing you.

> Two years before she was admitted to a nursing home, Mary gave $150,000 to a neighbor whom she trusted. The neighbor refused to return the money, claiming it was a gift, and it couldn't be proven otherwise. Medicaid was applied for, and denied. Mary was later admitted to the hospital; at first the nursing home refused to take her back but the hospital didn't have anywhere else to send her, and the nursing home felt obligated to take her back because it was afraid of affecting future referrals.
>
> The neighbor, a prominent member of the community, was accused of exploitation and later settled with the state for an undisclosed amount in fines (rumored to be substantially less than the amount Mary gave to her). It's interesting to note that the nursing home didn't receive any part of the settlement, even though Mary remained there for free until her death two years later. The neighbor, who claimed to love Mary as if she were family, never even visited the confused and disoriented nursing home resident.

Even though this example appears to be a blatant example of exploitation, it's difficult to prove that the patient didn't willingly give money away. There are many examples of people who exploit the elderly; they will work their way into the senior's life and are often considered part of the family. This places them in a position of trust, and they are able to gain access to the patient's money, personal possessions, cars, etc. The situation is often discovered years later, when the bank statements are reviewed for Medicaid eligibility. By that time, the money is usually spent and there's no chance of recovering any part of it to help pay for the patient's nursing home placement.

I was present when an unrelated couple brought an attorney, along with a notary, into a nursing home and attempted to have a patient sign over control of her finances (which totaled well over a million dollars). The police insisted that it was a civil matter. We called Adult Protective Services and, with their assistance, the best that we could do was delay the process until after 5:00pm when the banks were closed. The couple who orchestrated the event clearly stated that their plan was to discharge the patient from the nursing home and move her to an upscale rental (using her money), where they would care for her and provide her with physical therapy in the luxury pool located in the backyard. These scammers had no experience providing therapy – they simply thought they'd found an easy "mark."

Luckily, we had been able to contact an elderly cousin who was her power of attorney, and he immediately called the bank requesting that the accounts be frozen. He arrived with his own attorney a few hours later and had the patient sign her power of attorney back over to him. The next morning at 8:00am they successfully closed out the bank accounts to protect them from these people and arranged to move the patient to an undisclosed location. We were able to block this attempted fraud, but no one knows how many others this couple was able to orchestrate. The woman who was attempting to exploit the patient plays music as a volunteer in various group and nursing homes in a rural area, and since she hasn't been convicted of a crime she is allowed to continue to operate her often successful exploitation schemes. I saw her name included in an article in the local newspaper about a year ago; a nursing home was discussing the many activities it provides and she was one of their headlining acts.

There are many instances of people who ingratiate themselves into a senior's life via a common bond such as their religion. They become a trusted friend and then steal the victim's money; this is known as **Affinity Fraud**. This form of exploitation might not be discovered until the patient has been placed in a nursing home and the Medicaid application process uncovers the missing funds. It's the nursing home who is stuck, not the patient's family or even the person who exploited him. This is why nursing homes should be careful about whom they admit, but as long as there's competition the nursing homes will fall over themselves to get the patient referrals and worry about the money later.

Because there are so many different types of payment for nursing home placement, it's possible that patients or their families will become confused about which payment source that can be applied to their situation. It's important to discuss these issues with a knowledgeable person or agency to ensure that the patient's financial situation is addressed before he enters a facility. It's worth the cost to meet with an elder law attorney or other professional to determine whether the patient might possibly be eligible for Medicaid *even if someone tells you that the patient isn't eligible*. I've been in line in the grocery store and heard horror stories about seniors losing their home that simply made no sense, yet people seem to prefer to believe what they hear from a stranger in that setting rather than to listen to the advice of a professional. Most people with whom you'll have a casual discussion probably don't know what they're talking about, although they freely dispense advice to anyone who will listen. Beware of the private firms that apply for Medicaid on a patient's behalf; unless they are staffed by former Medicaid eligibility workers they might not be worth the cost. Regardless of their credentials, it's best to check references to ensure that these companies have had past success with Medicaid applications.

In some areas the local Medicaid office is able to perform pre-eligibility counseling; a worker might even tell the patient whether or not he's eligible, but he probably won't explain how to become eligible. Unless the application is a simple one, it's best to meet with an elder law attorney or other private Medicaid professional before the application has been submitted. Once the Medicaid office makes a determination that the patient isn't eligible it's an uphill battle to have the ruling overturned. If a professional is able to help with the process, it's best to have that assistance from the start in order to make it less confusing.

The Admissions Process

Once you've chosen the nursing home and have a good idea as to what payment source the patient will use, it's important to meet with the nursing home representative to have her help you get the patient admitted. Family members can meet with nursing home representatives no matter where the patient is currently located; if the patient is in the hospital, the nursing home might be able to act as the middleman to get the patient into their facility. Of course, it's not *that* simple to get the patient admitted; there are many issues to be addressed. Most nursing homes have a formal admissions process, with an admissions coordinator who will complete all of the steps necessary to get the patient admitted.

The admissions coordinator should try to do anything helpful to get the patient accepted rather than to look for reasons that the patient won't be admitted into the facility. If you get the feeling that this person is doing her best to discourage you from having your family member admitted, ask them why. It's a waste of your time to continue working with them if the patient has no chance of being admitted. Admissions workers often show their productivity to their supervisors by the amount of number of inquiries they have logged into their computer system. There's an incentive for them to inflate the number of patients that they are working with – whether or not they actually have a chance of being admitted.

There are many things that go on behind the scenes in order for a patient to be admitted into a nursing home; the process can take anywhere from a few days to several months depending upon the patient's payment source and physical needs.

When working with an admissions coordinator, it helps to develop a first-name relationship to personalize the admission. Hopefully she will work harder to get the patient admitted if she feels a connection with you. However, don't call her every day to the point that they grow tired of you. It's a fine line, but do your best to be respectful of their time and only call them when it's necessary. If they refer you to a Medicaid specialist or other worker, do you best to follow up with that person if at all possible. Let the admissions coordinator know if you are working with an elder law attorney or other professional so that they will have enough information to help the facility make a decision as to whether to accept the patient.

Some of the duties of the admissions coordinator are:

- **Meet with the Patient and/or Family Members** – she often gives the family a tour of the facility and obtains information about the patient. Since tours are usually pre-arranged, the staff has the opportunity to show the facility in a more favorable light. The admissions coordinator will probably have the patient/family sign a Release of Information form at this point in order to obtain information about the patient from his physician or other medical providers.

- **Obtain Information About the Patient's Physical Status** – if the patient is currently in the hospital or other acute facility, the admissions coordinator will contact the nurses or discharge planners to get information from the patient's chart. This includes a current ***History & Physical (H&P)***, discharge orders from the hospital or other facility, list of medications, therapy notes, the patient's face sheet (demographic information), and anything else that will give a clear picture of the patient's needs and ability to pay.

  Most nursing homes require that the patient's H&P be dated from within the 30-day period immediately prior to the patient's admission to the nursing home. If the patient isn't currently in the hospital, it's possible for the patient's doctor to send an older one and certify that the information is correct. However, if the patient hasn't been seen by his doctor in the recent past, it's possible that his physician won't update his H&P without seeing him. If the doctor isn't able to see him as quickly as the patient prefers, an H&P can be completed at a Quick Care facility that sees patients on a walk-in basis. Those patients who aren't able to leave the house for an appointment might possibly be seen by a doctor who makes house calls (usually this is a service that isn't covered by insurance), might possibly meet the doctor at the facility on the date of admission (as long as the facility will allow), or as a last resort the patient might make a trip to the emergency room. It's important to note that if the patient goes to the ER for this purpose, it's doubtful that his insurance will cover the cost of the medical care and ambulance charges.

  Regardless of where the patient is located, the nursing home admissions coordinator might be able to help with the process of obtaining an H&P and any other information that is needed for the patient to be accepted.

- **Ensure that the patient has received a chest x-ray within the past 30 days** – this is a requirement that is usually met during a hospital stay. If the patient is being admitted directly from his home he will need a chest x-ray. It's possible that a portable x-ray company can go to the patient's home for this purpose – usually the same day. The cost for a portable x-ray might possibly be covered by insurance, but if not the patient will be responsible for hundreds of dollars in fees. The chest x-ray is not optional; it proves that the patient is free of tuberculosis and without it the patient will not be accepted into the nursing home.

- **Obtain Information About the Patient's Payment Source** – once they know where the patient is located immediately prior to his admission, the nursing home staff will determine what his payment source will be (as discussed earlier). The admissions coordinator will verify that there are funds available for the patient's co-payments, deductibles and/or long-term placement so that a decision can be made as to whether or not the facility will accept the patient.

- **Obtain Insurance Authorizations** – for those patients whose insurance is a private commercial plan or a Medicare Advantage plan, the insurance company generally requires initial payment authorizations before the patient is admitted. Even if the patient has Medicare Part A, if the patient has a secondary (Medigap policy) via a Medicare Select plan it will be necessary for the nursing home to obtain an authorization number. This allows the insurance company the opportunity to review the patient's need and to approve or deny payment for the stay.

- **Review the Patient's Mental Health Status** – this is usually done by **PASRR** (Pre-Admission Screening and Resident Review). The first part of the PASRR is required for every patient who is admitted to a nursing home; the second level of screening will be administered to patients diagnosed with a mental illness or other condition that can affect the health or well-being of that resident or others in the facility. Some states require this paperwork be completed beforehand while others allow for the paperwork to be completed after the patient has already been admitted.

    If the patient has a severe mental illness with a recent display/onset of behaviors, it's possible that he will not be accepted into the nursing home. The facility must be able to meet the patient's needs, and it is doubtful that a nursing home is the appropriate setting to manage a patient's mental illness.

- **Obtain Facility Authorization to Accept the Patient** – the Admissions coordinator usually must provide all of the healthcare information to the Director of Nursing so that the patient can be approved medically. If there's any question as to whether the patient might be appropriate, the D.O.N. might visit the patient wherever he's located to perform a full assessment.

    In addition to the patient's physical status, the patient's payment source will be verified by the business office and a decision will be made as to whether the patient will be appropriate for either short-term or long-term placement. If the patient isn't accepted financially or medically, he will not be approved for admission.

- **Obtain Physician Orders** – each patient who enters a nursing home, either short or long-term, must have orders from a doctor that specifies the type of care the patient will require and prescribes medications that will need to be ordered from the pharmacy. If the patient is receiving services from a hospice agency, the nursing home will coordinate delivery of the medications between the hospice's pharmacy and the one that the nursing home uses to ensure that all of the patient's medications will be provided.

- **Coordinate with the Discharging Facility** – once the patient is approved, the admissions coordinator makes arrangements for a room to be ready. The nursing home staff might need to make arrangements for the patient to be picked up from the hospital (or wherever he is at the time of admission), and whether the patient needs oxygen or other *DME* (durable medical equipment) such as a specialty bed or therapeutic machine. Any specialty items should be present in the room when the patient arrives to ensure proper *continuity of care*.

- **Coordinate with the Patient and/or Family to complete the Admission Agreement** – the admission packet for most nursing homes is at often 20+ pages, and requires multiple signatures. Most nursing homes include a form that holds the patient's family financially responsible if the planned payment source fails to pay some or all of the charges. Each nursing home is different; some complete the intake packet at the time of admission, while others mail the packet long after the patient has been discharged. At the very least, the patient or family will need to sign a few forms granting the nursing home permission to provide medical care.

- **Provide Information about Advanced Directives:** the patient/family must be provided information about advanced directives upon each admission to a CMS funded facility. Even if the patient has already completed an advanced directive, it's necessary to provide this information to the nursing home every time the patient is admitted to ensure that the patient's wishes will be honored. Chances are the old ones won't be pulled forward and placed in the new patient chart; it's also possible that the patient completed a new power of attorney since his last admission. Providing the most recent power of attorney/advanced directive at the time of each admission ensures that the patient's wishes will be honored.

Most of the time, if any of the above information isn't available it's possible that the nursing home won't be able to accept the patient. I say "most," because in some rural towns patients are readily accepted and the facility works out the other issues later, especially if there is more than one nursing home in town with which they're competing. The hospital discharge planners often don't tell the nursing homes there might be a problem with the patient's finances because they want to get the patient out of the hospital as soon as possible – and the nursing homes don't ask questions. This can come back to hurt them later, especially if the patient lacks a long-term payment source.

Another exception to a lengthy admissions process are those nursing homes that have exclusively contracted with Medicare Advantage plans; they are contractually bound to accept almost any patient the insurance plan sends to them. Their goal is to get the patients admitted, provide as much rehabilitation as possible for the shortest period of time possible, and discharge the patient home.

Working with Medicare Advantage plans can be a problem for the nursing home when it comes to discharging a patient who has nowhere to go. There is an extremely high turnover in these nursing homes and they often develop a relationship with a less than desirable nursing home that accepts just about anyone. These facilities can be located hundreds of miles away from the area and it might be impossible for family members to visit. Unless the family remains vigilant and is willing to involve the ombudsman, patients are admitted to and discharged from facilities that simply aren't acceptable to family members.

l.e. green

Reasons for Denial

A nursing home has the right to refuse to accept a patient for any reason other than discrimination (which is difficult to prove). The standard excuse that facilities use when they refuse a patient is that they "don't have any beds available." While it's possible that they truly don't have any empty beds, what they often mean is that they choose not to make a bed available for that particular patient. If the nursing home denies your family member, you can call and speak to the administrator or possibly the parent corporation, but it's doubtful they'll change their mind.

There are many reasons that a patient might be denied admission in a nursing home:

- No beds are available (the facility is actually full).
- A Medicare bed is available, but the patient doesn't have a secondary insurance to cover copayments. If the patient appears to need more than 20 days of therapy, there won't be any payment to the nursing home for the copayment amount of $152 per day.
- The secondary insurance doesn't cover 100% of the costs of the copayments, and the nursing home suspects the patient can't afford the rest.
- The patient's HMO/PPO Insurance doesn't contract with the nursing home.
- The patient has been diagnosed with a serious mental illness and the state won't clear him to be admitted (or the facility doesn't feel able to appropriately manage the patient's illness).
- The nursing home believes that a patient is attempting to gain admittance under the Medicare rehabilitation benefit and will attempt to stay in the facility long-term via Medicaid – and they're not accepting new Medicaid patients. They might still accept the patient, but will attempt to discharge him after his therapy has been completed.
- The cost of the patient's care will e substantially more than the facility will receive from the insurance company.
- The nursing home doesn't believe that the patient meets the criteria for long-term placement, and he doesn't appear to have a viable discharge plan.
- The nursing home isn't able to provide the level of care that the patient needs, such as a ventilator, complicated wound care, etc.
- The patient is coming directly from home and will apply for Medicaid when he arrives. The nursing home might not accept "Medicaid pending" as a source of payment.
- The patient is receiving assistance from a hospice and that hospice doesn't have a contract with the nursing home.
- The patient is under the age of 60, and the nursing home prefers only to accept geriatric patients.
- The patient has a history of wandering, and the facility doesn't have the ability to monitor him to ensure his safety.

- The nursing home knows the patient and/or family, and for some reason doesn't believe that they are able to "meet their needs" (translation – the patient or family is too demanding).
- The patient has a history of checking in and out of nursing homes on a frequent basis, causing the staff extra work each time.
- The patient or family has a history of contacting the ombudsman or state bureau of licensure with concerns (even if they are legitimate). Healthcare workers refer to these patients as "having the State on speed-dial." These patients can be more trouble than they're worth.

Finding a Treating Physician

When the patient is being admitted to the nursing home directly from the hospital, the discharge orders from the hospital can either be signed by one of the doctors or specialists treating the patient, or by a ***hospitalist***. The term "hospitalist" describes a physician who specializes in coordinating patient care amongst all of the specialists, the case managers, and the patient's primary physician while the patient is in the hospital. He ensures that all of the providers are working together and that there are no duplicate tests ordered. However, in nearly every case the hospitalist doesn't follow the patient after he's discharged to a nursing home – and there needs to be a treating physician at the nursing home to sign the admission orders.

Depending upon the requirements in which the nursing home is located, the doctor who has been assigned to follow the nursing home patient is required to visit or see the patient either at the nursing home or in his office within 7 days of admission (or sooner). He is also expected to make himself available for calls at all hours of the day or night. This is why it's often difficult to find a doctor who is willing to follow patients in the nursing home. Even if the patient has a primary physician he sees when he's living at home, that doctor might not be willing to follow the patient in the nursing home. Whether or not the patient has a regular primary physician, the nursing home might have a list of doctors who are willing to take on a new patient in a nursing home. Hopefully that doctor will coordinate with the patient's primary physician to ensure the patient continues with the same treatments he received at home, but there are no guarantees that he'll be willing to do so.

> June falls down in her home and breaks her hip. She is sent to the hospital, where her hip is surgically repaired. She has developed an infection at the site of her incision, and also has a diagnosis of diabetes. June will require the services of an orthopedist for the surgery, a wound specialist for the wound care, a neurologist for follow up because she hit her head, and an internist for her diabetes. June is assigned a hospitalist to coordinate all of the care she receives in the hospital.
>
> Once June is ready for discharge to a nursing home, she'll be assigned a doctor to follow her at that facility. This doctor might be part of the medical group that treated her in the hospital, her regular primary physician, or he might be a doctor who has been randomly assigned by the nursing home.

In smaller towns, it's possible that patient's primary physician is willing to follow him in the nursing home, but this isn't always the case. The doctor might not want to make a house call in the nursing home, or he might not want to have the nursing staff call at all hours of the day or night. Even if he asks that they contact him at the end of the day, the nursing staff might not honor his request. It does make it easier for the patient if the physician who is following him in the nursing home is the one who has been providing his ongoing care, because he will be familiar with the patient's medical history. However, if he chooses not to follow the patient in the nursing home another doctor will be assigned to his case. This physician might not follow the patient's previous treatment plan and might possibly change a medication regime that has been working for years.

Having a doctor who visits the nursing home on a regular basis does make it easier on both the nursing home and the patient than to have the patient transported back and forth to his office. The doctor assigned to follow the patient in the nursing home might not be one that the patient prefers or even knows; the doctor is often assigned on a rotation basis by the nursing home front office. The patient will be told, not asked, which physician will be following him.

Patients do have the right to choose a specific physician to follow them, as long as he is willing to care for the patient and the nursing home allows for this to happen. In order for the doctor to physically visit and write orders for a nursing home patient, he must be credentialed (which can be a lengthy process). Depending upon the mindset of the nursing home, it's possible that the facility will make it difficult for new doctors to gain access to their patients; they often do this in order to please those doctors that they use on a regular basis.

The nursing home will reward the physician who cooperates with the requests of the administrator, such as delaying expensive tests and treatments until after the patient is discharged, by assigning more patients. Each time a physician visits a patient in a nursing home he receives the full Medicare reimbursement – and he learns to count on the revenue generated by these visits. If a physician is assigned 20 -30 patients in a nursing home, he can see them all in one day. Seeing patients in nursing homes can be a lucrative addition to the physician's bottom line.

Most nursing homes will want to work with as many doctors as possible in order to receive more referrals. However, if the doctor of the patient's choosing doesn't follow the nursing home's recommendations (such as the amount of therapy the patient is prescribed, the medications ordered or the date that the patient will be ready for discharge), the nursing home stands to lose thousands of dollars in revenue. Nursing home administrators often call doctors to ask them to change their orders, or might even ask the facility medical director to speak with an uncooperative physician in an attempt to discontinue expensive treatments. Many physicians don't allow a nursing home administrator to dictate the care that the patient will receive, which means that the nursing home won't want to work with the doctor in the future. If they want to continue seeing patients in that facility, they'll find a way to accommodate the administrator's requests.

This is not to say that every doctor who has a nursing home caseload is practicing according to the wishes of the administrator, but if he insists upon ordering treatments or medications that affect the nursing home's bottom line it's doubtful that he will continue to be assigned patients. The revenue stream created by a nursing home caseload can be a huge motivating factor in wanting to please the nursing home administrator.

Patients can always visit their preferred doctor in his office, but the nursing home can make this difficult. The facility might refuse to provide transportation and can insist upon following the orders of the physician that they have assigned (permission to have a doctor assigned by the nursing home is usually buried in the admission paperwork). A quick call to the long-term care ombudsman usually solves this problem, but if the nursing home insists upon dictating the patient's medical care it might be best to move to another facility that is willing to meet the patient's needs, if one is willing to accept him. The problem can be that the nursing home where the patient is currently located can block a transfer if they wish to do so, often by intimating that there is a problem with the patient.

Even if the patient prefers a specific physician, there is no guarantee that his wishes will be honored. The doctor himself might not want to follow him in the nursing home for any number of reasons. If the physician who has been serving a patient no longer wants to work him, he can send a 30-day notice to the patient requesting that he obtain another doctor. This isn't a common occurrence, but the physician has the right to provide care for whomever he chooses. Even though the family has the right to choose another doctor, if they're not able to find one the nursing home is ultimately responsible for ensuring that the patient has a doctor who is overseeing his care *whether or not the physician is paid for the service*. In these cases, it's usually the nursing home Medical Director who is stuck caring for the patient regardless of his ability to pay.

In a perfect world, the doctor assigned by the nursing home will provide excellent care and will continue to follow the treatment plan that was developed while the patient was at home. Unfortunately, when a patient is sent to the hospital he doesn't always receive the medications that he was prescribed before he was admitted. The hospital might not even be aware of certain healthcare conditions that the patient has. When he is discharged from the nursing home afterward, there might not have been any coordination with the patient's regular doctor. There's no great computer in the sky that contains all of the patient's healthcare information and it's possible that a serious healthcare condition will be overlooked. Even with the federal requirement that all medical providers must have electronic records systems in place by the end of 2014, these systems won't be able to freely access patient information from provider to provider without specific permission given. Unless someone is able to provide the name of the patient's primary doctor, it's possible no one will know his name or be able to access the patient's medical history. This is how serious conditions can go untreated for days, weeks, or even months.

Once the patient has been admitted into the nursing home, it's important for the family to speak with the doctor who has been assigned to his case in order to ensure that he receives appropriate treatment for all of his conditions. Bring a list of the patient's medications to the nursing home and be prepared to discuss the patient's goals. The patient might have been receiving a maintenance medication about which the nursing home has no knowledge. Be prepared to advocate on behalf of the patient; otherwise it's possible his needs won't be known (or met). Don't allow the nursing home to dictate the patient's care; this is the doctor's responsibility.

If a nursing home appears to be unresponsive regarding a patient's care, feel free to speak with the administrator, call the state regulatory agency or ombudsman. Feel free to speak with an attorney if necessary; patients have the right to be treated with dignity and respect, which includes a continuation of the treatment plan and medications they received at their home. It's not for the nursing home to decide what conditions will – or won't – be treated while he's inpatient.

Transportation to the Nursing Home

Once the patient has been accepted, the nursing home will help to arrange for the patient's transportation from his current setting. No matter what the payment source for the nursing home stay might be, most insurance plans (including Medicare) don't cover the cost of medical transportation from the hospital to the nursing home.

Medical transportation issues are confusing to many people. Medicare and most insurance plans only pay for a medical transport if the patient is admitted to a facility that provides a higher level of care and that level of transportation was medically necessary. For example, if a patient is at home and is transported to the hospital by ambulance, the bill will be paid as long as it can be proven that the use of the ambulance was medically necessary. An example might be an allergic reaction (anaphylactic shock) that requires immediate medical treatment or the patient is at risk of dying. Once the patient has been administered medications and is monitored in the emergency department, he might be able to go home without any further complications.

Even in those instances when it was vital that the patient be transported by ambulance, the insurance will often issue a denial of payment and the ambulance company will need to assist the patient in appealing the decision. Otherwise, the patient is stuck paying the bill out of his pocket (and the ambulance company risks not being paid).

It's not considered to be a medical need if the patient lives alone and calls an ambulance simply because he wasn't able to drive to the hospital by himself. The bill will be denied if the patient could have made it to the hospital by another method, such as calling a taxi. Payment will be denied, even if there is no taxi service available in the town in which he lives. Lack of available transportation is not a medical need, unless the patient would have been at risk of serious complications without the ambulance providing supportive services on the way to the hospital.

If the patient is in a hospital and requires specialty services in another hospital, his insurance will pay for this transportation whether by *medivac* (air transportation) or ambulance. When he's discharged, however, the patient is responsible for his own transportation back home, even if it costs him hundreds or thousands of dollars for airfare. I've seen families drive hundreds of miles in a rented van to pick up a patient who's been discharged because they couldn't afford to fly him back home. Sometimes hospitals have a transportation fund that can help patients return home, but not often. There have been cases of patients being discharged to homeless shelters because they had no transportation home (and no family to advocate for them).

Different rules apply when a patient is being transferred from a hospital to a nursing home. Care in a nursing home is considered to be a lower level of care and therefore medical transportation isn't medically necessary. Most nursing homes will pick up the patient in a van that is usually equipped to transport wheelchairs and *geri-chairs* (reclining chairs on wheels). If the patient isn't able to be transported in this manner, it's possible he'll have to travel by stretcher. In this case, the family or patient might have to pay for the medical transport out-of-pocket (or Medicaid will pay if the patient is already approved for the Medicaid program). Another option is for the family to drive the patient to the nursing home themselves.

If a patient is receiving care from a hospice, the hospice might be responsible for transporting the patient to the nursing home. Some hospice companies provide transportation in their own vans, while others contract with a medical transport company to move their patients. In order to avoid the cost of transportation, many hospices wait to sign the patient onto their service until after the patient has been physically moved to the nursing home. In cities with more than one hospice it's possible for the patient to simply sign onto the services of another hospice (or merely threaten to do so) and receive free transportation that way, rather than to pay for the transportation out of his own pocket.

There are many ways that patients can be moved out of the hospital when they're discharged, but most of the time hospitals won't pay for this transportation. If the patient has no safe transportation to his next setting, the hospital will either have to pay for the patient or keep him there until transportation has been arranged. On those rare occasions that they do pay for transportation, it's generally because every other option has been exhausted, and someone in the hospital's administration has approved the charges.

If the patient is transferring from one nursing home to another, in most cases the nursing home that's accepting the patient is responsible to make and pay for the transportation arrangements. If the patient is coming from far away, however, the patient or family will probably be responsible for providing the transportation.

Before the nursing home or hospital makes the arrangements for transportation, make sure that you know who is responsible for paying. If the patient will be responsible, it might be possible for the family to pick him up at the hospital and deliver him to the nursing home. There is no law that mandates medical transportation providers be used unless the patient's medical need can't be met in the family car (or van). Medical transportation for a couple of miles can cost well over $100, and if it's not medically necessary there's no reason why the family can't provide the transportation and save themselves the money.

Admission Day

Checking a patient into a nursing home can take several hours, as there will be paperwork, nursing assessments, and orientation to the nursing home. The patient will probably be weighed as soon as he enters the nursing home, and then returned to his room for the nursing assessment and to settle into his new surroundings. It's not necessary for the family to remain in the facility for the entire check-in process; once any paperwork has been signed and the patient's personal items have been logged in, the family can leave. This is the time that the patient will be oriented to the nursing home and his needs will be assessed.

What to Bring

If the patient is being admitted for short-term therapy services, it's best to bring clothing items that the patient can wear while he's participating in therapies. Sweatpants, comfortable shirts, and comfortable sleepwear are all good ideas. Don't forget to bring comfortable shoes that the patient can wear while working out, such as tennis shoes – but they should be comfortable shoes that the patient is used to, as he'll be wearing them for therapy. Most nursing homes recommend only 3-5 changes of clothing be provided, with each item clearly marked with the patient's name regardless of whether or not the nursing home will be doing the patient's laundry. Try to bring clothing that is easy to get on/off, with buttons or Velcro in the front. Pullover sweaters might be warm, but they're difficult to get onto a patient lying in a bed. If the patient is being admitted for a long-term stay, he will also need comfortable "everyday" clothing – and possibly something to wear at dinner in more formal facilities.

It's best to bring enough clothing to last a couple of weeks for long-term residents, so that there will always be something to wear. Remember that the patient will be spending most of his time indoors, so bring clothing to keep him warm in the summer (air conditioning can be very cool), and cool in the winter (facility heaters can be very warm). Bring enough items to allow him to dress in layers so that he can add – or remove – items according to his comfort.

Patients are usually welcome to bring their own shampoo, conditioner, soaps, shaving lotions and razors if they'd like (some nursing homes charge extra to provide these items). Patients might be prohibited from bringing in items that can be considered medication, such as mouthwash, vitamins, etc. Each nursing home has a written policy regarding items that might be brought from home. It's also permissible to bring favorite blankets, quilts, etc. although it's not necessary; the nursing home is required to furnish all of the items that the patient will need, including bedding and towels.

In most cases, patients aren't allowed to bring in extension cords, blow dryers, heating pads or other electrical items due to the risk of harming themselves or other patients. It's important to ask whether these items are permissible, because if they aren't allowed they'll either be confiscated or you'll be required to take them home. Don't leave these items if they're not allowed, once the nursing home staff removes these items from the room, it's possible they'll be lost forever.

Patients might be able to bring in their own television set, although TV's are provided in many nursing homes (at least in the Medicare-designated halls). Patients are also able to bring magazines, cell phones, laptop computers or other items, although if at all possible expensive items should be locked up so that they can't be easily stolen. It also might be possible for long-term patients to order their own satellite television service; they will be responsible for all of the associated costs (including installation) and might have to move to a different room that's equipped for satellite. If the patient wants satellite service, make sure that he orders it in his own name or you'll be stuck with a two-year contract if he moves to another facility or passes away.

It's possible that the patient will be provided with a refrigerator, or they might have to buy their own if they want one in their room. For additional information about what items might be appropriate to bring into a nursing home, please refer to the section *Patient Personal Items* in the chapter **Understanding How a Nursing Home Operates**.

Marking Items for Identification

Regardless of whether the patient will remain in the nursing home on a short or long-term basis, it will be necessary to mark every item with the patient's name. Using a permanent marker, clearly mark everything, including shoes, quilts, blankets, wall hangings, etc. Anything can become lost or stolen, so feel free to engrave the patient's name into large items like televisions. Do not mark the items with the patient's room number, because if he changes rooms it's doubtful he'll ever get his items back from the laundry. Don't assume that the patient will remain in the same room throughout his stay; because room transfers are a common occurrence in nursing homes.

Due to patient confidentiality rules, the nursing home staff members aren't allowed to write the patient's name on the outside of his clothing – but the family is free to write his name wherever they choose. The benefit to writing a patient's name on the outside of his clothes is that they can be easily identified when worn by another person; it also greatly increases the chance that the patient will be addressed by his own name, which is a dignity issue. Having a patient's name on his clothing will have the added benefit of helping to prevent medication or treatment errors. There are decorative paints or patches that can be used to identify the owner of the clothing, yet will look attractive. Many people are hesitant to write on their parent's clothing with a permanent marker, but no one else should be wearing the clothing so it really doesn't matter. There are multicolored permanent markers that can be used to mark anything from light to dark clothing. Feel free to be creative when marking your family member's clothing.

Even though patients are encouraged to bring in personal items, most nursing homes will do their best to keep from having to reimburse patients for lost items such as computers, DVD players, stereos, etc. In addition to marking these items with the patient's name, keep the original receipt and take a photo of the item in the nursing home when you bring it in. Always ask the nursing staff to add the items to the patient's inventory form in his medical chart, and obtain a photocopy every time the form is amended so that the nursing home can't deny the item existed. Remain proactive and look for the items every time you visit; if they come up missing, report the loss immediately.

If at all possible, have the dentist engrave the patient's name in his dentures, and have the patient's name pressed or engraved into the frame of his eyeglasses if at all possible. Engrave the patient's name into jewelry, and take a photo for identification purposes. Replace expensive jewelry with costume jewelry, or replace an expensive diamond with a cubic zirconia. A confused patient might not ever know the difference and a precious family heirloom will remain safe at home. Do your best to keep an eye on expensive items; the social worker's office in nearly every nursing home contains boxes of found items, along with rings, necklaces and wallets full of ID. Sometimes they attempt to find the family members in order to return the items, and sometimes they don't. Most of the time, there are no identification markings and precious items are never returned to family members.

Most nursing homes require that patients and/or their family members sign waivers that attempt to indemnify the nursing home from responsibility for replacing missing items. Even if such a statement is signed, the nursing home is generally responsible for items that staff members lose or ruin. This includes glasses that are broken while the patient is receiving care, dentures that are lost or broken, clothing sent to the laundry never to be seen again, or items that are misplaced when the patient is in the hospital. I've personally seen nursing homes replace laptop computers, smart phones, and miscellaneous other items that went missing after the patient was sent to the hospital.

Choosing a Room

In most cases, patients won't be allowed to choose their room. As much as nursing homes claim to "match" the residents, they usually place patients into the next empty bed without regard as to whether the residents will get along. Even if the patient has been given the opportunity to choose his room, the nursing home will place limitations on the choice. Payment source matters greatly; patients being admitted for Medicare Part A services might be offered a private room, because they will be receiving specialty services and are usually there for a shorter period of time. It can be difficult to meet their goal of recovering and returning home when sharing a room with a patient who yells all night. Those nursing homes that only provide shared rooms usually group patients by the type of service they'll receive (long-term versus skilled services). In most nursing homes, Medicare rehabilitation rooms often are located on halls that have their own entrance and a dining/activity room that is separated from the long-term care patients. These patient rooms are usually located near the rehabilitation department so that they can quickly access the gym, and are nicely decorated compared to those in the long-term halls. Nursing homes do whatever they can to cater to the patients whose payment is the highest source of profit.

Long-term care patients generally are housed on separate units from the Medicare patients. They're often assigned rooms according to their level of care; patients who are more **alert & oriented** are housed in one area, while those who are confused or require maximum assistance with their ADL's are cared for in another area. Some nursing homes offer locked units for patients who wander with no sense of purpose; these units generally offer specialty activities that are geared toward the patients' level of functioning. Other nursing homes offer doors that lock down when a patient wearing a wander guard bracelet gets near, allowing patients to wander through larger areas of the nursing home without being in danger of escaping. Still other nursing homes have doors that are always locked and visitors must use a code or buzzer to get through the doors.

If you're fortunate enough to be able to choose a room for your family member, some people believe that a room near the nursing station is the best choice. While it might be easier for staff to hear if the patient needs help and can get to the room quickly in case of a fall, it's also possible that the room will be louder due to the activity around the nursing station. Not only do patients tend to congregate around the nursing station, this is the area where the nurses hang out and the phones are ringing. The call light system will be located at the nursing station, meaning that the alarms will be loudly ringing at all times of the day and night. The area will be well lit 24-hours per day, making it more difficult to sleep. If the patient is hard of hearing, these issues might not be a problem for them (although the bright lights at the nursing station might remain a problem). These are just a few reasons why a room closer to the nurse's station doesn't necessarily translate into better care.

It's possible to avoid the activity around the nursing station by shutting the door to the room, but most nursing homes discourage patients from shutting their door because it's difficult to see inside the rooms and check on the patients as staff members pass by. It's also harder to hear if a patient is calling out for help when the doors are shut. However, patients do have the right to shut their doors if they choose as long as all of the residents in that room agree. If the nursing home staff won't allow your family member to keep his door shut, speak with the administrator. You also have the right to call the ombudsman or state licensing agency without fear of retaliation.

Many nursing homes have bathrooms located inside each patient room, meaning that the bathroom will only be shared by the residents of that room. However, if the bathroom is shared by two separate rooms, there could be a long wait to use the toilet, and the restroom might not be as clean and private as the patient might prefer. If the bathrooms include showers, there could be an additional delay for the other residents if they need to use the restroom. Even if there are showers located in the patient rooms, it's possible that patients will be showered in a common shower room located down a long hallway.

The room assignment also depends upon the patient's diagnosis; if the patient is being isolated for some type of infection such as *C-diff* or *MRSA*, it might be necessary for him to be placed alone in a room or with another resident who has the same infection. The Medicare benefit pays the nursing home an extra premium for those patients who require isolation while Medicaid does not; the same patients who required a private room while receiving therapies under the Medicare benefit will be moved to a shared room the moment that their Medicare benefit has been exhausted. This is an excellent example of how a facility can manipulate Medicare in order to receive the highest possible payment.

A room change such as the one described above can happen whether or not the patient still has an active infection, severely compromising the health of the patient in the next bed. Even if the patient doesn't get out of bed, anyone who touches the patient and then touches *anyone or anything* can transmit the infection. It can also be transmitted in the bathroom when the staff members touch the faucet as they wash their hands. One way of identifying whether a patient has an infection is to observe whether the staff is required to don gowns & gloves before entering the room; this might not be a problem if the patient is bedbound and is only contagious with physical contact. With appropriate hand-washing and isolation, an infection might well be under control. However, if the staff must wear masks and eye protection before treating your family member's roommate, request a room change and call the state regulatory agency if he's not moved immediately. If you believe that your parent is sharing a room with a patient who's been diagnosed with a communicable disease, speak with the administrator, call the ombudsman, or speak directly with the state licensing agency.

Personalizing the Patient's Room

Nursing home rooms are normally furnished with hospital beds and matching, well maintained furniture. Patients aren't required to use the nursing home's furniture, however. Those patients who have been admitted for long-term care and are able to use a regular bed should be able to bring in their own bed as long as it fits into the room and doesn't infringe upon anyone's space. Remember that there usually isn't a lot of room for extra furniture; if your family member is in a shared room he'll only be able to bring items that fit on his side of the room and don't interfere with anyone else's personal space. Any furniture that is brought in must also allow for patient care to be performed for both the patient and his roommate.

If the patient requires assistance getting out of bed, or personal care while lying in bed, he will need a hospital bed that rises and lowers so that staff members don't hurt their backs attempting to lift him. Patients who own their own hospital bed might have the ability to bring that one from home as well, although it might be necessary for an employee from the nursing home maintenance department to check it out to ensure it's in working order and meets the safety requirements. Any furniture that's brought in remains the property of the patient and should be returned to his family when he discharges or passes away.

Hospital beds have come a long way in their design but can be very uncomfortable; if the nursing home staff offers to switch out the mattress, chances are good that they'll replace the mattress with the exact same model and the patient will remain in pain. If your family member isn't comfortable, speak with the nursing home administrator about the issue. There are specialty mattresses that can be ordered that will be more comfortable; however, if the patient is paying privately the nursing home can charge hundreds or thousands of dollars per month for a specialty mattress. Buying a specialty mattress would be well worth the cost and would pay for itself in a couple of months. If the patient remains in pain and his payment source is Medicaid, the nursing home must find a mattress that is comfortable to him. Remember that even though they might do their best to deflect a problem onto the family, the nursing home is ultimately responsible to ensure that the patient remains comfortable. Any specialty mattress they're forced to buy cuts into their profits.

Visiting Hours

All nursing homes are required to post their visiting hours, but in most cases families are able to visit 24 hours per day as long as they are respectful of staff and other patients. Although it's not common, some nursing homes offer trundle beds or comfortable chairs for the family members of patients who are actively dying. The nursing home might also be able to bring extra chairs into the room so that all members of the family can be comfortable during their visit. Although the staff will (hopefully) do their best to accommodate for a dying patient, it's important to be respectful of the other residents in the facility. For the most part, nursing homes don't have areas for family members to hang out.

Most nursing homes will not allow family members to stay the night in an extra patient bed that happens to be in the room, or to shower there. This is because the nursing home can be held liable if the patient or family slips and falls. It's possible that the nursing home will attempt to place a restriction on the number of visitors, but as long as they're not disturbing other patients or visitors there shouldn't be any reason to do so. If it appears that the nursing home is restricting a patient's access to visitors, speak with the administrator or feel free to call the ombudsman.

Photographing for Identification Purposes

Nursing homes usually have the patient/family sign a release in the intake packet that allows the nursing home to take the patient's photograph for identification purposes (and also for promotional purposes or during group activities). Patients and/or their family members do not have to give permission to be photographed, but that does mean that if the patient meets a certain milestone such as her 100th birthday, the facility doesn't have permission to print this information in the facility newsletter or allow a human interest story from the local television station or newspaper.

If permission to be photographed isn't given, the nursing home can still take the patient's photo but only for identification purposes. Most nursing homes use the photos for their *medication administration record (MAR)*, which is the book that nursing homes use to record medications given to patients during the times that they are *passing meds*. The idea is that the nurse will look at the photograph to ensure that the patient listed on the form is the same person that's taking the medications, although this doesn't always happen. It's a good idea, though.

Signing the Intake Packet

The date that the patient is admitted, he will be asked to sign several forms. These include a *Permission to Treat* (without that form, the nursing home doesn't have the legal right to provide any medical care for him), consents for psychotropic medications (such as anti-anxiety medications, anti-depressants, or any other mood altering medications), and permission for flu and pneumonia vaccines to be administered. The vaccines can be declined, but the other consents must be signed in order for the patient to receive his medications. If he isn't able to sign these medications, it's possible they will ask the family to sign them. It's vital that you read the forms that they ask you to sign and ask any questions you might have before signing them.

Within the first few weeks of admission, a nursing home representative will contact the family and present them with a rather daunting intake packet for their signature. Even if the patient is able to sign on his own behalf, it's common for the nursing home staff to ask the family to sign on the patient's behalf. Make no mistake about it, this is a formal contract that the nursing home's legal counsel has developed in order to protect the nursing home, and certainly not the patient or family. They're asking you, as a family member, to sign the packet because they would like to make you financially responsible for the patient in the event that his insurance won't pay the bill.

For the patient who is being admitted for a short-term respite, the nursing home might have a streamlined admission packet that they ask you to sign, although in most cases they will still ask you to sign the full packet. They often mail the packet weeks or even months after the patient has been discharged. Feel free to sign the packet – or not. The facility is required to present the packet for signature, but there is no law that requires the family member to sign the packet. It can be upsetting to receive a large packet in the mail months after the patient has already been discharged home that repeatedly states that the patient/family was responsible for the charges when the patient was admitted by the hospice or other agency, and they paid for the admission. *If the nursing home has pre-dated the admission packet and you sign any part of it, cross out their date and write in the actual date that you signed.* Photocopy the forms before you send them back and save the postmarked envelope for your records. It's illegal to falsify medical records, including back-dating signatures.

Don't be overly concerned about the date issue; if audited, the nursing home business office will say that it was an oversight and that they had written in the date that they completed the packet. You are merely being honest when you sign and date the forms. If there is any type of lawsuit or the nursing home attempts to collect money years later, the back-dating issue can help to support the family's claims that the nursing home has been less than honest in its dealings. In every case, always keep a copy for your records.

Don't be afraid to refuse to sign the packet and to ask them to speak directly with the patient. CMS requires that the nursing home make every attempt to have the forms signed, but it doesn't matter if the patient signs with an "x" or with his full name. The family can't be forced to sign on behalf of a patient; if a nursing home threatens you because you refuse to sign the packet, contact your attorney. Even if the patient has named you as his power of attorney, in most instances you aren't personally responsible for his bills.

I've known of nursing homes that threatened the family with a referral to the public guardian's office simply because the family refused to sign the intake packet. The only way that a public guardian will be appointed is if the patient lacks the capacity to make his own decisions and he is in eminent danger due to the lack of family intervention. A judge wouldn't even entertain appointing a guardian simply because a patient and his family member won't sign an admission packet. The parent corporation would probably be angry if they were to find that their staff members were bullying patients and their family members, although it's also possible that the staff was merely following facility protocol.

The packet has many, many forms (20+ in most cases!) that require a signature, such as one that accepts financial responsibility, another that grants the nursing home permission to bill insurance on a patient's behalf, and an agreement to participate in binding arbitration that effectively waives the right of the patient/family to take issues to court. With so many forms to sign, it's almost impossible to understand each one unless you take extra time to do so. In most cases the clerk is busy and will schedule half an hour or less for the patient's packet to be signed; she probably doesn't even understand most of the forms, but it's her job to get you to sign them anyway. If you don't feel that you have enough time to comfortably read the packet, don't sign it. Make sure that you obtain a copy of every form in the packet for your records *immediately after you sign them* before they're able to alter them. Most of the time, the nursing home won't attempt to alter the forms, but if there's any problem later on, the first thing that will be reviewed is the intake packet and permissions to which that the family agreed.

Be cautious when you accept responsibility on the patient's behalf, because you might be held personally responsible for his bills at some point in the future. If at all possible the patient should sign his own intake packet, or the family member should write the statement "*I am not personally responsible for my mother's bills*" on the financial responsibility form. It's also possible to sign for the patient by writing "*Mary Doe* for *Mr. John Doe*," or "*Mr. John Doe* by *Mary Doe*." If the nursing home won't accept this, walk away. The patient has already been admitted and they can't throw him out because you won't sign the packet. If you feel that they're forcing you to sign, feel free to ask them to fax a copy to your attorney for his review.

The packet will contain an intake sheet that provides the nursing home with demographic information in order to create a ***face sheet*** for the patient's medical chart that provides all of the information that the facility will need, including the patient's religion, marital status, choice of mortuary, etc. This is the form the nursing home sends to every doctor's appointment, pharmacy, and other medical provider. The patient himself should be listed as his own responsible party, because any family member listed as the responsible party will be billed for copayments, deductibles, and bills not covered by insurance such as dental care or eyeglasses. Ask to review the worksheet they use to complete the patient's face sheet, and verify that the information is correct a few days later (after it's been placed in the medical chart). Remember that holding the power of attorney doesn't automatically make you financially responsible for the patient; you should be listed under next-of-kin or power of attorney and not in the box designating you as the responsible party.

Nursing homes rarely have an in-house pharmacy; the intake packet will include a billing form from the professional pharmacy that delivers medications to the nursing home. It's vital that you provide the requested billing information, but you don't have to sign the form. By doing so, you might be promising to pay for those medications not covered by insurance. Don't sign it unless you truly intend to be responsible for the bill out of your own personal funds. If you must sign the form, sign "*John Doe* by *Mary Doe*," and add the phrase "*I am not personally responsible for this bill*." Again, only sign the form if the patient isn't able to sign.

It's also possible that the doctor who will be treating the patient in the nursing home will include his billing forms in the nursing home intake packet. Again, don't sign them unless you truly intend to be personally responsible for the patient's medical bills. If the patient isn't able to sign for himself, they can remain unsigned.

Make sure that you provide all of the patient's insurance cards, including pharmacy coverage and photo identification, at the time the patient is admitted. Don't let them out of your sight; have them photocopy the cards and return them to you; you may need them in the future so be sure to store them in a safe place. Always keep the originals and allow the providers to take photocopies.

The bottom line: if there are any forms that you don't understand, don't sign them. The patient has already been admitted, and it's the nursing home's problem if they're not signed. Provide as much information as possible so that the patient's insurance will pay for his bills, but don't sign any form accepting personal responsibility for the patient unless you intend to pay the patient's bills out of your own pocket. Feel free to speak with an attorney if you have any questions and have him review the forms before they are signed, although the cost of an attorney might not be necessary. Remember that the forms are there to legally protect the nursing home and certainly not the patient or his family.

The Nursing Assessment

Nursing plays a key role during the admission process, because the patient has been admitted for skilled nursing care. The patient will be weighed in order to monitor the patient's weight gain/loss during the nursing home stay. For patients who retain fluids from diseases or conditions that are kidney or cardiac related, weight gain is an excellent measure of the patient's healthcare status. Because excess fluid can mask the patient's true weight, it's also possible to gauge whether the patient is gaining/losing weight by measuring the circumference of his arm or thigh. The nurse or an aide will take the patient's vital signs and record them for comparison later.

The nurse will also complete a full-body assessment, which provides an overview of any sores, rashes, or wounds that the patient might have. This can be embarrassing to the patient, as the nurse must view his entire body. Although the nurse has been trained to make the patient feel comfortable, it's also possible to ask for a different nurse if the patient becomes embarrassed. The nursing home is usually able to accommodate this request.

The nurse documents everything about the patient's physical status, including dentures, hearing ability, visual ability, whether the patient is able to walk independently, etc. The nursing assessment provides a *baseline* for later comparison, which helps to show a patient's improvement during his stay; the nursing home must justify the patient's physical status and improvement to the insurance company. Even if you provided this information to the front office, you can help the nurse complete her assessment by providing a list of medications that the patient took at home (which might indicate any conditions he has); it's also helpful if you provide the name of all of the doctors who were treating him while he was at home.

Follow up later on to ensure that the nursing home has discussed the patient's home needs with the doctor. If a patient has a chronic disease that was overlooked in the hospital, it's important that the condition be treated before it becomes life-threatening.

Medication Issues

After the patient arrives, the admitting nurse will review the medication orders that were sent with the patient from his previous setting. She will either manually or electronically (or both) log in all of the patient's medications on the ***Medication Administration Record (MAR).*** If the patient arrived with any medications, they will be counted and logged in on the MAR as well. In most instances patients don't bring their own medications, because nursing homes have strict regulations and policies that they must follow regarding the delivery and storage of medications. However, patients who are being admitted from other facilities or even from home might arrive with enough medications to last until the commercial pharmacy is able to make the regular delivery.

There are generally three options for medication delivery in nursing homes. The first is for an on-site pharmacy, which is expensive and is a rare occurrence except in those nursing homes that are attached to hospitals. When a patient arrives in a nursing home with an on-site pharmacy, his medications are ordered and administered immediately. The main drawback is the cost of the medications; if the nursing home is hospital-based, the cost of the medications can be astronomical. This is only an issue if the patient is paying out-of-pocket for his medications, because in every other instance the medications will be billed through the patients' healthcare insurance plans. Unless these pharmacies are open to the public, they're not cost-effective.

There are also automated delivery systems, where the medications are filled by a pharmacy into an on-site delivery system. Medications are delivered to the dispenser on a regular basis – so essentially they never run out – and the nursing staff enters the medication orders into the computer system. The appropriate amount of medication is dispensed immediately, meaning that there is no delay in the delivery of medications. Not only are patients able to quickly receive their medications, these systems only charge for the actual amount of medications that are used, saving the nursing home (and patients) thousands of dollars each month in medications that would otherwise be destroyed. There are several different types of automated delivery systems; they are expensive and the nursing homes must bear the entire cost of purchasing (or leasing) and maintaining the systems.

The most common method of medication delivery in nursing homes is the use of commercial pharmacies. These pharmacies make millions of dollars each year serving nursing homes, hospices and other medical providers by delivering medications twice a day – or by sending a runner on a specialty run, if warranted. When the patient arrives at the nursing home, the procedure is for the nurse to enter the medications into the MAR, then fax or email the medication orders to the pharmacy and wait for the next scheduled delivery. Once they are delivered to the nursing home, the medications will need to be logged in before they are actually administered to the patient. Because the medications must be ordered, processed by the pharmacy, delivered and then logged in, it's a distinct possibility that a patient will have to wait several hours in pain while the nursing home meanders through its medication ordering process. Commercial pharmacies are the most cost-effective for the nursing home, as facilities are rarely charged delivery fees. The nursing home does have to pay for those medications that were ordered and never given to the patients, which can be thousands of dollars each month.

Patients don't always have to wait for pain medications; depending upon the state and local laws in which the facility is located, it's possible that there is an e-kit (emergency medicine kit) on premises that provides for a limited amount of "comfort" medications to be administered while the regular medications are en route from the pharmacy. The patient will still need to have a prescription for these medications and the supply for the entire facility is limited to a few doses.

One of the reasons that the medications take so long to be delivered to the nursing home is that they are only ordered after the patient has arrived at the nursing home, and not a moment before. This is because the nursing home is ultimately responsible to pay for all of the medications that have been delivered. If the medications are ordered before a patient arrives and he never makes it, the nursing home will be charged hundreds or thousands of dollars for the unused medications (the nursing home is responsible for the cost of all medications while patients are receiving services under the Medicare benefit). An example of a patient never arriving would be the patient who decides to discharge home or chooses another facility at the last minute.

Another reason that the delivery of pain medications (or other controlled substances) are often delayed is that they require an original, signed prescription in order to be filled. Since nursing homes rarely have physicians in-house, the usual procedure is for the doctor to give verbal orders over the phone and sign the orders later. This procedure impedes the nursing home's ability to obtain controlled substances. Some pharmacies will allow the prescription to be faxed in, and allow the delivery person to return the original to the pharmacy. This still requires a signed physician's order, but at least it allows for expedited delivery of the medications.

The best way to work around this regulation is for the nursing home to coordinate with the discharging facility and to request a signed prescription be sent with the patient from the hospital. Doctors are on-staff at the hospital, and in most cases they personally sign the discharge paperwork prior to the patient leaving. In most cases, doctors write short-term prescriptions for patients who are being discharged home so this request is nothing out of the ordinary. A simple phone call from the nursing home to the hospital case manager can alleviate a patient's pain and suffering and allow sufficient time the nursing home to obtain a longer term prescription. The patient will still have to wait until the medications are entered on the MAR, delivered and logged in, but it won't take as long as it would have without the signed prescription on-hand.

It's possible that a patient will arrive at the nursing home in intractable pain or distress and will require his medications immediately, only to find out that there is no such thing as "immediately" when it comes to pharmacy issues in a nursing home. Even though the nurse might be doing everything within her power to obtain the medications, it's simply not good enough for the patient who remains in distress.

Mrs. Smith arrives at the nursing home at 4:00 pm, and after she's check in the list of her medications is faxed to the pharmacy at about 5:00 pm. However, she has been prescribed a narcotic medication that must be accompanied by an original signed prescription. Luckily, the fax made it to the pharmacy before the runner left so the first round of her medications is delivered at 6:00 pm. However, her pain medications weren't included in the initial order due to the lack of a prescription. The charge nurse calls the doctor's office and asks him to fax a prescription to the pharmacy, but he has already left his office for the day.

The doctor promises to stop by after dinner to leave a signed prescription, but he is delayed until after 7:00 pm. When he arrives, the nurse is in the middle of passing her evening medications. Mrs. Smith's pain medication order isn't faxed to the pharmacy until after 8:30 pm, which is less than half an hour before the pharmacy closes. The prescription sits on the fax until the next morning.

The next morning, there are several medication orders ahead of Mrs. Smith's and they're processed on a first come, first served basis – so her pain medications don't make it on the 10:00 am medication run. The end result is that Mrs. Smith's pain medications finally arrive at 6:00 pm the next evening, over 24 hours after she was admitted to the nursing home.

Several hours can seem like forever to the patient who is laying in agony, counting the seconds until his medication is delivered to the nursing home. Once it arrives, it must be logged in and then administered. If the nurse lacks compassion (and I've met many that do), she won't rush the process once the medications have been delivered. This can further delay the administration of the medications up to an hour or more. If the family is present and the nurse is angry with them because of their constant interference (asking several times when the medications will be delivered), she might deliberately slow down; unfortunately it happens all of the time. It won't help if the family complains about her, because in most instances the nurses will protect each other.

The good news is that there are ways to ensure that your family member doesn't encounter this problem, starting with a request that he be sent to the nursing home before noon. This leaves sufficient time for the medications to arrive before the patient's bedtime, long before the pharmacy closes. *Before he leaves the hospital*, make sure that the nurses administer all of those medications that are due (including those "prn" or "as needed"), and ask if the doctor can write a prescription for a few days worth of pain medications to be sent with the patient. If the patient's transfer time can't be better coordinated, bring his medications from home in the original bottles to the nursing home and insist that they be administered to the patient. The medications must be listed on the admission orders that the doctor has signed; if the patient was taking a certain medication at home that isn't listed on the orders, it won't be given to the patient even if it's in his original prescription bottle. If it's something important, feel free to stand in front of the nurse and ask her to call the doctor for a telephone order; once the doctor gives a verbal order for the medication, the patient will be able to receive the medication you brought.

To ensure that the patient receives the medications, stand there and wait until they have been administered. Be sure to only bring enough to last until you anticipate that the medications will be delivered; even though these medications belong to you it's standard practice for nursing homes to destroy medications that family members have brought in. If you bring a full bottle into the nursing home, it will not be returned to you, meaning hundreds of dollars in unnecessary replacement costs. Those medications will surely come in handy when he returns home, and *they belong to the patient*. That's why it's important that you only bring enough medications into the nursing home to give the pharmacy sufficient time to deliver a two-week supply.

If the patient doesn't receive his medications as ordered within a reasonable amount of time, ask for a supervisor, call the director of nursing, the administrator, or 911 if you need to. I was present in a nursing home when a patient lay in agony while the nurse took her sweet time administering the medications that had just been delivered; after repeated requests, the patient's daughter called 911 from her cell phone. The look on the nurse's face was priceless as the paramedics rolled through the front doors, and the patient chose to be admitted to a different nursing home when he was discharged from the ER. This lack of action on the nursing home's part cost them tens of thousands of dollars in lost revenue.

Another way to help ensure that the patient's medications will be available to him is to sign him onto a hospice program (as long as he's not receiving rehabilitation services via the Medicare Part A benefit). Generally speaking, medications are ordered directly from the nursing home's professional pharmacy. However, hospice patients who are being admitted for a respite stay might be able to bring their medications with them at the time of admission. It's possible that the medications will need to be bubble-packed by the commercial pharmacy so that the nurses can easily count and record them. They will be kept locked in the medication cart or a medication room that is accessible only to nursing staff. The hospice will do their best to ensure that the medications are available to him; if the patient has a difficult time receiving his medications in the nursing home, call the hospice and ask to speak with a supervisor.

Remember that the nursing home has ordered the medications from the list that the doctor wrote, and he received his information from the last facility where the patient was located. The medications might not be the same as those he took while he was at home. Feel free to bring a handwritten list of the medications he took at home, or go to the pharmacy you use and ask them to print a list of his medications so that you can compare them to the ones he'll be given in the nursing home. If there is a discrepancy, ask to meet with the director of nursing or the physician. Don't allow the nursing home to bully you when it comes to the patient's medications, and don't allow the patient to remain in pain. Nursing home staff members often appear to believe that they're more knowledgeable about medications than the patient & family, and make statements such as "patients might become addicted." It's none of their business as long as the doctor orders the medications; the only thing that matters is the patient's comfort.

In many cases, nursing homes hold back on "prn" (as needed) pain medication, refusing to give narcotics unless the patient specifically asks for them. Even then they're reluctant to give medications because they don't believe that the patient is in "enough" pain. Remember that the patient's medications are prescribed by the doctor, and that the nursing home is required to give them regardless of the nurse's opinion. If you believe that your family member isn't being medicated correctly, feel free to speak with the doctor and ask for the medications to be administered according to a schedule. You should also feel free to meet with the facility administrator or the nursing home ombudsman about the nurse's lack of compassion regarding pain medications.

PASRR Screenings
There is a federal requirement that each patient being admitted to a nursing home must be screened for mental illness, mental retardation and developmental disabilities. This screening is called the ***Pre-Admission Screening and Resident Review (PASRR)***. The purpose of this screening is to ensure that severely mentally ill or disabled patients aren't being admitted into facilities that aren't able to meet

their needs, and to make recommendations about specialized plans of care that these residents will receive. If a nursing home admits a mentally ill patient who isn't appropriate to be there, it's possible that fines will be levied against the facility.

There are two parts to the PASRR; Level I is completed for each patient entering the nursing home regardless of his need. Level II is completed if the patient has a diagnosis of a severe mental illness or developmental disability that might possibly require specialized services, such medication management, day treatment programs, or counseling programs.

Each state has a different procedure for the PASRR process; some require that the patient be approved before his admission, while other states allow the nursing home to complete the paperwork after the patient is admitted. The PASSR only affects the patient or his family if the state won't approve his entry into the nursing home, which in most cases is a situation reserved for the severely mentally ill.

Some states require that patients who are admitted with traditional Medicaid be assigned a level of care prior to being admitted to the nursing home. If so, this paperwork will be submitted by the nursing home before the patient is ever admitted. In most instances, the patient and/or his family will never interact with anyone regarding his PASRR or his assigned level of care. This is strictly a federal compliance issue, and the PASRR process rarely translates into additional care for the patient.

Departments within the Nursing Home

There are several departments within the nursing home. Even though each department has specific responsibilities, the duties often overlap with those of other departments. The departments work together to address all of the patients' needs:

- *Activities* is responsible for providing programming that stimulates the patients' minds and keeps them occupied. It's more than just playing "Bingo," it's an opportunity to keep busy and socialize. The activities department coordinates volunteers, invites bands and other groups to perform for the residents, and celebrates birthdays and holidays. The department is required to develop a calendar of events that includes special programming designed to meet the needs of residents who are confused and have lower cognitive functioning. The activities department offers books, videos/movies, and puzzles that can be brought to patient rooms if they're unable to get out, and brings patients their daily mail. The activities department also takes people out of the facility on shopping trips, to movies and other places in the community. Without the activities department, residents would have nothing to do all day and life for the residents would be unbearable. The activities department head is not a well-paid position and generally doesn't require a college diploma; these workers must be licensed or certified in accordance with state laws.

- *Admissions/Marketing* is in charge of marketing as well as coordinating all of the information required for a patient's admission. It's their responsibility to visit hospitals, physicians and other medical providers in order to gain as many patient referrals as possible. The nursing home is competing with all of the other nursing homes and rehabilitation facilities in the area, and the competition can be fierce. Once the nursing home receives a referral, the admissions coordinator works quickly to ensure that the patient is medically appropriate, has the ability to pay, and that the facility can meet his needs. She ensures that the nursing home will be ready for him when he arrives, and often arranges the patient's transportation to the nursing home. The admissions director is not a licensed position and there are no specific education requirements.

- The ***Business Office*** is in charge of accounts payable and receivable. The office manager rarely has autonomy; most nursing homes are owned by a large corporation and the role of the business office is to submit paperwork to the corporate office for processing. For example, the business office might collect and deposit payments, but the corporate office will apply the payments to the proper accounts and perform collections for the nursing home. The business office is required to maintain and update patient financial files. The business office manager coordinates with insurance providers to ensure that patients' medical bills are paid, and assists with insurance-related issues. This includes working with Social Security, SSI, private insurance plans, the Veteran's Administration, banks, the local Medicaid office and other financial entities on behalf of the patients. The business office might also employ a person whose job it is to file Medicaid applications on behalf of the patient and/or family. It is also the responsibility of the business office to maintain the patient trust account and provide patients access to their funds during regular business hours.   The business office manager is not a licensed position and there are no specific education requirements.

- *Central Supply* is where all of the supplies and specialty equipment are stored; the director orders the supplies that keep the nursing home in business. This includes gloves, briefs, medical supplies, oxygen, specialty mattresses, etc.   All of these items are billed to private-pay patients as they're used, although the nursing home is required to provide them to Medicaid patients at no extra cost. The central supply department ensures that all of the supplies are available by delivering them to the medical floor as they are needed. The director of central supply is not a licensed position and there are no specific education requirements.

- *Housekeeping/Environmental Services* is responsible for cleaning and every area of the nursing home, and ensuring the facility remains as germ-free as possible.   Housekeepers are also responsible for cleaning and monitoring the temperature of all refrigerators and kitchen areas.   They disinfect every area using state and federal approved cleaning supplies, and maintain current *MSDS* (Material Safety Data Sheets - information about specific products) for every chemical used in the housekeeping department. Most nursing homes have housekeepers available during the day only; nursing staff tidies up rooms after hours and waits for them to be deep-cleaned until the housekeeping staff arrives the next day.   The director of this department is not a licensed position and there are no specific education requirements.

- *Dietary Services* is the common name for the kitchen/food service department. In most nursing homes, the kitchen staff prepares meals and sets them onto meal carts to be served by floor staff, although in some facilities the food is served buffet-style. Regardless of the manner in which the food is served, staff members ensure that there is food available that is able to meet the specific dietary needs of each patient (dietary services works with a Registered Dietician to ensure that each patient's nutritional requirements are addressed). The kitchen staff must keep a record of patients' food preferences and allergies, and ensure that the patients are provided with meal choices. The kitchen and floor staff monitor the amount of food that each patient eats, and ensures that snacks are available at all times. It's difficult to keep costs down in the kitchen, but there is a strict budget to be adhered to (usually less than $10 per patient per day). Patients often complain about facility food, which is rarely of restaurant quality. The director of this department is not a licensed position and there are no specific education requirements.

- *Human Resources* is required to maintain personnel records for each employee, including verification of their licenses and certifications (such as remaining current on CPR certification). The director of human resources ensures that each employee passes a criminal background check. The director of this department is not a licensed position and there are no specific education requirements.

- *Education Department* is an important part of the nursing department; the Director of Staff Development is responsible for ensuring that every staff member is screened for tuberculosis, is up-to-date on shots & vaccinations, and is provided with all of the training that he needs to perform his job. The DSD ensures that the staff is all kept current on all pertinent laws and regulations, and coordinates training schedules for the nursing staff. The director of this department is a licensed position (R.N. or L.P.N.), with the education requirements required for the license that they hold (1-2 years).

- *Maintenance* must be able to perform a variety of tasks, from electrical work to painting and plumbing. The director's job is to ensure that all systems of the nursing home are kept in working condition, coordinates with the fire/smoke alarm company, maintains the back-up generators, and ensures that the facility will pass multiple inspections required by state and federal law. The requirements of this job are many, and it takes an extremely capable and flexible person to be able to maintain the physical plant of a nursing home. They must be able to fix anything from a call light to a hospital bed. The director of this department is not a licensed position and there are no specific education requirements.

- *Medical Records* is responsible for all patient charts, both current and those of patients who have been discharged. This department is responsible for obtaining physician signatures and performing chart audits to ensure that all departments are submitting their paperwork in a timely manner. Medical records will request the patient's past medical records from other providers as needed and copies medical records for patients and their families upon their request. Although there is such thing as a certified Medical Records Technician, most nursing homes don't hire professionals because it's not required. Generally speaking, nursing homes don't want to spend the extra money to hire a professional when they could hire someone for half the cost. The director of this department is not required to be a licensed position and there are no specific education requirements.

- *Nursing* is headed by the Director of Nursing, also called the Director of Nursing Services. The D.O.N. is responsible for all of the nurses, nursing aides, medications, medical supplies, staff development, and coordination with anything medical. This is the largest department in the facility and therefore has the highest labor costs. The nursing department is also responsible for the task of MDS reporting to Medicare and providing case management authorizations in order to ensure that patient care is reimbursed. The D.O.N. must have a minimum of two years of nursing education and be a Registered Nurse.

- *Pharmacy Services* Most nursing homes contract with a professional pharmacy to provide the patient's medications, which means that there isn't a pharmacy on-site to provide the medications. In most cases, pharmacies make their deliveries to nursing homes twice each day. This gives the nursing home the opportunity to order only the amount of medications that patients need, which cuts down on amount of medications that are wasted (thrown away). The nursing home is required to have a pharmacy consultant who reviews patient charts and makes recommendations about medications, dosage and frequency in order to better meet each patient's needs. The pharmacist keeps the nursing home current on the requirements and laws that apply to nursing homes. It's important to note that pharmacy consultants might recommend a change in a patient's medications, but the physician and the patient have the final word in any changes. The consultant must be a licensed pharmacist, with all of the licensure and education requirements of the Pharmacist profession for the state in which the nursing home is located.

- *Social Services* coordinates with all other departments to ensure that the patient's needs, both medical and non-medical, are met. They often go shopping for patients, investigate lost items, coordinate room changes, participate in and act as mentor to the Resident Council, and perform many tasks that enhance patients' lives. They also make discharge planning arrangements, such as helping the patient develop a plan as to where he will go when he is ready to leave. Social Services ensures that the patient will have the follow up he needs after discharge by ordering medical equipment, home health care, transportation, and meals-on-wheels for a patient's use after discharge. Social services is responsible for ensuring that the patient and families have information about *advanced directives* (planning regarding end-of-life issues) and assist in filling out the forms when necessary. The licensure requirements for social service workers vary from state-to-state, and depending upon the size of facility, may not be required to provide licensed social workers. They're able to hire resident advocates or social service assistants who work in the social services department but aren't required to have a license or education of any type. If a social work license is required, the social worker must generally have a minimum of a four-year degree.

l.e. green

The Billing Office and Financial Issues

Understanding how the billing office works will make it much easier to build a good working relationship with the nursing home. Every nursing home operates under the same federal laws and guidelines, but there are some differences in state laws regarding management of patient financial affairs. Additionally, each nursing home or parent corporation manages its business office differently, and applies different rules to the patient's personal monies. Regardless of the way it's managed, every nursing home is required to allow the state access to its financial records upon request, and must have numerous checks and balances in place in an attempt to keep patients safe from financial exploitation.

The Billing Office Manager's responsibilities include:

- Processing patient payments

- Billing Medicare, Medicaid, the Veteran's Administration, Private Insurances, State or County Programs and Patients.

- Processing accounts payable & receivable

- Collecting monies due

- Data entry and medical coding

- Maintaining the patient trust account

The billing office manager is an unlicensed position that requires no financial background whatsoever, and it's up to the company (and each nursing home administrator) as to what qualifications the position requires. While the billing office manager might extensive experience in medical billing, she probably has little or no experience at all and might have been promoted from a lesser position, such as receptionist. The office manager might receive support and training from the corporation in order to succeed, or she might be attempting to find her way in the position. Unless she is trained in the finer points of state and federal laws, she might attempt to make arbitrary rules that affect patients. If you believe that the office manager is making inappropriate decisions that affect your family member, you should discuss your concerns with the administrator or parent corporation. You also have the right to call the ombudsman or to file a complaint with the state licensing agency.

The checks and balances that are in place don't necessarily mean that it's impossible to steal from a nursing home, or from the patients themselves. There have been thousands of incidents of employee theft, from small amounts to the theft of hundreds of thousands of dollars – it is a reflection of the administrator's ability to manage his staff when a worker is able to steal large amounts from a facility over a long period of time. A small amount might not be caught, but when a worker is able to steal tens or thousands of dollars from a nursing home, it might be in the patient's best interest to find another nursing home more closely monitors the actions of their employees.

If such a theft is discovered, the nursing home will complete an audit to determine how much money was stolen. It is possible that a nursing home might attempt to bill the patients long after the fact in an attempt to recover any monies they possibly can. Even if the patients were billed and had paid in a timely manner, it's possible that the money was never applied to their accounts and the nursing home will attempt to collect from patients – or their families – long after the fact. They'll be told that it's their responsibility to prove that they paid; this can be difficult if the checking account was since closed out or if the payment was made in cash. This is an example of why it's important to keep proof of any payments made to the nursing home for several years.

The nursing home can bill a patient at any time; it doesn't matter whether or not the patient is a current resident of the facility. It can be distressing when a family member receives bills long after a patient has died. A nursing home administrator can be extremely intimidating when it comes to account collection – but after a person's estate has been settled it's doubtful any monies can be recovered. If you are contacted for a bill that was incurred and the patient has since passed away, it would be best to consult an attorney before making any payments on the patient's behalf. The nursing home won't want the publicity of a lawsuit, nor will they want to pay the cost of hiring an attorney to file such a suit.

Even if the patient is a current resident, it's possible that the nursing home won't be able to recover any money long after the fact. It's a simple matter to resolve if you are able to present a copy of a cancelled check or receipt from the nursing home. However, if the nursing home is attempting to bill for charges that they overlooked, there might be several reasons that the bill will never be paid. For example, a patient who is now indigent and Medicaid is paying for his room & board in a nursing home won't have any money available to pay and the family isn't responsible whether or not they signed a personal letter of guarantee. Another reason could be that the statute of limitations has passed, and the nursing home can't legally bill for the items. A really great reason that the nursing home won't want to push the issue is the desire to avoid publicity about the matter. A quick call to the consumer advocate at the local television station, or local newspaper, can often help make the issue go away. Even if such an employee theft has made the local papers, the nursing home would just as soon not have the general public know that they're trying to collect on their losses from the patients.

In the case of one nursing home where I worked, the administrator and parent corporation were willing to write off any amounts they weren't able to collect rather than to suffer any negative publicity after the billing office manager stole well over $100,000. They retroactively billed patients thousands of dollars, and attempted to force family members into paying for charges that had never been billed. The administrator told the families that the corporation was forcing her to collect on these long past due charges, even though she told her staff that the corporation was willing to write off the amounts rather than to pursue it in court.

In fact, in most cases the administrator has the discretion to write off bills of any amount, although they don't want you to know this. I've seen administrators negotiate bills in excess of $150,000 down to less than $50,000. Regardless of the situation, if you receive a billing long after the fact it would be best to check with an attorney before making any payments. According to collection laws, if you make a payment on a long-past-due bill you are accepting that the billing is legitimate and might become responsible to pay the amount in full – even if the statute of limitations has passed.

In addition to processing patients' payments, the nursing home billing office is responsible for coordinating the billings for doctors, dentists and podiatrists who visit patients in the facility. If the patient is a veteran who is receiving care though the VA medical system, the billing office will need to coordinate with the nursing staff to ensure that his medications are ordered via the VA pharmacy rather than for the patient to pay thousands of dollars out-of-pocket for medications that are otherwise covered. If the billing office doesn't understand the system, it's possible that the patient (or more likely, the nursing home) will be on the hook for thousands of dollars in pharmacy charges. Even though the errors are due to the nursing home's billing practices, they will do everything possible to pass along their losses to the patient and/or his family.

In many cases, the billing office manager will be working directly with patients' personal monies and has the discretion of making certain financial decisions on the patient's behalf. Don't trust that she is acting in the patient's best interest; she might not understand that the patient's medications can be covered cheaper though the VA or that a hospice program is paying for his durable medical equipment. Feel free to question any decisions that the facility makes on the patient's behalf, and speak with the administrator or the appropriate state agency if you disagree with her.

The Resident Trust Account

All nursing homes are federally mandated to offer a ***resident trust account*** for the use of every patient, regardless of the payment source for his room & board.

The trust account is like a bank that's located in the nursing home that the patient is able to use to gain access to his funds. In most cases, the nursing home must provide a bond or other guarantee to ensure that the patients' money remains safe from employee theft. The account exists solely for the convenience of the patients, because it's difficult for them to get to the bank to access money for incidentals.

It's a personal choice as to whether a patient wants to deposit his monies into the trust account; the nursing home is required to offer the account, but the patients have the right to continue to use their own personal checking or savings accounts if they choose. The nursing home can't require that a patient open a trust account, even though some nursing homes state in the intake packet that it's a requirement. Patients have the right to continue to manage their money in whatever manner they wish.

The money in the trust account belongs to the patient and/or his family, and he has the right to use it for whatever purpose he chooses. If the nursing home staff members are concerned about the way the patient is spending his money, they have the right to contact the ombudsman. I knew of a patient who received $90.00 from the Veteran's Administration every month, and he paid a woman to bring him vodka every month. The facility wasn't able to limit his access to his own funds, because the patient was alert & oriented and able to make decisions on his own behalf. Eventually the patient was evicted for non-payment (he refused to pay his share of his nursing home costs).

The benefit of using a patient trust account is that the patient has immediate access to his money if he wants to buy snacks or go on an outing with the nursing home activity department. It's not a good idea for a patient to hold cash in his room, as it could be lost or stolen and he won't have any recourse. Using the trust account might also alleviate the need for patient's family members to provide bank statements every month, but each situation is different. The disadvantage of using a trust account is that the patient/family is at the mercy of the facility's rules unless he contacts the ombudsman to ensure his rights aren't violated.

According to federal requirements, the nursing home must pay the patient interest on any balance over $50.00 and is required to provide quarterly statements to the patient or his representative. They must also provide a current accounting upon request. Many states have a cap on the amount that can be held in the account to keep the nursing home from holding thousands of dollars of the patients' money.

Patients' family members often go shopping for them; some nursing homes prefer that family members spend their own money on the patient and present the receipt for reimbursement rather than to allow them to withdraw cash to go shopping with. The nursing home must be realistic with these requests; for example, it's not reasonable to expect that the family spend hundreds of dollars out of their own pocket for a flat-screen television and wait to be reimbursed. If the patient or his representative is willing to sign a request for the money, the nursing home <u>must</u> provide it immediately. The nursing home can ask for a copy of the receipt to prove where the money went, but they can't make this a requirement. Ultimately it's up to the patient if he wishes to access his own funds.

If the nursing home business office won't allow him access to his funds in the trust account, ask to speak with the administrator. If this doesn't work, call the nursing home ombudsman or the state bureau of licensure; when contacted by these agencies it's amazing how quickly the nursing home staff can change their mind. It might be worth considering a transfer to another nursing home if the administrator won't work with you on such a basic issue. Patients have the right to manage their own funds regardless of what the nursing home administrator says.

If the patient's monthly income is sent directly to the nursing home, the general procedure is for the money to be deposited into the patient's trust account. The nursing home then writes a check out of the trust account for the patient's liability (share of cost). This is an arrangement that is set up by the nursing home, but if the patient refuses to allow the nursing home to access his funds, they can't withdraw anything from his trust account. It can be frustrating for a nursing home to have the funds sitting in his trust account, but he has the right to use his money for whatever he wishes. The nursing home can call the ombudsman in an attempt to negotiate an agreement, but the patient still has the right to refuse them access to his funds. Obviously, this is an extreme case, but it does happen and the nursing home must then go through the legal process to evict him if he refuses to pay his share of cost. A nursing home eviction is a long, drawn out process.

Patients whose room & board are paid by Medicaid must pay their entire income, less about $30.00 per month, as their share of cost. This amount, called the patient's *personal needs allowance*, can be used for whatever the patient would like. The amount that the patient is allowed to keep varies from state-to-state and is determined by that state's Medicaid program. The amount is so small because almost everything is provided for patients on Medicaid, except for cigarettes, candy, daily newspaper, money for outings (going to a restaurant, or ordering out), hair appointments, etc. (The personal needs allowance also varies according to whether the patient is married and his spouse remains out in the community).

Obviously, the personal needs allowance isn't enough to cover many items and it's possible for family members to help out by paying for certain items such as newspapers, etc. However, due to Medicaid rules it's probably best to provide the assistance in the form of gift subscriptions, cartons of cigarettes, etc. rather than to deposit money into the trust account. The patient whose payment source is Medicaid must be able to explain every miscellaneous deposit and withdrawal out of both his patient trust account and personal bank accounts, if any. The Medicaid program might view the money as ongoing income, and count it toward the patient's share of cost in the nursing home.

Those patients whose room & board are paid by Medicaid and are either veterans or the spouse of a deceased veteran might qualify for an additional $90.00 per month from the Veteran's Administration Aid & Attendance program; this helps if the patient's personal needs cost more than the Medicaid allotted amount. However, this amount can quickly add up if not spent. (Veterans whose room & board are paid by other means – not Medicaid – might also be eligible to receive up to $1,758.00 per month (widowed spouses are eligible to receive up to $1,130.00 to help offset the cost of the nursing home room & board). For additional information about Aid & Attendance, please visit www.veteranaid.org or www.va.gov.

Nursing home billing office managers often attempt to make arbitrary rules as to how the patient's money can be spent. One nursing home for which I worked had an office manager who limited trust account withdrawals to $35.00 per day. A patient wanted to give his daughter a wedding gift of $500.00; even though he could well afford to do so, the office manager wouldn't allow it. He asked to speak with the administrator, but the office manager refused to allow him this. He called his daughter and asked her to help him with the matter.

When his daughter attempted to intervene, neither the office manager nor the administrator were interested in discussing the matter any further. In fact, they told the patient that he wasn't allowed to give away any of his money and that his family must present a receipt before any money would be given to them for reimbursement. The office manager had held that position for less than a year and was under the impression she was the ultimate authority as to what patients could do with their money. The nursing home administrator, who was later fired for actions such as this (and many more), incorrectly believed that she was the ultimate authority on how patients were allowed to spend their own money. However, the daughter did not receive her wedding gift due to the arbitrary rules imposed by nursing home staff members.

The amount of money held in the trust is considered to be the patient's asset, and in most instances he's free to either save or spend it however he chooses. However, if his payment source for room & board is Medicaid and the trust account is his only asset, he can't allow the account to build to the point that it exceeds $2,000. Once a patient's total assets exceed $2,000, he is no longer eligible for Medicaid to pay his room & board. Not only will the patient will have to spend all of his savings on his care, he (or his family) will probably have to suffer through the Medicaid application process all over again.   The nursing home might lose out on the difference between what the patient owes and the amount he has in his trust account for that month.   All of this can be avoided by keeping the patient's assets, including the money held in the trust account, below $2,000. The nursing home will often monitor the amounts in the trust account and will even purchase items for the patient if the family isn't able. Anything that is purchased out of the patient's funds belongs to the patient and, once he passes away, to his family.

The resident trust belongs to the patient as long as he's alive, but once a patient dies the nursing home must follow state regulations regarding disbursal of funds. In some states, that means that any money in his account will be refunded to Medicaid if that program is paying his room & board.

If the family had intended to use the money in the account for the patient's burial, they might have to find another way to pay for it. The best plan is to keep the patient's trust account down to a minimum amount and pay for his burial ahead of time; however, don't allow the facility to choose a burial plan without discussing the matter with you first. After all, the patient might prefer to be buried in another state which can substantially increase the costs. All of this can be prearranged and monthly payments can be made well ahead of time (for additional information, please refer to the section on *Burial Plans* later in this chapter).

Representative Payee vs. Guardianship

Many nursing homes prefer that their patients' income be sent directly to the nursing home, rather than to have their families continue to assist with their finances. This is because the nursing home will be guaranteed that the patient's bill is paid every month. Although the nursing home can request that this be the case, they can't make it a requirement in order for a patient to remain in the facility. For the patient who will be remaining in the nursing home on a long-term basis, a change of address might not be an issue. However, if the patient is only there for a short period of time (such as for rehabilitation), a change of address can take weeks or months to process. After he leaves the nursing home, his income will still be sent there until another change of address can be processed.

Many nursing homes will process a change of address immediately upon admission, regardless of the patient's wishes (the change of address form is often included in the intake packet). It's best to read all of the paperwork in the admission packet to ensure that one of the forms you're signing doesn't give permission to change addresses or allow the nursing home to become responsible for the patient's funds without discussing it first. If they don't discuss a change of address with you, bring it up yourself.

Even if the patient's income is sent directly to the nursing home, he still has the discretion as to how his funds will be spent. As I mentioned before, a patient can refuse to pay his share of cost even if the money is deposited directly into his trust account. But there is a way for the nursing home to circumvent the possibility of not being paid; they can apply to become the patient's **Representative Payee** though the Social Security Administration, which allows them to manage the patient's social security income. It doesn't allow them access to any other income, such as retirement income, nor does it allow the nursing home to make any other financial decisions on a patient's behalf.

The Representative Payee program was created for those patients who aren't able to manage their social security income, and becoming representative payee is a fairly simple process. A person (such as a family member) or company (i.e. the nursing home) completes an application promising to be responsible for paying the patient's bills with his income. The person or entity appointed as the representative payee, also referred to as *payee*, is not automatically the patient's power of attorney and has no authority to make decisions on the patient's behalf, nor is he required to subsidize the patient's income out of his pocket. The payee's sole responsibility to the patient is to help to manage the social security income. The payee must keep accurate records and submit a report every year that details how he spent the patient's money. Becoming the representative allows the nursing home access to his social security income, which is usually the largest source of income for a nursing home patient.

In many instances, it's helpful to the patient for a payee to be appointed. For example, a family member who is payee can ensure the bills are paid while a patient is in the hospital and is too sick to make financial decisions or even sign a check. In some cases, such as in the case of drug or alcohol dependent patients, the SSA will require that the patient have a representative payee in order to ensure they remain housed in a safe environment. The representative payee can be anyone as long as the social security program approves him. There are companies that will act as representative payees for a price, but the charges must be reasonable or Social Security won't allow it.

It's important to understand that, once a representative payee has been appointed, it's probable that the SSA will require the patient always have one unless he is able to prove that his original reason for having one no longer exists. If he doesn't like the person or business that was appointed his payee, he can request that another payee be appointed (the SSA doesn't have to approve the new payee that the patient has chosen and can require that another candidate be located). Simply stated, if the patient ever intends to leave that particular nursing home, he shouldn't allow the facility to become his representative payee or even allow them to process a change of address to the nursing home. It is much harder to leave the facility when they have a hold on his finances. It's best to make this clear to the nursing home so that there will be no problems later on.

Nursing homes often apply to be appointed Representative Payee without informing the patient or his family. Regardless of what they claim, the nursing home administration can't require that the patient or family allow the facility to become the representative payee, nor can they demand approval over monies spent on the patient's behalf. That is clearly overstepping their fiduciary boundaries. The patient or his family has the right to continue to manage the finances if they wish. The only time that the nursing home should apply to become payee is when the patient intends to remain in the facility on a long-term basis and there is no family member willing or able to accept the responsibility. If a nursing home has a stranglehold on your family member's finances, you have the right to contact Social Security and inform them of the problem.

It's becoming more common for patients to file a protest when a Representative Payee is appointed without their knowledge, because some nursing homes have made it a habit of applying to become the Representative Payee upon every patient's admission. The application requires a doctor's signature, and sometimes that still isn't enough. The Social Security Administration has become increasingly suspicious of such applications and is often requiring the patient's permission or a psychiatric consultation before they will appoint a Payee.

A facility for which I worked applied to become the patient's representative payee and the patient called Social Security to stop it; this went back & forth several times until it was determined that the only way that the SSA would allow the nursing home access to the patient's funds would be for the facility to obtain a court order. The patient was alert & oriented, and the nursing home was never able to access his funds. He actually remained there for over a year, rent-free.

If a patient with substantial assets doesn't have anyone to help with his finances (or family members are fighting over control of his money), it's possible that a court will appoint a family member as ***conservator*** or appoint a ***guardian*** to ensure the patient's funds are used appropriately for his care. The person appointed as conservator must be a resident of the state in which the patient resides; if not, the family member can be a co-conservator but there will have to be a local person or entity that is legally responsible for the patient. If there are multiple family members vying to become guardian, it's possible that the courts will appoint a temporary conservator until the issue can be resolved. The courts will appoint a third party, but they rarely appoint the nursing home as conservator due to the fact that the nursing home has a financial interest in any decisions that are made on the patient's behalf.

There are public agencies that act as patient guardians; however, they often have long waiting lists and won't become involved unless the patient is in some type of danger of either becoming homeless or being financially exploited. For those patients who have the ability to pay for a guardian, there are often private guardianship companies that are able to quickly and efficiently apply for guardianship and work with the patient's family to ensure his needs are met. The court will approve a schedule of fees regardless of whether the patient has been appointed a private or public guardian.

Sometimes the facility won't recognize a family member as the legal representative, and it will become necessary for the patient to be appointed as decision-maker in a legal capacity. A conservator is able to act on a patient's behalf to obtain refunds when a facility won't recognize a family member as the patient's legal representative. In one case I knew of, a nursing home required a confused patient to sign a check in an amount exceeding $50,000 and held it in his patient trust account to ensure that the facility was paid every month. When his daughter, who lived out of town, was made aware that the patient had been placed in a facility, she brought him to his home and provided the patient with 24-hour care. The nursing home refused to give the family any information about the finances, citing patient confidentiality. Instead, they called Adult Protective Services to investigate the patient's home situation. APS stated their belief that the patient was receiving appropriate care at home and no further action was taken.

The nursing home held the patient's money hostage for nearly a year without his daughter even knowing about it, until she filed a petition with the courts to become his legal guardian/conservator. It was during the proceedings that it was discovered the money sitting in the patient's trust account in the nursing home. The nursing home office manager fought turning over the money to the family, stating her belief that the patient would someday return and the money guaranteed that the facility would be paid. The courts ordered the nursing home to immediately return the funds (plus interest) or face theft charges – and the patient remained at home until he died, surrounded by his family. This isn't a common occurrence, but it does illustrate what can happen when a nursing home arbitrarily makes financial decisions on a patient's behalf.

Financial Exploitation

It's possible for a facility employee to exploit a patient financially while he's in a nursing home. As I mentioned before, the facility is required to offer a trust account for patients and the state can audit the account without notice; it only follows that these accounts should be safe from theft. However, it's possible for the person in charge of the account to embezzle from the patients for years without being caught. The state doesn't closely monitor trust accounts, and if the administrator or parent corporation doesn't perform random checks it is possible that the patient trust account will be used for an employee's personal use.

The business office manager can apply payments to any account (including her own bank account) and claim that payment had never been made. Unless the family is able to prove they've paid, they might be presented with a huge retroactive bill and aggressive collection techniques. This is why it's vital that patients and their families keep a record of every payment made to the nursing home. Several years down the line, you might need to prove that you paid the bill.

Another way that a patient can be financially exploited is by a facility employee taking the patient's credit card from his wallet when he's admitted. They can charge thousands of dollars worth of items, and if the employee intercepts the patient's bills no one will find out (it's difficult to prove that the patient didn't authorize the charges). The credit card company will end up writing off the bill, with no one the wiser. It's best to cancel all cards when your family member is admitted to the nursing home; if the patient is confused and insists that he carry a credit card, give him a blank that is sent in the mail for advertisement. Since he won't be using it, he will never know that it's not real. Remember that most people carry money their entire lives, and even though they've been admitted to a nursing home, they still have the desire to continue managing their own finances.

One reason that financial exploitation often goes unreported is that nursing homes don't want bad publicity, nor do they want the state investigating their financial dealings. The issue isn't simple; once an employee has been caught exploiting a patient, the legal proceedings can take years before the case is resolved. One tactic that attorneys often use is to delay the process with multiple filings, so that by the time the case goes to court the patient has died. Since people have the right to face their accuser, the charges will be dropped because technically there's no longer a victim. This is a common legal ploy used to ensure that the thief does little or no jail time, even if they confessed to the crime.

It's unfortunate, but just like physical and mental abuse, financial abuse can be hard to prove. Family members can head off potential abuse by managing the patient's money themselves, rather than to allow the nursing home to do so. Make sure that the patient only has a few dollars on his person and $200 or less in his trust account at any time, and remove all credit cards and ATM cards from his wallet before he's admitted. Keep a copy of any money deposited into the patient's trust account and ask for monthly accountings to ensure that the patient has access to his own money.

If the patient has the ability to manage his own finances, there should be no problem with his doing so. It's possible to ask for a lock on the patient's drawers or bring a file cabinet so that he has a safe place to place any paperwork he might have. Even if he's competent when he's first admitted, he will probably decline with age and it's important to review this issue at least annually. A trusted family member can provide help if and when the patient requires assistance. The bottom line is, don't trust anyone with the patient's finances; a nursing home isn't a prison and can't require that the patient allow them to manage his monies.

Burial Plans

Nursing homes are required to ask which mortuary a patient has chosen and to have this information listed on his face sheet. This doesn't mean that a formal burial plan must be in place, it only means that this is the mortuary that the family intends to use when the patient dies. However, paying ahead for a burial plan is an excellent way to spend the money in a patient's trust account to ensure that he remains eligible for Medicaid.

If at all possible, choose the mortuary on your own. Mortuaries heavily market nursing homes, because they have a patient base that will likely need their services within a short period of time. The salesperson makes a healthy commission, and he will do whatever he can to get the nursing home to refer as many patients to him as possible. The staff isn't allowed to accept financial gifts, but he might bring lunches and promise to do all of the legwork necessary to ensure their patients' needs are met. This can include selling them items they don't need and can't afford. In many towns, there is more than one mortuary and it's possible to get a better price than the one offered by the nursing home's favorite company.

Burial plans can be expensive; a simple cremation can cost anywhere from $300 to $2,500, while burials can start at around $1,200. The mortuary's mission is to get you to pay as much as possible by mentioning the tribute that you're paying to the deceased, and adding on extras such as casket, chapel, viewing, flowers, personalized programs, dressing the body, headstone, etc. Many of these costs can be dramatically decreased by shopping around. Most mortuaries offer packages that discount their services, but some will drastically increase their prices if you add or remove items (such as buying the casket elsewhere). With a product mark-up anywhere from 100% to 1,000% or more, mortuaries will do everything possible to preserve their profit margins. According to federal law, all mortuaries must provide pricing information upon request, so feel free to shop around to all of the local mortuaries.

One tactic that the mortuary will use to increase revenue is to tell you that their caskets have to meet certain industry standards, and imply that any other casket won't perform the same. Although this may be true, it might not matter to most people if the casket begins to deteriorate immediately once it's in the ground, because it will probably never be seen again. The burial vault and/or grave liner is another way that they can make extra money; these items might not be required by state and local laws and the mark-up on these items is huge Remember that the mortuary is counting on your lack of knowledge and emotional state to dramatically increase their profit.

Buying the burial plan ahead of time helps to cut back on the effects of the emotional sales tactics many mortuaries use. It's a personal choice as to whether or not to make pre-arrangements, but it's a good idea to shop around to ensure you receive the service that you would prefer. Prices vary quite a bit between mortuaries. Using the one that advertises the most can cost thousands of dollars more than the patient or family intended to pay. Be realistic about the services the patient will need at the time of his death.

If the burial plan is being purchased for a nursing home resident whose room & board are paid by the Medicaid program, it's vital that this be discussed with the mortuary. Many burial plans are actually insurance policies, and the cash value that accrues counts toward the patient's $2,000 asset limit (the asset limit is higher is some states, such as New York). Some states will allow for the patient to irrevocably assign the cash value of the policy to the mortuary, but other states won't allow for this transfer. That's because even though the cash value has been "irrevocably" assigned to the mortuary, the cash value can be reassigned back to the patient (or to another mortuary if the patient moves from the area). The policy itself might possibly be gifted to a family member, but that can be viewed as divestiture of an asset to become eligible for Medicaid. The mortuary probably has experience with this issue; if not, discuss the issue with the nursing home business office or contact an elder law attorney.

Nursing homes are places where patients are provided room & board – not where they are held hostage. It's important to remain vigilant when it comes to dealing with the patient's finances. Don't pay any bill unless you are certain that it is the patient's responsibility, and don't allow the nursing home to order expensive items without first discussing them with you.

Don't assume that the nursing home is acting in the patient's best interests – if your family member needs to spend some money in order to remain eligible for Medicaid, you have the right to help him with this spend-down. You probably know the patient much better than the nursing home staff; even if you don't live locally and aren't able to go shopping, you are welcome to provide input as to what they will buy for him. Anything that the nursing home buys for a patient with his own money belongs to his estate after he passes away, and family members are free to keep or donate items such as televisions after he's gone. Don't allow the nursing home to convince you to donate a big-ticket item – such as specialty equipment or an expensive television – unless this is truly what you want to do. Whether or not the nursing home is operated for-profit, it's possible that the nursing home will increase its revenue by charging the next patient who uses these items.

l.e. green

Understanding How a Nursing Home Operates

Nursing home operating procedures are different than most people would imagine them to be; it's much easier to maneuver through the system when you have a working knowledge of how nursing homes are operated. Even though the patient and his family members are oriented to the facility at the time of admission, it's simply not possible for the nursing home to explain everything at that time (and for the family to remember it all).

After the patient has been admitted, a family member might be able to ask a question of any staff member and receive pretty much the same (correct) answer. However, it's also possible that they'll receive different answers from the various staff members they encounter. This might be because the staff members are attempting to hide information, but in most cases it's because they don't know the answers. Every department views the information from the perspective of the department that they represent – and most staff members don't understand the system themselves.

In some nursing homes, the departments are territorial and are in competition with one another; when a staff member is asked a question, she might be attempting to sabotage another department or employee by promising that to pass along a message (and then purposely not following through). The internal politics can be difficult for patients and families to understand – this is much more common than the nursing home industry would like to admit. When asking questions, families never know whether the staff members are guessing at an answer or are attempting to sabotage another department. The nurse might be angry because the social worker complained about a patient left in pain, or the physical therapist might be angry because a nurse complained about their lack of cooperation with the nursing department. Not all nursing homes have this problem, but if you find that you aren't able to get a straight answer it might be best to speak with a department supervisor or the administrator about your issue.

Nursing homes aren't allowed to control their patients' actions, although many will try. Patients have the right to make decisions about what they want to do with their day, how they want their finances managed and who to allow access to their medical information. Unfortunately, many nursing homes attempt to make arbitrary decisions regarding patients' needs and abilities. Staff members are there to serve the patients, not the other way around. If your family member is being treated with anything but respect, discuss the issue with the charge nurse, administrator, ombudsman or even the state licensing agency. Most of the time, issues can be resolved without involving the state – but family members must advocate for the patient to ensure that he is treated with dignity and respect. Whether or not the allegations are true, if the patient's perception is that they aren't being treated with the utmost respect *it's real to them* and should be investigated.

If you do have a formal meeting with the nursing home staff, don't allow them to bully you or the patient; bring a witness with you or openly record the meeting. Consult the ombudsman or the state licensing bureau if you believe that the patient's rights are being violated – you even have the right to consult an attorney if you wish (although it rarely escalates to this point). Feel free to move your family member to another nursing home if the nursing home won't work with you.

Responsible Parties

At the time of admission, the nursing home staff members will probably decide who it is that they will consider to be the responsible party, and this might forever be the person to whom they will send the bills. The nursing home staff will also decide to whom they'll release information, with whom they will speak, and who they will allow to make decisions on the patient's behalf. The nursing home is legally required to honor powers of attorney, and can't arbitrarily decide who's responsible or to which family member they'll speak. If you or your family members are having difficulty dealing with a nursing home, a quick call to the ombudsman or your attorney might be warranted.

Patients have the right to name someone as their power of attorney (see the section on *Powers of Attorney* in the chapter on **Advanced Directives**). This doesn't mean that the power of attorney is the responsible party – only that the power of attorney is able to make decisions when a patient isn't able to do so. If a patient is no longer able to complete the forms, each state has laws in place that designate which family member is able to make decisions on his behalf. The nursing home can't arbitrarily designate a family member for this purpose, nor can Family members have the right to make decisions when patients are no longer able, and the nursing home can't pick & choose which decisions they'll honor.

I worked in a facility where an overzealous nursing home administrator informed a dying patient's family that they weren't allowed to make end-of-life decisions because she hadn't completed a power of attorney. Even though there were multiple family members who agreed that they didn't want to put the patient through more procedures, the administrator told them that they had no right to make choices on the patient's behalf because they weren't listed as the patient's responsible party. Had the family contacted an attorney or the ombudsman, they would have found that they had the legal right to make a decision to withhold treatment for the patient. Instead, the patient was sent to a sister facility to have the feeding tube inserted, then returned to the nursing home where Medicare paid handsomely until her death about a month later. This was extremely distressing to the family, but the corporation made tens of thousands of dollars in profit as a result of a decision made by the administrator.

Since the person designated as a patient's responsible party will be held accountable for his bills, it's always best to have the patient sign his own admission packet and let him accept full financial responsibility for his own care. If he's not able to do so, sign the forms "*John Doe* by *Mary Doe*, or *Mary Doe* for *John Doe*," and at the bottom of the form write "*I am not personally financially responsible for this bill*," and sign your name to *that*. If at all possible, the face sheet should list the patient as his own responsible party – but that doesn't mean that family members aren't able to make decisions when patients lack the capacity to do so themselves.

Patient Personal Items

Patients are able to bring personal items into the nursing home; as mentioned in the section *Admissions Day*, any items that are brought into the facility should be marked with the patient's name. This applies to everything from dentures to refrigerators.

Some nursing homes offer refrigerators in patient's rooms; if not, ask the admissions coordinator if you can bring one in so that the patient will have refreshments in his room. If you buy one, make sure it's an actual refrigerator that can keep food at the proper temperature (33-38 degrees, or in accordance with the state regulations). Many of the small personal refrigerators that are sold in department stores are actually coolers that keep food at about 20 degrees below the ambient room temperature; these are not acceptable according to food safety standards. They're represented to be refrigerators, which can be confusing, but the way to identify a true refrigerator is that most refrigerators have freezers, even if they're tiny, and the compressor takes up quite a bit of room (the fridge compartment is smaller due to the size of the compressor). Nursing homes are required to follow certain state and federal regulations regarding refrigeration of food, and these regulations are not negotiable. The nursing home will probably place a thermometer in the patient's fridge in order for the staff to monitor the room temperature, and if the refrigerator fails it will either need to be repaired or replaced.

It's important that you make sure that every item that's been brought in has been logged into the nursing home computer system or on the inventory sheet. Ask for a copy – and any items that are brought in after the patient has been admitted should be added to the inventory. If the item comes up missing, ask for it to be replaced. If the nursing home refuses, speak with the administrator or parent corporation. If necessary, speak with the ombudsman or consult an attorney.

Expensive items shouldn't be left in nursing homes without the ability to lock them up. Laptop computers come with locks, and the keys can be kept on the patient's person or they can be secured with a combination lock. Patients should be given a key to a locking drawer or they should be able to bring a file cabinet where they can keep personal items. Items should be locked up whenever the patient leaves the room, whether it's for supper or to complete rehabilitation. It's vital to keep cell phones on the patient's person or locked in the patient's room.

Remember that patients who are medically fragile might require immediate medical help – if the staff is performing CPR, they will throw everything out of the way to get to the patient. While they might be responsible to replace a stolen laptop, it's doubtful that a judge would hold a nursing home responsible for an item broken when the staff was administering emergency treatments. Try not to have expensive items sitting around so this will become an issue – or buy replacement insurance. It's worth it.

Physicians and Medical Care

Every patient who is admitted into a nursing home must have a physician who directs his overall care. This is the doctor that the nursing home will call for orders about the patient's general care at any time, day or night. Additionally, the patient might also have one or more specialists who are following a specific condition, such as an orthopedist who follows a broken hip or a nephrologist for kidney issues. It's truly in the patient's best interest to have a general practitioner following his care to ensure that there are not duplicate medications and that that serious conditions aren't left untreated.

Depending upon the patient's healthcare condition, he might need to see his doctor as often as every month. Due to the fact that many physicians don't make nursing home visits, patients often must be transported to their doctor's for appointments. It is the nursing home's responsibility to ensure that patients make it to their appointments, whether they provide the transportation themselves or set it up with a medical transport company. As long as the patient is in agreement, family members are welcome to attend these visits. There are also doctors who visit their nursing home patients, although they usually work these visits around their regular office hours. This makes it difficult for the family to meet with a physician at the nursing home.

There are several different methods by which the physician who will follow the patient might be assigned:

- The nursing home will assign one from a rotating list, or
- The nursing home will assign its Medical Director, or
- A doctor was assigned at the hospital (before the patient discharged), or
- The specialist who performed a surgery follows the patient and there is no general practitioner, or
- The patient's primary physician at home agrees to continue treating him while he's in the nursing home, or
- The family chooses a doctor, or
- If the patient is on hospice, the hospice medical director can take over the patient's care.

Regardless of whether or not the doctor visits the nursing home, most of the time communication between the nurses and physicians occur over the phone. The nurses will call the physician and report what they see, then ask for treatment or medication. It's up to the doctor as to whether he will prescribe the requested medication or treatment. The doctor is responsible for the patient's physical care and it's up to him as to the treatments he prescribes. However, he will only know what the nurse tells him; if the nurse doesn't provide sufficient information, the patients can suffer.

There is no great computer in the sky that holds every patient's information, and facilities only know what they've been told. If the nursing home patient was admitted directly from the hospital, it's important to understand that the medical history contained in the nursing home's medical chart will be the one that was provided by the hospital. If the treating physicians in the hospital weren't aware of any previous healthcare issues, these conditions might continue to go untreated in the nursing home. There can be huge gaps in the historical information available, and a serious condition that's been successfully treated for years might go untreated at the hospital and nursing home. This is an excellent reason as to why a doctor who already knows the patient might be the best option for his care in the nursing home. For example, a patient who has lupus might be sent to the hospital and treated for complications from an auto accident; her lupus might be left untreated until she is able to verbalize her needs to the staff. The pain medication that is normally prescribed for broken bones will be tapered off, while the pain from her underlying condition (lupus) will continue until the patient or a family member provides information about the patient's medical history.

Some nursing homes will insist on assigning the patient's doctor, rather than to allow for the patient to be sent out to his preferred doctor. There could be many reasons that they would do so, but the most likely is that this physician physically visits the nursing home and cooperates with most of the facility's requests. The problem with this can be that the facility's doctor might disagree with the patient's normal regimen and completely change the medications that have been working for years. It could take months to get the patient back to his baseline after such a drastic change has been made, during which he could remain in pain or severe distress.

Patients have the right to choose their doctor, as long as the doctor will accept the responsibility of treating him in the nursing home. The patient's chosen physician doesn't have to visit the facility – he just has to be willing to direct the patient's medical care and see the patient in his office. As long as the nursing home staff remains respectful of the doctor's time and limits their calls to office hours (unless there's an emergency), many physicians are willing to follow their own patients when they're admitted to nursing homes.

Many nursing homes use electronic medical records, but it's possible that the nursing home's electronic system and the hospital's system aren't compatible. In this case, the hospital will need to print the patient's records and send them to the nursing home to ensure that the patient has continuity in his care. The primary doctor's system – as well as the records system of all of the specialists he's seen – might not be compatible and will also need to be printed off for the nursing home. This doesn't always happen; important medical records aren't always available and the treating physician isn't able to develop a clear picture of the patient's physical status. Patients who appear healthy but have a painful underlying condition might not receive their medication, causing an exacerbation of their disease process.

The doctor's care is only as good as the nurses who are calling for orders; the doctor relies on the nurses to provide all of the information that he needs in order to make appropriate medical decisions. He trusts that the nurse has checked the patient's chart to ensure that the patient doesn't have allergies or adverse reactions to the requested medications. It's possible that the pharmacy might catch an error (as long as the information is listed on the patient's face sheet), but often this information wasn't available at the time that the intake forms were completed. In most cases, the doctor doesn't have a copy of the patient's chart in his office (or wherever he is when the nursing home calls him) and it's vital that the nurses provide accurate information.

It's important that family members ask questions and demand accountability for patients, because the doctor directs every aspect of the patient's care *with the assistance of the nursing home staff*. The patients are at the mercy of the nurses; if their assessment is that the patient isn't in pain, the doctor won't increase the patient's pain medication. I've worked in several nursing homes where patients were moaning in pain and the nurses ignored their pleas for medication; there is absolutely no reason why this should occur, but it does. Nurses might equate the pain that they feel with that of the patient, and everyone is different. I've been present when nurses tell physicians that they believe that a patient might be "addicted" to pain medications, even though the patient was diagnosed with an extremely painful condition. I've also seen patients who are prescribed strong pain medications because the nurse believed that the patient's pain was much greater than it actually was. If the doctor is prescribing medications based on one nurse's opinion, patients can easily be over or under medicated.

Many nursing homes don't appreciate it when family members ask questions, and might view their actions as interference. The nursing home staff might prefer that the family stay out of the medical care part of the patient's business in the nursing home. However, family members know patients better than the nursing home staff who just met them; this is precisely why family members should remain involved. If your family member complains of pain or if other symptoms don't appear to be resolving, feel free to speak with the doctor and the director of nursing. It's difficult for patients to recover when they're uncomfortable.

The nursing home must adhere to certain state and federal laws regarding the frequency of physician visits; often the patient must be seen by a doctor within 24-72 hours to dictate a history & physical and complete an initial assessment, and then he must be seen once every 30-60 days thereafter (this includes hospice patients). As mentioned before, some physicians make nursing home visits while others require their patients be transported to their office. If the physician who is treating the patient in the nursing home isn't his the doctor who treats him at home, ask his primary physician to follow up with the nursing home. It's important that there be continuity of care between the patient's primary physician and the treating physician in the nursing home. Make sure that you alert the nursing home as to any appointments that you make on behalf of the patient, and don't be surprised if the nursing home asks that the appointment be delayed until after the patient is discharged. Depending upon whether Medicare is paying for the patient's stay, the facility might be responsible to pay for any physician visits related to the patient's primary diagnosis.

If the patient (or his family) doesn't like the physician that the nursing home assigns, he has the right to choose another doctor. All that must be done is to find another doctor who is willing to treat him, and to have the nursing home make an appointment with that physician. Make sure that the physician's name is added to the patient's chart and that he is listed on all of his paperwork. It's best if you call the current doctor's office to advise him that you'll no longer require his assistance. Speak with the nursing home administrator if the staff won't coordinate with the doctor of your choosing; he will probably need to be "credentialed" in order to write orders for the nursing home. Again, if the nursing home steers most of the patients to certain doctors, they might have a problem with a patient choosing his own physician. If the nursing home refuses to coordinate with your family member's primary physician and they won't resolve it with you, feel free to call the state licensing agency to complain.

Patients have the right to seek the services of a specialist if they choose. The only exception to this rule is that the patient might be responsible for a specialist's bill if the patient is receiving services under the Medicare Part A benefit (either rehabilitation or hospice services) and the appointment isn't preauthorized. It's best to check with the nursing home billing office or charge nurse before you make an appointment with another doctor if the patient is receiving Part A skilled services.

Depending upon the nursing home's operating policies, patients who are prescribed certain medications might receive a consultation from a psychiatrist. While it might be helpful to have a psychiatrist review the patient's psychotropic medications, it's also possible that he will change a drug regimen that has worked for years. The patient and his family have the right to refuse medication changes; if this happens to your family member, don't sign or allow the patient to sign the consent form until you speak with the psychiatrist or primary doctor. Remember that this doctor has a large amount of patients to see in an extremely limited amount of time, and that he receives all of his information from the facility staff – in most cases, the psychiatrist will spend less than 10 minutes with each patient. The patient might be responsible for co-payments and deductibles, even if he didn't want the psychiatrist's intervention.

Most nursing homes have agreements with podiatrists, who schedule a monthly visit to the facility. There's usually a list at the nursing station, and all that the patient or family must do is ask to be added at the next available podiatrist visit. Just as with other physician visits, there will be copayments or deductibles. It's possible that these fees can be paid out of the patient's trust account, or that the doctor will send a bill for these amounts.

Some nursing homes also have agreements with dentists who visit their patients, so that patients can receive necessary dental care. Most health insurance policies don't cover dental care, so these fees will need to be paid out of pocket. In many states, Medicaid doesn't cover dental care, although patients who are dual eligible (have both Medicaid & Medicare) and sign up with an HMO often have dental coverage.

Each nursing home has policies as to how often a patient must be seen by a doctor, and for the most part these policies must be followed. However, patients have the right to participate in the development of their treatment plan. They have the right to request changes of medications and to be seen by a specialist if their needs aren't being met. Most nursing homes are willing to accommodate such requests – but if not, patients have the right to discuss their concerns with the state licensing agency. Remember that as the patient's representative you, not the nursing home, are in control of his medical care. Don't allow the nursing home to bully you into accepting treatments that the patient doesn't want (or need) in order to increase their profits.

Transportation to/from Appointments

In most cases, the nursing home is required to ensure that its patients have transportation to medical appointments. Depending upon the area in which the nursing home is located, Medicaid might pay for its patients transportation, or the patient/family might be asked to assist with transportation. Some Medicare Part C Advantage plans also provide transportation to doctor's appointments. Regardless of the patient's payment source, it is ultimately the responsibility of the nursing home to ensure that the patients make it to their medical appointments.

Most nursing homes offer a van for patients to be transported to physician appointments; if so, they must provide this service to all of their residents. It can be viewed as discrimination if they only provide transportation for certain residents – such as Medicare patients – unless there is a specific reason that the patient can't be safely transported in the facility van.

It is the nursing home's responsibility to ensure that the patient is seen by a physician according to state & federal regulations. It's best to coordinate all appointments with the nursing home to ensure that they are able to arrange for the transportation. The transportation department can be very busy, and it's possible that they will ask that non-emergent appointments be made once the patient returns home. The nursing home might attempt to refuse to transport a patient by saying that they provide transportation as a courtesy, but the bottom line is that they assume responsibility for the patient's medical care when he is admitted and are required to get him to/from necessary appointments.

Medication/Pharmacy Issues

As mentioned before, most nursing homes don't have a pharmacy on the premises. The medications are prescribed by the doctor (usually over the telephone); the nurse records the order and faxes it to the pharmacy. The pharmacy delivers the medications on a schedule, generally twice a day. The nursing home must have a documented physician's order for every medication, even if the patient has a prescription for the medication at his home. In most cases, the doctor will prescribe a requested medication for the patient to use in the nursing home as long as the request is reasonable (the doctor might not have known that the patient has been using a specific medication if he just met the patient). He might also refuse to prescribe a medication – if this is the case, it might be necessary to call the doctor to discuss this issue. The doctor assigned by the nursing home is under no obligation to follow the treatment plan that the patient followed at home under the direction of his primary doctor. If the physician assigned by the nursing home won't work with you, find one who will.

In most cases, nursing homes will require that medications are provided them in *bubble-pack* form (also known as *blister-packs*). The pharmacist places the separate pills on a card that has individual compartments, where they can be easily counted. All medications are tracked and accounted for, and bubble-packing makes it easier to do so. If the patient's medications are provided by outside pharmacies – as in the case with the VA or part D plans that provide medications in 3-month supplies – the medications are sent to the commercial pharmacy that serves the nursing home, where they're bubble-packed for a few dollars. The nursing home must pay the cost of the bubble-packing if the patient's room & board is paid by Medicaid; otherwise the patient will have to pay for the bubble-packing out-of-pocket.

Controlled substances (medications) such as pain medications often require an original signed prescription from the physician. This can be difficult for the nursing home, as the general procedure is to call the doctor and record the prescription as a *Telephone Order* (also known as a *T/O*). The pharmacy might have an agreement with the nursing home to send a few days' worth of medications until a signed prescription can be sent over – but if not, the patient might remain in distress until the procedure can be followed.

Depending upon the applicable state and local laws, some nursing homes have emergency medications on-hand in an *e-kit* (also known as an emergency kit). The nursing home doesn't have the ability to administer those medications to just any patient, in every case the patient must have an order (prescription) for the specific medication before the kit can be opened. This allows the patient to start his medications without delay and gives the pharmacy enough time to deliver a full prescription amount at the next scheduled delivery time. An e-kit holds a minimal amount of medications which are closely monitored by the pharmacy and director of nursing.

It is possible for the nursing home to have medications delivered at times other than during the pharmacy's scheduled delivery; generally there must be an emergent need such as the patient being in pain or an antibiotic that must be started immediately. The medications might be delivered by a runner from the pharmacy, or they might be picked up by a worker from the nursing home. This does allow for some flexibility – but this type of service isn't provided everywhere.

Most commercial pharmacies aren't open 24-hours, so if the doctor prescribes a new medication at 2:00am the patient won't receive it until the pharmacy opens in the morning, or possibly even later in the day due to the time it will take for the pharmacy to process the medication. For medications such as antibiotics, such a delay can be painful or even life-threatening.

Every medication administered in a nursing home, including those that are available over-the-counter, must be prescribed by a physician. This applies to vitamins and other supplements – for each medication the nursing home will call the doctor and request an order. It's possible that the family can bring over-the-counter medications into the facility in order to save money, rather than to allow the nursing home to order them at a substantial mark-up. If the doctor orders medications that the patient doesn't want, he has the right to ask for a medication change or to refuse to take certain medications altogether. All the nursing home must do is call the doctor and obtain a change order, then fax it to the pharmacy to be filled that day (unless the family brings them in). Many physicians return their calls in the late afternoon; if the requested change isn't requested "stat" by the nurses, the medications won't be available until the following morning or possibly even the next afternoon.

The doctor must prescribe all medication changes, such as an increase or decrease in dosage or the frequency that the medications are taken. Patients who are in pain have the right to ask for a higher dose, or to take the medications more often. If the nursing home doesn't call the doctor quickly enough, the patient and/or family have the right to call themselves and ask for a medication change.

Although it might make the nurse angry when the family calls the doctor themselves, sometimes it's the best way to get their attention (and for the patient to receive the medication). It really doesn't matter what if the nurse is angry as long as the patient receives his medications and his needs are met.

Method of Ordering Medications in a Nursing Home

- The patient presents a need (either by request or symptoms)

- The nurse calls the doctor's office, requesting to speak with the doctor. He is busy and will call her back.

- The doctor returns the call (hopefully) within a couple of hours, and gives a verbal order for the medication.

- The nurse documents the doctor's order, then faxes it to the pharmacy to be provided on the next medication run

- The medication is received by the nursing home 8-12 hours later

- The nurse must then log the medication in, and provide it to the patient. If she is busy, this could take another couple of hours

- If the medication is a controlled substance, the process can take longer because of the need for a signed prescription; a runner might be sent to the doctor's office or it's possible that they will send a 3-day supply; enough to get the patient started while the signed original prescription is being delivered to the pharmacy.

Nursing homes must follow strict rules regarding medications; if the doctor orders a medication be *PRN* (as needed), the patient will usually have to ask for the medication when he needs it. Because there are nurses who don't believe that patients are in pain, they might refuse to give the patient pain medications even when asked. It's unfortunate that this occurs, but if it does happen to your family member speak with the director of nursing, administrator, or the doctor. If the issue isn't resolved, call the ombudsman or state regulatory agency. Move to another nursing home if necessary. I've witnessed nurses who refuse to call the doctor because, in their opinion, the patient shouldn't be feeling as much pain as they claim to be. Since everyone is different, medications work differently and it's impossible to compare one patient's pain to that of another patient.

Medications that are ordered PRN don't always work in nursing homes, because in most cases the patient must be able to ask for them. Those patients who aren't physically able to ask for PRN medications are at the mercy of the nurses; hopefully the nurses can adequately assess whether the patient needs the medication, but if not the patient's pain might not be managed very well. Patients aren't always monitored closely; a bedbound patient might not see a staff member for several hours and if they aren't able to ring their call light, they can remain in pain for hours. To ensure that the patient's pain or anxiety doesn't get out of hand, ask the physician for the medications to be administered according to a schedule (such as every four hours). If the medications aren't given as prescribed, meet with the administrator to address your concerns.

Another problem with PRN medications is that nursing homes are often required to discontinue and destroy them if the patient doesn't take them for awhile, generally within 30 days. This can be a problem with medications such as those for anxiety, a condition that comes and goes. It's possible that the patient won't require the medication for weeks or months, yet after 30 days their pills are dutifully destroyed and the prescription is discontinued. When the patient feels a panic attack coming on, he'll have to wait until the doctor calls back with an order and the pharmacy arrives with its regularly scheduled delivery. The patient might endure eight or more hours of hell before he receives the medications, during which time the situation can become critical and the patient might be sent to the ER to be treated. The way to ensure that this doesn't happen is to have the patient ask for an anti-anxiety pill every week, needed or not. The facility is just following federal law, but the laws aren't compassionate when it comes to patient care.

The same rule applies to all PRN medications, including those prescribed for pain; if they're not used on a regular basis CMS requires that they be discontinued. The only way around this is for the patient to request the medications once a week or so. It's unfortunate that the patient has to manipulate the system in this manner, but the nursing home is required to follow federal regulations.

Pain medications can be tricky; if the patient has been prescribed pain medication and the nurse doesn't believe that the patient is in pain, he/she isn't legally allowed to give the medication. There are many nurses who believe that they understand their patients' pain better than the patients do and will refuse to administer the medications because they don't think that the patient is experiencing "enough" pain. Having medications administered according to a schedule can cut down on this problem – although as mentioned before, nurses can still refuse to give the medications. If this happens to you or your family member, ask to meet with the doctor or nursing home administrator.

Many nurses are conservative with medications and will assume patients are exaggerating their pain levels in order to get more medications (aka ***drug seeking***). The problem is that nurses often base their assessment on their own life experiences and not on the patient's claims of pain or discomfort. Everyone reacts differently to pain; some patient's pain can be alleviated with lesser medications while others require morphine for the same problem. I've known many nurses who don't understand disease processes and accuse patients of attempting to get a "buzz" from their medications rather than to give them as ordered. I've even seen them go so far as to call the doctor and request a change of medications because they don't believe that the patient is in pain. The doctor might discontinue the medications based on the nurse's report.

If any of these events happen to you or your family member, call the doctor immediately and also feel free to report this to the state agency that regulates nursing homes. The trend in medicine is to believe the patient and to treat the pain; there should be no exceptions to this rule but each nurse is different. It's inhumane to allow a patient to remain in pain because the nurse doesn't think that the pain is bad enough to warrant taking medication.

The nursing home is required to *attempt* to give all medications as ordered. Patients have the right to refuse to take a single dose or can refuse to take the medications at all. Families have the right to give their input, and can refuse to provide consent for medications if they're the power of attorney and/or the patient can't make his needs known. The nurse will make a note that the patient has refused, and if this continues the patient might be sent to the doctor to ensure that the patient is aware how refusing the medications might jeopardize his care. The nursing home might require a care conference, but ultimately the patient has the right to choose.

> I worked for a nursing home where it was reported to me that, after a patient refused to take her medications, a nurse crushed the patient's medications and drew them into a syringe; she then forced the syringe into the patient's mouth. I was told that the patient attempted to fight off the nurse, but she wouldn't allow it.
>
> The nurse then held the patient's nose until she swallowed the medications. The patient was a very high risk for aspiration (inhaling the medications into the lungs which can lead to the patient's death). When I reported the situation to the administrator, the nurse was fired but was never reported to her licensing board.
>
> The administrator told me that if I wanted to report it myself, I was welcome to do so. However, I wasn't present when the incident occurred and the proof was held by the administrator – so I wasn't able to report the incident. The nurse is still practicing three years later. The appropriate action would have been for the director of nursing and administrator to file a formal report of the incident to the Board of Nursing.

Patients also have the right to refuse treatments if they wish. The best that the nursing home can do is to explain the risks and benefits of their choices and to document the interaction. If your family member refuses to take his medications, it's possible that he'll agree if someone explains to him how the medications will benefit him. In most cases, the physician and/or nursing home can't force the patient to take medications against his will. There have been court battles over mentally ill people who refuse to take their medications; if they took their meds they might possibly be stable enough to stand going to trial for their actions, yet the courts are rarely able to force the medications upon them. Forcing medications or treatments upon a person is considered to be a form of physical assault.

Sometimes a nursing home will claim that a patient is a danger to himself or others when he refuses to take his medications, and attempt to send a patient to a psychiatric unit. Refusing to take a specific medication doesn't mean that a patient is crazy and requires hospitalization unless he is acting out inappropriately or attempting to harm the staff. If the nursing home calls to tell you they are sending your family member to a psychiatric unit and you don't believe that the admission is appropriate, you have the right to refuse to allow the patient to be sent and to ask for additional information. Unless the patient is truly a danger to himself or to other residents, they must honor your wishes.

If a patient complains about being in pain even though the staff is reporting that he is receiving his medications as ordered, it's possible that he might not be receiving his pain medications at all. There have been many cases of staff members who steal patient medications and there are multiple methods that this can be accomplished. In most cases, medications are usually stolen from the most vulnerable patients, such as those who are confused or unable to speak. The general method of medication distribution is for the nurses to dispense the medications into cups, and then give the pills to the patient. It's possible for the nurse to remove some of them from the cup before the patient takes them, or to write in the medical record that the patient refused the medications. Then, instead of destroying them, the nurse can take whichever medication she wants. All the while, the patient remains in pain or distress and it's possible that no one will notice. If your family member appears to be in pain or his symptoms haven't improved, speak with the director of nursing or his doctor.

Pills aren't the only types of medications that can be stolen, pain patches are easy for a staff member to steal and the only way it's known is if the patient is able to communicate that his pain isn't relieved. **Transdermal Patches** dispense the medications directly through the patient's skin and are usually changed every 72 hours. They can easily be removed while they still contain medication and replaced with older patches that contain no medication. The standard of care is to write the date & time the patches were placed on the patient with a permanent marker, but it's possible to erase the writing or replace the patch with one that has expired. Almost any staff member from the housekeeper to the administrator can remove a pain patch; a quick Google search turns up thousands of incidents of stolen pain patches. Even though they're extremely effective in providing long-acting pain medication, many nursing homes limit the use of patches because they are so difficult to monitor.

One indicator of medication abuse is when a patient claims that he's not receiving his medications or appears to be in constant pain, yet the nursing home records reflect that he is receiving every dose. If speaking with the administrator isn't helpful, you can call the ombudsman or state licensing agency and file a complaint. You are also free to call the police and file a complaint, although this can be distressing for the patient (probably not as distressing as going without medications). Be careful about discussing this with the floor nurses or other staff members; much of the time the nursing home staff members will do their best to protect each other and might be covering for each other. Even if they're not stolen for self-administration, pain patches and other medications can easily be sold for profit.

Cutting Down on Medication Costs

For those patients who are receiving services under the Medicare Part A benefit, all of their medications and treatments are provided by the nursing home. The nursing home receives a daily rate out of which they must pay for all of the services the patient receives. It's common for a nursing home to accept a patient with full knowledge of his medication regimen, and then immediately ask the doctor to change his medications to something less expensive. While the nursing home has the right to ask for a less expensive equivalent, it might not always be in the patient's best interest to change to a different medication. This is a gray area, ethically speaking. If asked, the nursing home will deny responsibility, saying that the doctor changed the medications when in fact it's the nursing home that requested the change. The nursing home should not dictate the care that the senior is receiving, but this happens more often than one would imagine.

An example of cost-saving measures nursing homes might attempt is when patients are prescribed chemotherapy drugs used to treat cancer. Most skilled nursing facilities won't accept patients receiving these expensive medications, because they can cost over $1,000 per day. If the patient is accepted, as soon as he has been admitted the nursing home administrator or another staff member might ask the physician to change his medication to something substantially cheaper. They might even ask the doctor to delay his treatment until he is discharged home from the facility. For the patient who remains in the nursing home for the 100 day maximum, such a delay in treatment might hasten the patient's death. Patients and family members have the right to refuse changes in medications, and the nursing home is obligated to provide the medications as the doctor originally ordered. The nursing home can't discharge the patient because they're not making the profit that they hoped to. Medical decisions should be between the physician and the patient, not the nursing home administrator and his/her budget.

I was present at a meeting when the administrator attempted to force a family member into agreeing to change a patient's medication regimen; the family refused and the administrator became angry. She threatened to discharge the patient to the hospital and also threatened to call the ombudsman; the family insisted that the patient receive the medications as ordered. The patient remained in the nursing home for 2 months, and the nursing home lost tens of thousands of dollars on his care. The facility never should have accepted the patient in the first place if they hadn't intended to provide the medications as prescribed. An issue such as this can make it more difficult for a nursing home to be located in the first place, but once a nursing home has accepted him they're responsible to administer his chemotherapy in accordance with the treatment plan developed upon admission.

Once the patient is no longer eligible to receive skilled services under Medicare Part A, the patient and/or family are responsible for paying for the medications. The pharmacy will bill the patient's Medicare Part D benefit, but this can still result in thousand of dollars in copayments and deductibles. This can be extremely expensive for patients who don't qualify for Medicaid and are paying privately, but there are ways to cut back on the patient's out-of-pocket costs.

As long as the patient is receiving services under the Medicare Part A skilled nursing benefit, the nursing home will order 1-2 weeks worth of medications at a time. This is because the nursing home is responsible to pay for the medications and therefore will do its best to hold down costs. Once the patient is no longer receiving services via Medicare, medications are normally ordered in 30-day increments because most pharmacy benefits will pay for a one-month supply.

Just because it's the usual way for things to be done, medications don't have to be ordered in 30-day increments. It's possible for the family to request that all new medications be ordered in one-week increments until it can be seen how they affect the patient. That way, if the patient isn't able to use all of them he or his insurance saves 75% of the normal cost of a month's prescription. If every nursing home did this with new medications, it would save the Medicare Part D program (and the patients) millions of dollars each year. The pharmacy will have to fill the prescriptions more often, but since they deliver to the nursing home twice a day it's not an inconvenience to them (although it would significantly decrease their profits to provide the 30-day supply). Other than the pharmacy having to work a little harder, there is very little downside to ordering new medications on a weekly trial basis. Remember that the nursing home is required to destroy unused medications; you would be amazed at the thousands of dollars of medications that are destroyed by nursing homes every day.

Prescription plans don't pay 100% of pharmacy charges, so the potential cost to the patient/family can be thousands of dollars *each month*. The doctor generally orders medications without considering the cost to the patient, and the pharmacy is required to fill that prescription exactly as written. Every medication doesn't necessarily have a generic equivalent, and even generics can cost hundreds of dollars. New, expensive medications are introduced onto the market every day, and pharmaceutical representatives push their medications as the latest & greatest treatment for all sorts of conditions. Doctors have to try these medications on *someone*, and it could be your family member – but you don't have to accept this. A doctor serving a patient in a nursing home might not realize that the medication is not affordable to the patient; if he were to be told that the option is either not to take the medication or to take a less expensive equivalent he might change his order.

It would significantly hold down costs if family members were to insist that the nursing home contact the patient or family for approval of every change of medications. If the patient and/or family don't believe that a change is necessary, they don't have to allow it. Nursing homes often don't like to do this, because it takes extra time to educate the family as to the need for the medication, and the family might refuse (causing more work for the nursing home). However, this simple request can save the patient/family thousands of dollars each year.

There are drug company assistance plans that might be able to help provide medications for a patient; a quick search of the specific medication on the internet might turn up a program that can help a senior in a nursing home afford his medications. This step isn't necessary for patients who are receiving services via Medicaid or the VA – but if they're paying out of pocket, the cost of medications most certainly can deplete the patient's finances.

Medicare Part D plans don't cover all types of medications; if the patient is paying privately for his room & board his potential cost for certain psychotropics (such as antidepressants, antipsychotics, and anti-anxiety medications) can be prohibitive. Considering that it could take six or more weeks before a psychotropic takes effect, the potential cost to the patient could be thousands of dollars for a medication that might not even work. This can be particularly distressing, considering that the patient/family might not have even wanted a medication change in the first place. Ask that the doctor prescribe a common medication that has a generic equivalent, rather than the latest, greatest medication. If he won't do so, ask if he can provide samples until the medications are working. Then, ask if there is assistance through the corporation that makes the medications.

Every nursing home uses a contracted pharmacy, and normally the cost to the patients for their medications is quite high. This is true especially if the commercial pharmacy that the nursing home uses doesn't work with the patient's Part D plan. However, every Part D plan has a mail-order pharmacy that can send medications in 90-day increments, with a discounted co-payment. It's possible to ask that the nursing home order 90 days worth of medications from a mail-order pharmacy at a deep discount, and have them mailed to the nursing home. In most cases, the nursing home then sends the medication to their contracted pharmacy to be specially packaged in bubble-packs for less than $10 per prescription. This can be substantially cheaper than buying the medications through the nursing home's pharmacy.

If the patient is eligible for the VA to pay for his medications and there is a clinic nearby where the patient can be seen, it's worth the time and trouble to get the patient registered with the VA and to have his medications sent to the nursing home. The co-payment is negligible and the patient is benefitting from a program set up to help veterans such as him. When the medications arrive at the nursing home they will dispense them to the patient as-is, or send them to the pharmacy to have them bubble-packed. It's possible that the VA will mail the medications to the patient's house; if the VA sends your family member's medications to his home, bring them into the nursing home as soon as possible. It's between you and the nursing home as to whether you should bring in a month's supply at a time or all 90-days worth at once. Some facilities prefer that the package not be opened and brought into the nursing home as soon as it is received.

The rules are different for Medicaid recipients; neither the pharmacy nor the nursing home can legally bill the patient for non-covered items. The pharmacy closely monitors the medications to ensure that they don't lose money by ordering non-covered items, and by waiting to refill the medications until they'll be approved. In most cases, medications are filled in 30-day increments and if the nursing home attempts to order the prescriptions before the 30 days are up, the pharmacy will send a notice of non-coverage to the nursing home.

Patients who are receiving assistance from hospice programs are able to save the cost of medications that are related to the patient's terminal diagnosis because the hospice is required to pay for these medications. Patients are also able to save the cost of medical supplies; cost saving is but one benefit of choosing hospice for the terminal patient who is paying privately for his nursing home placement. The medications that the hospice covers can be a "gray" area, so it's best to ask if the hospice can cover a medication before paying out of pocket. The hospice often "manages" the medications whether or not they are covered and can help to get them ordered or discontinued. Some medications that are considered to be long-term such as statins to reduce cholesterol, or dementia medications such as Aricept & Namenda, aren't going to help a patient whose life expectancy is cut short by a terminal disease. Whether or not the patient is paying for his medications out-of-pocket, he or his family should ask to discuss this with the hospice case manager or physician. If a medication isn't going to help a patient, he has the right to ask that it be discontinued.

Call Lights

Each patient bed has access to a call light system in order to summon staff members to their rooms, and on the day of admission the patient and family will be oriented as to how that particular nursing home's system works. There is usually a button next to the patient's bed, and another in the bathroom that summons assistance when the patient presses the button. Most call light systems have lights outside the patient's room that can be seen down the hallway (from the nursing station), and are also connected directly to the nursing station where they will eventually set off a buzzer or high-pitched noise if not answered immediately. This is why a room near the nursing station might not be the best choice; multiple call light buzzers can disturb patients in the rooms nearby at all hours of the day and night.

There are many different types of call light systems; some have intercoms that allow the nurses to answer through a speaker from the nursing station, while others have pager systems that track the amount of time the call light has been on without being answered. Generally speaking, call lights should be answered within 5-10 minutes, with anything beyond that considered excessive. Workers are able to manipulate this system by walking into the room, deactivating the call light and returning much later to actually assist the patient (or never returning at all). While meeting the technical definition of being answered, the patient doesn't receive the assistance he requires. Sometimes the patient must hit his call light multiple times before being assisted, which can be distressing when he needs to use the bathroom and isn't physically able to get there on his own. Lack of prompt toileting can lead to chronic constipation, rashes or even decubitus ulcers (aka bedsores).

Regulations require that call lights be accessible to the patients at all times when they're in their room, whether or not they're mentally or physically able to ring the alarm. There are special pads with light-touch sensors for those patients who aren't physically able to press a call light button; every nursing home is required to accommodate for the needs of such patients.

If your family member has been in the nursing home for awhile and he tells you that the staff never comes when he rings his call light, it's best to meet with the nursing director or administrator to discuss this issue. They might be able to print a log if the nursing home is equipped with such a call light system, or you can ask them to have a staff member do spot checks. It's also permissible for family members to monitor the call lights themselves by visiting the patient and ringing the call light, then documenting how long it takes for staff to respond. If the staff consistently takes an excessive amount of time answering the lights and administration isn't interested in taking action, you have the right to call the ombudsman or other state agency to discuss this issue.

The biggest problem with call lights is that often there aren't enough nursing assistants to assist the patients; those nursing homes that are staffed with the absolute minimum requirements often have one C.N.A. to a hallway filled with 20 patients. Nurses often sit at the station while their C.N.A.'s are going crazy answering call lights, when all that some of the patients wanted was a drink of water or something that would have been simple to obtain. The aides are the lowest paid of the patient-care staff, yet they do all of the physical work. Nursing home corporations are often willing to put profits ahead of patient care; it's difficult to comprehend why they would rather pay a fine to CMS for substandard care than to hire a couple of more staff members per shift.

Don't allow the nursing home to make excuses as to why they're not answering the call light for your family member; this is a focus for the Centers for Medicare and Medicaid Services (CMS) due to the problems that can occur as a result of their not being answered in a timely manner. Speak with the supervisor, the director of nursing, administrator or call the state regulatory agency if the call lights aren't answered and patients' needs aren't being addressed within 10 minutes.

Cameras/Recording Devices

Taking photographs of your family member with their favorite staff member is allowed, but you may not take photos of other residents without their permission. This is a confidentiality issue, and these same rules apply to other people taking photos of your family member. There are often activities where pictures are taken to be later placed in scrapbooks, but the resident doesn't have to allow his photograph to be taken if he doesn't want to. If the local news station comes to the nursing home and airs a human interest story on a particular event, the release that was signed at the time of admission allows your family member to be filmed for this purpose. Carefully read the information that you are signing on your family member's behalf, and consider his feelings about being filmed or photographed.

Some people bring personal recording devices into nursing homes, so that the patient can tape staff members if they are concerned that the patient is being abused (these recorders can be hidden inside a stuffed animal or artificial flowers, etc). This is okay as long as the patient gives permission to be taped; there are cameras that run on batteries and can record all day long. There have also been recent instances of state licensing agencies videotaping patient rooms, with the patient/family's permission, of course.

Another very real example of nursing home negligence is the patient whose husband visited often, and who was helping the C.N.A. with transferring his wife from her bed to a wheelchair. She was morbidly obese and her arm caught behind her, causing the bones to snap in two. The husband later told me that he immediately reported the sound of the snapping of his wife's arm as well as her increased pain to the nurse, but no x-ray was completed until the next day. The nursing home administrator told the patient's husband that he was at fault because he was helping when he shouldn't have been... but this simply isn't true. C.N.A.'s often asked for his help due to their being consistently understaffed. Had he recorded this conversation, or the many that followed, he would have been able to force the nursing home to change their procedures in order to care for the patients appropriately. Not only should the patient have been transferred from her bed to her chair by two nursing home staff members at all times, a nurse should have immediately completed an assessment and called the doctor to report the incident. This would have saved the patient from over 24 hours of excruciating pain as well as the trauma of a broken arm.

Her husband told me that the reason he didn't record the staff's apathetic reaction was due to the possibility of retaliation from the staff. Regardless as to whether or not he had recorded the event, he could have consulted an attorney in order to force the nursing home to hire sufficient amounts of staff members to safely transfer its patients. It's not appropriate for a nursing home to accuse a family member of being at fault when the staff asked for his help on a daily basis.

> In early 2010, fourteen workers at a nursing home in upstate New York were arrested for neglecting patients as a result of a video sting conducted by the Attorney General, while eight others were arrested in a western New York nursing home for neglect. In both cases, the staff members were accused of falsifying the patient record to cover up their actions. The thought of such a sting is terrifying to nursing homes. The workers in nursing homes are human and do make mistakes, but if they are mistreating patients or acting in a negligent manner they shouldn't be allowed to continue the offending behaviors.

I can't stress enough that most patients are safe, and most nursing homes are proud of being successful in their mission to provide excellent care to their patients, but there are exceptions. If you suspect that your family member is being abused, take photographs with the date stamped so that you can document what you've found. If the room is consistently filthy, take photos. You are able to take photos of your family member at any time, and if a staff member demands that you surrender the camera, call the police *and* the nursing home ombudsman. You have the right to take photos as long as you aren't infringing upon anyone else's privacy.

Refusing Treatments

Patients and families have the right to refuse treatments for any reason, and most of the time the doctor will understand. For example, if you were to explain that the expensive order tests or treatments he ordered aren't covered by insurance, he might suggest a less expensive alternative to diagnose the patient's condition. Finances aren't the only reason a test might not be in the patient's best interest; if the patient has a diagnosis of end-stage lung cancer an expensive test for another condition won't change his course of treatment. It might take a trip to the doctor to explain to him what the issue might be, but it's worth it if the patient is able to receive the treatment that he prefers rather than to simply comply with the doctor's orders (or the nursing home's wishes). Even if his doctor insists that the treatment is necessary, he still has the right to refuse.

If the patient presents with the symptoms of a particular disease or medical condition, it might be possible for the doctor to order medications to start treatment right away rather than to wait for the results of expensive tests to confirm the diagnosis. If the patient improves, the tests might not be necessary. It's worth discussing this issue with the doctor, especially if the patient has had that particular symptom before and it was alleviated with medication.

Doctors don't always get along with patients and families; if they continually disagree or refuse to follow the treatment plan, the doctor has the right to refuse to treat the patient any longer (in the same way as the patient has the right to find another practitioner). The doctor can serve the patient a 30-day notice and the patient will have to find another doctor. However, if the patient isn't able to find another doctor who'll treat him in the nursing home, his physician will have to continue treating him until one can be located. It's considered to be patient abandonment if he stops treating the patient without another physician who can assume his care. Sometimes the nursing home medical director will take over, but not always. The medical director is paid to provide support to the nursing home but isn't automatically obligated to accept every patient that's been assigned to him.

Patients who refuse a recommended life-extending treatment might be referred for hospice care. The patient has the right to accept or reject the services of a hospice; people die every day in nursing homes, comfortably and pain-free, without hospice care. It's often easier for the nursing home when the patient signs onto a hospice program, because the treatment focus becomes comfort care rather than a fight to keep the patient at his current level of functioning (required by CMS). Choosing hospice can save the patient or his family quite a bit of money (see the sections on hospice), as well as the ability to benefit from the combinations of medications that hospices use for comfort. If the patient chooses to elect the hospice benefit, he also has the right to choose which agency will serve him as long as the hospice has a contract with the nursing home. Some nursing homes will only work with a few hospice agencies, rather than all of the ones in the area. If the patient/family insists upon using a non-contracted hospice agency, he may have to go to another nursing home to receive that care. It depends upon the nursing home administrator; he might be willing to develop a one-time service agreement with a non-contracted hospice rather than to have the patient moved to a nursing home that does work with the hospice he prefers.

Patients who have been prescribed radiation and chemotherapy services while in a nursing home under Part A Medicare are often sent to one specific nursing home in town that will accept them. Most facilities won't admit patients who require these expensive treatments because the nursing home is required to pay for the treatment out of the daily rate they receive from Medicare, which cuts significantly into their profit margin.   Those nursing homes that do provide radiation therapy will use a contracted provider (rather than the one preferred by his primary physician), which is fine as long as the patient receives the treatment he needs. However, it's possible that the nursing home will attempt to decrease the number of treatments to save money. Just as with chemotherapy, patients and their families have the right to refuse changes in their treatment plan and the nursing home isn't allowed to bully the patient or family into changing the treatments simply to save money. If this happens to your family member, speak with the administrator or call the state licensing agency. If the nursing home accepted the patient knowing that he had expensive treatments prescribed to him, they can't force him to decrease them for the benefit of the nursing home.

Because chemotherapy and radiation treatments are so expensive, the nursing home might try to force the senior to participate in the maximum amount of therapy no matter how poorly he feels. The nursing home's goal is to bill Medicare at the highest rate possible in order to offset the cost of the chemotherapy and radiation. If the nursing home is able to pull this off, Medicare will more than cover their costs. While encouraging a patient to participate in as much therapy as possible can be therapeutic, it's unethical for the nursing home to threaten the patient with a discharge if he won't work harder. I worked for a nursing home where the administrator threatened a patient with discharge if she didn't complete 3 hours per day of therapies, so she attempted to do so even though she was weak and vomiting the entire time.   A quick call to the nursing home ombudsman and the state regulatory agency helped to resolve these issues. I can't stress enough that many nursing homes are acting in the best interest of the patient and wouldn't act in such a manner, but it's important for family members to remain vigilant in order to ensure the patient isn't mistreated.

Refusing Care
It's possible that the patient will refuse care such as showers, and the nursing home will send in different staff members in an attempt to convince him to accept the care. If the patient continues to refuse, the nursing home might call his family or the ombudsman. The nursing home might serve the patient a 30-day notice if his behaviors offend others, but it's rare for the nursing home to succeed in discharging a patient unless he is clearly a danger to himself or others. More often than not, the patient will at least allow a bed-bath even if he doesn't want to shower.

Refusing care can be an issue when the nursing home is attempting to bill Medicare for the treatment; each time the patient refuses to participate in therapy it places the facility's ability to bill the Medicare program for therapy in jeopardy. If the patient continues to refuse therapy, it's possible that the Medicare program will not pay for his continued room & board. The nursing home might not be thrilled at the prospect of losing thousands of dollars in revenue because a patient is refusing care, but he has the right to refuse and must suffer the consequences of his actions (such as discharge to home, or ending therapy services before he believes that he is ready). The bottom line is that the patient has the right to refuse treatment, medications, and patient care without fear of retribution.

Patient Showers

Our skin becomes more fragile as we age. Most nursing home patients are only showered 2-3 times per week, because more frequent showers can dry out their skin. Showering isn't always the best part of a patient's day, especially if the patient is schlepped up and down a crowded hallway to be showered in a common area rather than in the patient's room. Another reason that shower time might not be the favorite part of a patient's day could possibly be the time that the patient is being showered. Considering that C.N.A.'s are required to shower 8-10 patients (or more) each day, someone will be waking up at 6:00am or earlier to shower. The shower rooms are cold, the water might not be as warm as the patient prefers, and patients are showering in front of staff members. What's not to like?

Many nursing homes utilize designated shower rooms, which means that patients will be transported down busy hallways wrapped in nothing but a sheet. Some nursing home patients don't mind this; but others feel embarrassed, especially in those cases when the sheet doesn't wrap completely around the patients and various parts of their body are in full view as they pass by. It's undignified, to say the least, when a patient is wheeled down a busy hallway wearing next to nothing by a C.N.A. who isn't even acknowledging him. It only takes a few extra minutes to dress a patient in a robe and to treat him as though he were going to a spa, and it makes all of the difference to the patient – but it's rare to find patients who treated in such a manner.

In many cases, the shower rooms are huge tiled rooms that aren't warm and inviting, and they are rarely disinfected between patients. Diseases such as athlete's foot or plantar warts can be easily passed from patient to patient. Nursing home admissions staff members might have shown off their fancy bathtubs during their tour, but most patients aren't able to benefit from a bath due to the extra time and staff that it takes to perform a bath versus a shower.

Regardless of where the patient is showered, make sure that his preferred bath products are available so that he will be as comfortable as possible during his designated shower time. It's often a nursing home policy for a C.N.A. to stand by while even the most independent of patients are showered; this means that patients might not be bathed according to their preferred schedule. If your family member prefers to be showered in the mornings, ask that this be part of his Care Plan in order to ensure his wishes are met if at all possible.

Patients with dementia are often afraid of being showered and might fight the shower aide or scream the entire time; this is a normal occurrence and isn't an indication of abuse. It often takes two aides to shower patients with these behaviors in order to ensure that no one gets hurt. It can be distressing for a family member who is present in the building at the time of her mother's shower, but if it is explained to her what's happening and she is provided with literature about dementia she might feel better about the entire situation.

The showering process can be so much more pleasant when the patients are treated with dignity, and not felt as if they're being rushed. It's an often overlooked event, but patients feel more comfortable if they're allowed to choose the time of their shower and treated with respect by the nursing home staff members.

Restraints

Restraints are anything that restrict or restrain a patient's movements. They can be belts, vests, specialty chairs, bedside rails, secured (locked) units or even medications that make it difficult for patients to function and move about freely in their usual manner. According to federal rules, restraints must be used only to keep a patient safe and must be medically necessary; they can't be used for the convenience of the staff or as punishment for patient behaviors. Patients and their families have the right to refuse to allow the use of restraints, even if it makes it harder for the nursing home staff to work with the patient.

Every nursing home is required to have a policy regarding restraints, whether or not they are being used to keep the patient from hurting himself. These policies must include procedures that address how often physical restraints must be released, repositioning of the patients to keep them from developing bedsores, and the use of ongoing assessments to determine that the patient continues to require the restraint. Improper use of restraints can result in multiple problems, including decubitus ulcers (bedsores or pressure sores), lethargy, and depression due to restricted movement.

Nursing homes have the right to refuse to allow certain types of restraints to be used in their buildings. For example, bedside rails are a form of restraint that can keep a patient from falling out of bed, but they can also cause a patient to crawl over the rail and fall from a greater height than if there were no rail. Patients can become stuck in the bedrail when trying to climb out of the bed, resulting in a fractured arm or leg. Many nursing homes do not allow more than one bedside rail to be in the up position at any one time. Those patients who might climb out of their beds are usually placed in a lower bed with protective mats placed on the floor around it, so if he falls it will only be a few inches rather than a foot or more. Nursing homes are more likely to use half-rails, which cover only half of the bed rather than full side rails that restrict movement from the patient's head to his feet.

Patients with the potential to fall out of wheelchairs might have a soft harness to keep them from falling, but they can't be belted (or tied) into the chair. There are special "lap buddies" that provide a soft surface for the patient, yet fit tightly into the chair in such a manner that the patient isn't able to get out of it easily. Some restraint usage leads to the necessity of other restraints, such as using psychotropic medications to make the patient more manageable. If the patient is overmedicated, he might need to be tied into his wheelchair to ensure he doesn't fall out. The danger becomes that he can try to get up and become tangled in the wheelchair. This is one of the reasons that nursing homes aren't allowed to medicate a patient in order to make it easier for the staff to deal with him. There are many laws that address restraints in nursing homes and this is often a focus of state investigations.

There are horror stories out there, such as the true story of the facility that placed a patient in an adult-sized "crib" that was more like a cage from which he couldn't escape. When questioned, the administrator's explanation was that he was already in the crib when she started working there a few years before. She had chosen not to change his torturous situation; it's interesting to note that the facility received a huge fine, yet the administrator wasn't held personally accountable for her lack of action nor was the general public ever made aware of the incident. In fact, much of what goes on in nursing homes is never known to the public.

In another case, a patient who was alert & oriented and used a motorized wheelchair left a nursing home to go to a nearby store, which was a common occurrence. His chair ran out of power and he was forced to wait for help from strangers. When he returned to the nursing home several hours after he was expected, he was placed on the secured unit with dementia patients because he was an "escape risk" and denied the use of his telephone charger. He remained there for two days until I returned to work after a long weekend and was able to have him transferred back to his original room. Had he called the state regulatory agency, the facility would have been fined for their actions. This was a blatant case of misusing a restraint to limit a patient's ability to move about the facility.

Psychotropic Medications

Psychotropics are medications such as antipsychotics and antidepressants that affect a patient's mind, mood, or behaviors. Anti-anxiety medications can also be considered psychotropics. These types of medications are used to treat mental or emotional disorders and can be considered to be a type of chemical restraint due to patients becoming less functional when taking them. They aren't supposed to be used to control patients behaviors or restrict their movements, but these are side effects of the medications. Nursing homes aren't supposed to use psychotropics to make it easier to manage their patients, but it happens.

The use of psychotropics must be monitored by the nursing home to try to ensure that they are being used to benefit the patients and not to sedate them into submission. Patients who are administered these medications are monitored for adverse side effects such as being overly sedated, tardive dyskenesia (excessive movement of the tongue & mouth), involuntary muscle movements, weight gain/loss, and memory impairment.

Federal laws mandate that physicians and nursing homes work together to attempt to decrease the dosage amounts of these medications in order to make sure that patients aren't overmedicated. The way that this is accomplished is by a pharmacy consultant or nursing home staff member reviewing the chart of every patient who is prescribed psychotropic medications in the nursing home. If a patient isn't displaying any symptoms or behaviors, the recommendation will be to decrease or taper off the medications altogether. The problem is that quite often the staff member or consultant will make these recommendations without ever having laid eyes on the patient; chances are that they don't know the patient's long-term history at all. Sometimes their recommendation is the best thing for the patient, but it's also possible that the reason that a patient isn't displaying any behaviors is because the medications are working correctly. Any change in the regimen can affect a delicate balance of medications that have been working for years.

To further support the decision to change their patient's psychotropic medications, many nursing homes have interdisciplinary psychotropic committees that meet on a regular basis to review patient charts. While these staff members might have extensive experience in dealing with mental illnesses, it's possible that they have no experience at all. There's no educational requirement to sit on one of these committees, even though these people are helping to decide which medications will be administered to the patients to enhance their psychosocial functioning. I've personally seen "committees" that consisted of a nurse who completed the forms and then presented them to staff members to sign without further discussion. When I refused to sign the form, I was dropped from the committee.

Regardless of who makes them, the recommendations will be sent to the doctor for his signature. They'll probably be buried in a stack of paperwork, and once he signs the recommendation the changes are made. The patient and his family are rarely notified, even though these modifications in the patient's mediation regimen can be distressing for the patient who has been stable for many years. Remember that the changes are usually made because a patient is doing well, not because there's a problem. Even a slight change in a patient's medications can throw off the delicate balance that allows him to function. Once the changes have been made, he might start to display behaviors and suffer months of emotional trauma before he returns to his former level of functioning. This can result in a roller coaster of behaviors and medication changes, which are not only distressing to the patient and his family but also can be very expensive.

Even though federal law mandates that the nursing home *attempt* to decrease the use of psychotropic medications, it's not mandatory that the patient/family allow them to do so. Patients and families aren't told that that the staff's recommendations are actually suggestions; instead they are given a blanket consent form to sign that authorizes the nursing home to make changes at any time. Patients and families don't have to sign the consent form, and have every right to approve or deny any recommended changes to the patient's plan of care. Nursing home staff members who just met the patient might not be the best judge as to how to adjust a patient's medications. The staff might be unhappy when family members refuse to sign a blanket permission form, but it's important to remember that this isn't about the nursing home – it's about the patient's needs.

Following the death of her husband and daughter in 1995, Julia was diagnosed with depression and anxiety. After several years of fine tuning her medications, her doctor was able to stabilize her symptoms. She took the medications in this manner for more than 10 years without any problems.

Julia was admitted into a nursing home in 2007. The psychotropic committee noticed that she didn't appear to be depressed or anxious, and they recommended a decrease in the dosage that had worked for years. Within a week, she began exhibiting severe anxiety when left alone and would refuse to leave her room. This issue was discussed during the next scheduled psychotropic committee; they changed her medications with no results. They later recommended increasing her medications back to their former levels but there was no immediate effect. It took about six months of adjusting her medications until she appeared to be stable again. Once the committee noticed that she wasn't exhibiting any behaviors, they attempted to decrease her medication dosages again.

This time her family was ready for the recommendation. They contacted the nursing home, doctor and pharmacy and refused to allow any medication changes without their permission. The psychotropic committee made a note that the patient's family refused the recommendation and moved on to the next patient on their list.

Some nursing homes work with a psychiatrist, and refer every patient who is taking psychotropic medications in order to ensure that psychotropic medications are being administered in the best interest of the patient. This consultant bills the patient's insurance, and there will be a copayment involved. If your family member is taking psychotropics, discuss the parameters of the consulting physicians with the director of nursing to ensure that a psychiatrist doesn't attempt to change his medications without your permission; you are even able to refuse to allow the patient to be seen by a psychiatrist if you wish. At the very least, family members have the right to request a meeting with the psychiatrist to ensure that the patient's needs are being addressed and his psychotropics aren't changed without your permission.

The best way a family can ensure that the medications aren't arbitrarily changed is to make sure that no responsible family member sign a blanket consent form; if it's not completed or isn't specific enough don't sign it! Feel free to discuss the issue with the doctor, the director of nursing, and the administrator if necessary. You can also request that a notice be placed in the front of the chart insisting that the family be consulted before any and all medication changes are made. Many nursing homes consider this to be family interference, but that's their problem. A well-managed nursing home will welcome the family's input and view the family as a part of the patient's care-giving team.

Oxygen and Related Equipment

In order to administer oxygen to their patients, nursing homes must monitor the patients' oxygen saturation levels (*O^2 sats*). Usually the rates must be 89% or less, and the oxygen can only be given to patients with a physician's order. Although some nursing homes have oxygen piped into the walls, most will contract with a medical equipment company to provide *oxygen concentrators* to their patients. These concentrators are about the size of a nightstand, and can come with 50 feet or more of tubing, which allows patients to walk around their room without restriction (although the tubing can cause a tripping hazard). These concentrators can put out a lot of heat and are quite loud, which is why it's best to have them placed several feet away from the patient's bed.

For patients who are mobile, most nursing homes offer portable bottles so that patients can be moved about the facility or to doctor's appointments without an interruption in the oxygen. These bottles can be placed in a holder on the back of the patient's wheelchair, or in a small cart that the patient can push beside him. There are smaller, refillable bottles that can be provided to patients, but they're rarely used in nursing homes due to the time it takes to refill the bottles.

There are also small, battery powered concentrators available that provide patients with freedom to move around the facility without attempting to manage a huge oxygen bottle, but most nursing homes don't provide these because they're substantially more expensive than the bottles. In fact, many insurance companies don't cover the cost of these concentrators; if a patient wants one they might pay $6,000 or more out-of-pocket. These concentrators are also approved for airline travel; generally they're rented for a short period of time in order to accommodate for the flight and then are shipped back to the oxygen provider.

Nursing homes provide the oxygen free of charge for patients who are receiving services under the Medicare Part A benefit (including hospice patients), Medicaid or whose room & board are covered by the VA or private insurance; however, it's a different story for the patient who is paying privately for his room and board. The private-pay patient will be charged out-of-pocket for his oxygen at a monthly rate that can easily exceed $100.00. There are exceptions; if the patient received oxygen from a Medicare certified provider prior to being admitted to the nursing home and is staying for long-term-care, Medicare will pay for it to continue and he'll be responsible for the same copayments he paid before he arrived. However, if the patient wasn't prescribed the oxygen while he was at home, he'll have to pay 100% of the charges for his oxygen. All oxygen must be provided by a licensed medical equipment company to ensure that it's safe and well maintained; in other words, it's not possible for a family member to bring in an old concentrator they have laying around.

Nursing homes must also follow certain guidelines regarding BIPAP (bi-level positive airway pressure) and CPAP (continuous positive airway pressure) machines; these are used to treat patients diagnosed with sleep apnea. In order to qualify for these items, it's possible that the patient will need to have a sleep study that involves being monitored while he sleeps. There are other types of devices that might assist patients, such as SVN (small volume nebulizer) machines that administer breathing treatments; all of these machines are either paid out of the Medicare/Medicaid, VA benefits, ordered through patient insurance plans, or the patient must pay out of pocket for them (considered to be specialty equipment).

Another method of obtaining oxygen and related equipment at no cost to him is for the patient to sign onto a hospice program. Patients who are receiving hospice care will have this equipment provided by the hospice company (oxygen is considered to be a comfort measure) at no cost to the patient. Obviously, a need for oxygen doesn't qualify a patient for hospice but if he does have a terminal condition, the program can save him the cost of oxygen as well as the cost of other equipment. Patients who are receiving hospice care don't have to qualify (have 0^2 sats of 89% or less), because the hospice has the discretion of providing oxygen regardless of the patient's oxygen levels.

Miscellaneous Supplies and Specialty Equipment

Nursing homes are able to charge their private-pay patients for supplies and specialty equipment. These are the same supplies that the nursing home must provide free of charge to patients receiving services under Part A Medicare, Medicaid, or the V.A. Patients who are receiving hospice care services often will have supplies and specialty equipment provided by the hospice at no cost to the patient. This is yet another reason why electing to receive hospice services can be beneficial to a nursing home resident.

The most common type of supply is incontinence briefs and pads. Nursing homes can either charge by the brief or can charge a per diem rate. The mark-up is usually several hundred percent. However, the nursing home is required to allow the family to bring in the items if they wish. If you choose to decrease your out-of-pocket costs, you can purchase them in bulk from many discount retailers. It's important to ensure that the nursing home staff isn't using the briefs that you bought for other residents simply because they were convenient. The best way to do this is to either request that they be locked away at the nurse's station or bring them in one package at a time (if you visit often enough). It's possible to save hundreds of dollars each month by buying them yourself, and these products are often of better quality than those provided by the nursing home.

Long-term patients who require specialty wound care services and supplies (including a **Wound Vac**) can cost upwards of $4,000 per month in addition to their base costs, an amount that isn't covered by Medicare or most insurances. When you consider that the patient is already paying $6,000.00 each month (or more) for room & board, the added cost of wound care can break the bank. The same equipment is provided at little or no cost for a patient who lives in his own home or an assisted living facility.

Another type of specialty item for which nursing homes charge handsomely is an air mattress overlay. There are many types of air mattresses, which are designed to keep patients from developing decubitus ulcers (bedsores). Air mattresses range from the simplest models to those that are extremely complicated, and they can cost as much as $8,000.00 to buy. Nursing homes charge up to $100 each day for these items, but if the patient will remain in the nursing home on a long-term basis it's definitely cheaper to buy one of these mattresses outright. It's possible that a local medical equipment company will be able to provide an air mattress at a deep discount, but even if they charge full price the patient saves money after a month or two. Items such as this should only be purchased from a medical equipment provider, because the warranty doesn't transfer between private parties and it can be expensive to repair air beds. You might end up paying for an expensive piece of equipment that can't be repaired.

If the patient's bed is uncomfortable, it's possible for him to use an egg-crate mattress over his regular mattress. As long as the patient isn't leaking fluids (such as being incontinent or having weeping legs due to edema), this mattress can be much more comfortable than the standard mattress. The nursing home might not tell you that you can bring in your own egg-crate mattress purchased at a discount store, because the one that they provide from a medical supplier will be marked up several thousand percent in order for the facility to make a profit. If your family member tells you that his bed is uncomfortable, discuss this with the nurse or her supervisors. Sleeping in an uncomfortable bed can lead to bed sores, lack of sleep, irritability and other issues.

Patients have the right to bring in their own beds and mattresses as long as they don't interfere with the patient's personal care or encroach on his roommate's space in the facility. Hospitals bed mattresses aren't the most comfortable to begin with, and if the patient complains about his discomfort the nursing home will probably replace that mattress with an identical mattress. In most instances, the nursing home uses the same model of mattress for all of its beds and they tend to break down under the wear & tear received in a nursing home.

Durable Medical Equipment

Nursing homes are required to provide all of the equipment necessary for the patient to receive appropriate care while he is in the facility. This includes wheelchairs, walkers, hospital beds, bedside commodes, specialty beds, overhead trapezes and Hoyer lifts. It doesn't matter whether the patient is there under Medicare, Medicaid, or the VA, it's usually the responsibility of the nursing home to ensure these items are provided.

The patient who is paying privately will have to rent these items from the nursing home (which can quickly add up), or can buy them outright and bring them in. If they have the equipment brought in, everything should be prominently marked with the patient's name to ensure they remain his property. In most cases, Medicare and other insurances will buy them before a patient is admitted but don't provide medical equipment for the patient who resides in a nursing home. If the patient doesn't own them already, the choice will be to rent them from the nursing home or buy them outright.

Durable Medical Equipment for Discharge

When planning a patient's nursing home discharge, Medicare and other insurance plans have their limitations regarding medical equipment. Medicare will pay for a regular front-wheeled walker or for a portion of the cost of a four-wheeled walker with a seat, but it won't pay for both. It will pay for the walker or a wheelchair, but not both; Medicare also does not pay for a shower chair (this is considered to be a non-medical item). Medicare will pay for a bedside commode, hospital bed and overhead trapeze if the patient needs them; in most instances the medical equipment company will take care of any paperwork and preauthorizations that might be required. All of these items must be prescribed by the doctor following a face-to-face visit and the patient must demonstrate a need for the item. This can be confusing; speak with the social worker or discharge planner about the items that you will need upon discharge and she will help to obtain them.

For patients who have been discharged, Medicare doesn't pay for a recliner/lift chair although it might possibly pay for the lift mechanism itself. The patient is responsible for the actual cost of the chair, because a recliner is not a piece of medical equipment and the Medicare program doesn't pay for household furniture items. Once these items have been purchased, they have little resale value because the warranty doesn't transfer between private parties. Medical equipment companies often resell these items on consignment for patients who are no longer able to use them.

Again, patients who are receiving hospice care will have all of the regular equipment that they need provided by the hospice company when they are discharged from a nursing home. Hospice does make it easier for the patient & family, but the patient must qualify as "terminal" in order to receive hospice care.

Motorized Wheelchairs

Patients who aren't able to independently propel a manual wheelchair might benefit greatly from a motorized wheelchair, and most nursing homes will allow patients to use one as long as the patient is able to safely maneuver throughout the facility. A motorized chair or scooter can be purchased via the Medicare benefit while the patient lives at home, but after he's been admitted into the nursing home the Medicare program won't pay for either of these items. A new wheelchair can easily cost anywhere from $6,000 to $10,000 depending upon the patient's physical needs, and there is a 20% copayment required. Most Medigap policies will cover the out-of-pocket costs, but once the warranty expires on these items, the patient is responsible for the cost of any repairs. These wheelchairs are usually heavy duty and can last for years as long as they are properly maintained. Once a wheelchair is out of warranty, it can be expensive to fix.

Depending upon the state in which the recipient lives, the Medicaid program might purchase a motorized wheelchair for him as long as truly needs it. It can take months to obtain the authorizations necessary for a motorized wheelchair to be provided to a patient. Once the warranty expires, Medicaid will usually pay to repair motorized wheelchairs that were purchased with the assistance of the Medicaid program. In most cases, the Medicaid program will not bear the cost of repairs for a wheelchair it didn't buy. This includes replacing of batteries, which generally go dead after 2-3 years of use. Since most nursing homes aren't willing to pay $300 or so to replace the batteries for their patients' wheelchairs (and patients only have about $35.00 each month to spend), it's possible that when the batteries die the patient will no longer be able to use his wheelchair. This is unfortunate, as it severely limits the patient's ability to freely move throughout the nursing home.

Many private-pay patients will choose to discharge home for a day in order to have the Medicare program pay for a motorized wheelchair, and then readmit to the nursing home the following day. This is a huge inconvenience for the nursing home; a new patient chart will have to be started and all of the paperwork, including consents from patients/families, will have to be completed all over again. It can also be difficult for the patient, especially if he has to arrange for caregivers at his home for even one day. It is a viable option, albeit inconvenient, even though it is a manipulation of the system in order to receive a piece of equipment that would greatly enhance the patient's life. Once the patient has obtained a motorized wheelchair, the company from which it was purchased is required to provide repair service as long as the wheelchair is under warranty regardless of where he lives (nursing home or at his private home).

Just as with other types of specialty equipment, it's always best to buy a brand new wheelchair from a medical supplier because the warranties don't transfer between buyers. Once the patient dies or no longer requires the motorized chair, many family members will try to sell them only to find that they have little resale value. The resale price of a like-new $6,000 wheelchair is in the $500 range, although I've seen them sell for as little as $250. Many charitable foundations won't accept motorized wheelchairs as donations due to the potential liability if the chair breaks and hurts someone.

People have been able to qualify for scooters and wheelchairs for many years, whether or not they actually needed them. The advertisements for these items claimed that anyone could qualify for them, and for the longest time, pretty much anyone could. This is the reason that the Medicare program is closely monitoring the companies that provide scooters and motorized wheelchairs, and some are suffering financially as a result. The Scooter Store, which led the nation in sales of scooters and motorized wheelchairs, filed bankruptcy after an FBI raid led to a $19 million dollar fine for chairs issued to patients who didn't appear to qualify for them. Motorized wheelchairs can be wonderful tools to provide patients with the mobility that they're lacking, but if the patient is able to walk it's important that he use his body as much as possible or he will ultimately lose his ability to walk.

MDS Assessments

Nursing homes are required to provide ongoing patient assessments to the Centers for Medicare and Medicaid Services (CMS); these assessments begin on the date of the patient's admission and continue at regular intervals until the patient dies or is discharged. This computerized form is called an **MDS** (**Minimum Data Set**) and the assessments it contains reflect the needs of each patient. The form also tells CMS the amount of time that the patient participates in physical, occupational, and speech therapy services and sets the amount that Medicare will pay the nursing home for his skilled services. There is an assessment team (part of the nursing department) whose job it is to gather the information and transmit it to CMS.

Patients and their families rarely interact with the MDS Coordinators and are rarely privy to the information that's been gathered. They don't need to know the reporting deadlines and the assessment doesn't really affect them. The patient's only interaction regarding the MDS will be with a social worker who asks them questions on the **BIMS** (Brief Interview for Mental Status) and **PHQ-9** (Patient Health Questionnaire); these provide input about the patient's cognitive status. Most of the information in the MDS will be obtained by reviewing the charting that's been completed by the various departments. Please note that the MDS process can't be changed and that the staff members are required to ask the same questions each time the assessment is completed. This is irritating to the patients, but unfortunately it's a federal requirement that these questions be asked time after time (sometimes a few days apart).

The Medicaid program also uses the MDS assessment to evaluate the average level of care of all the patients in the nursing home. This is the way that the Medicaid program negotiates the rate that it will pay the nursing home to care for each specific patient. The greater the overall need of the patients, the greater the amount that Medicaid will pay to the nursing home. An evaluation of the average level of care for the patients is generally conducted every year.

The MDS coordinators must transmit the required information at specific intervals that are determined by CMS; if the information isn't submitted in a timely manner the nursing home will be fined. The MDS is truly a collaborative effort between the departments, and is extremely important to the nursing home's financial well-being. It is also a time consuming task, taking away precious time that staff would otherwise be able to spend with patients.

When the initial MDS has been completed, the program prints a report that identifies potential problems (*Care Area Assessments,* or *CAA's*) that must be explored further. The staff is required to develop an approach to deal with each of these issues, and to add the approach to the patient's care plan. The *plan of care* (usually referred to as care plan) must correspond to the MDS assessment and also must be changed every time a new problem is identified.

Again, most patients don't know (or care) about the MDS assessments, CAA's or care plans. The only way that the assessment affects the patient is that, if he is in the facility receiving physical therapy via the Medicare Part A benefit, he will be encouraged to participate in as many minutes of therapy as possible in order to hit the highest level of payment that the assessment allows.

Care Plans

Every medical or patient care facility is required to develop and follow an individualized *plan of care* for each of its patients. This applies to hospitals, rehabilitation centers, hospices, home care agencies, assisted livings, etc. Every care plan is developed by members of the *Interdisciplinary Team (IDT)*, and is signed off by the doctor. It's important to remember that everything in a facility is performed at the direction of a physician, and the care plan is the proof. Every change to the patient's treatment plan involves a change of the care plan. The care plan is reviewed at least quarterly and must be discussed with patients and their families at any time if they request a review.

IDT/Care Plan Meetings

The *Interdisciplinary Team (IDT) Meeting* is another part of the care planning process. The team, consisting of the nursing, dietary, activity and social service departments, meets with the patient and/or family. These meetings, also called *Interdisciplinary Group (IDG) Meetings* or *Care Plan Meetings*, are usually held soon after the patient has been admitted into the nursing home, and then every three months thereafter (unless there is a specific need to be addressed in between those times). They usually take 15-30 minutes, unless the patient and his family have multiple issues to resolve. Many patients/families don't attend every IDT meeting, as the information rarely changes from month-to-month.

In most cases, the nursing home IDT has an agenda they follow to keep the meeting on track. While it's important that the facility staff have enough information to ensure that patients' needs are met, this isn't a forum for the family to recite the patient's life story. Please remember that the nursing home will be meeting with other patients and families, and anything that the family can do to keep the meeting moving forward is greatly appreciated by the staff. Provide the necessary information, and if you wish to speak with the nurse or social worker feel free to ask to meet with them after the meeting.

IDT Meetings can be helpful and informative, or they can appear intimidating to patients and families. It depends upon the attitude of the facility administration, including the director of nursing, as to whether the care planning process is a collaborative process or merely fulfilling federal and state requirements that mandatory meetings be held. I've seen it happen both ways; it actually works the best for staff when the family participates as a part of the caregiving team. However, those nursing homes that discourage family involvement might view the IDT meeting as a necessary evil in order to obtain the family's signature so they can move on to the next patient's chart.

Those nursing home patients who are also receiving services from a hospice will have the option of attending IDT meetings with a member of the hospice team. The hospice can help to clarify and resolve any issues that the patient, family or nursing home might be experiencing.

It's important to remember that patients and/or family members can ask to meet with the facility staff on a regular basis; they can also meet with the administrator and director of nursing at any time. If they are experiencing unresolved problems with the facility, they can also report it to the state agency listed on the bulletin boards in the public areas of the building or to the ombudsman. If they wish, families and patients can ask an ombudsman to attend IDT/Care plan meetings in order to ensure that the patient's needs are met.

Therapy Services

Nursing homes reap the majority of their profits from Medicare Part A services, including physical, occupational and speech therapies. Patients who are receiving services under the Part A benefit usually have larger – or possibly even private – rooms. In most instances, every effort is made to ensure that these patients are happy because nursing homes want the patients have such a satisfying experience that they will tell their friends & family, and will return every time they're discharged from the hospital. Once the patient has recovered or has used every day of the maximum 100-day Medicare benefit, his therapy services will end and he will probably be moved to another room. While he will be monitored to ensure that he doesn't backslide, he will no longer receive therapy (whether or not he needs it). Any further progress will be the patient's doing, because his payment source has dried up.

After a patient has completed his therapy under the Part A benefit, he can still use the gym and workout equipment. However, it won't be at the direction of a therapist (unless the family pays privately for the service). Most nursing homes offer patients the opportunity to use the gym during those limited times that it doesn't interfere with those patients receiving physical therapy. However, the therapists aren't able to provide professional assistance with patients using the gym on their own, nor are they required to motivate patients as they work out.

It's the responsibility of the nursing home to ensure that he maintains his current level of functioning once his therapy benefit has been exhausted. This is the case even if the patient is in his 90's and doesn't feel like moving around much. Nursing homes attain this goal by providing **Restorative Therapy**. The nursing aides who provide the care are specially trained to work with patients at the direction of the physical therapy department. They are the staff members you'll see walking with residents and providing them with **range of motion** exercises. However, these aides can only do so much, and if the patient appears to be backsliding he will probably be referred for additional therapy under the **Medicare Part B** benefit.

Medicare Part B provides for therapy that is designed to keep a patient at his highest level of functioning; it has its limitations, with a maximum amount of $1,900 available for physical and speech therapy combined, and another $1,900 allotted for occupational therapy. There are copayments and deductibles that apply, which often must be paid out of the patient's personal funds unless he is a Medicaid recipient. Because physical therapy provides the highest profits for nursing homes, nursing home staff (usually therapists, nurses and possibly the administrator) will conduct "walking rounds," to identify patients who might benefit from the additional therapy paid for under Part B. Therapists will then screen the patients to see if they require therapy (which often lasts as long as the payment, regardless of the patient's actual need), and the therapy will often begin without the patient and/or family even being aware.

Patients might be told they're going to the gym to work out when in reality their insurance is being charged for professional services; the therapy department doesn't have to obtain specific written permission in most cases because a blanket permission form was signed with his admission packet. It can be a surprise to patients or family members when they open their monthly bill and find charges for therapies being provided without their knowledge.

Therapy isn't necessarily a bad thing, but the nursing home's need for revenue isn't more important than the patient's or family's right to refuse to participate in therapy. The family might not notice a difference in their family member after weeks of therapy have been provided, and the patient might not enjoy having to perform the required tasks. It's important to insist that the nursing home obtain your permission for each service it provides, rather than to allow them to do what they believe is in the patient's best interest and bill you later. Remember that the services that they are claiming are in the patient's best interest are revenue producing; even if they're not in the patient's best interests, they're definitely benefitting the nursing home's profit margin.

Hospice patients rarely receive therapy; Medicare will not directly pay for the service, and the hospice agency must authorize the payment in order for therapy to occur. In most instances, the hospice will pay for a physical therapy consultation and provide teaching & training to care-givers, but comprehensive therapy might not benefit the patient whose life expectancy is six months or less. I've been present in nursing homes that recommend that patients revoke from hospice in order to receive physical therapy, and then sign back onto the hospice program. If this would benefit the patient and allow him additional quality of life, that's okay – but not if it is more for the benefit of the nursing home.

Medicare 2-Day Notices (NOMNC)

Patients who are receiving skilled services via the Medicare benefit must be notified in writing a minimum of two days prior to the end of the services. The notice is called a ***Notice of Medicare Non-Coverage (NOMNC)***. The 48-hour notice allows the patient time to make an appeal while he continues to receive the therapy; if the appeal is decided in his favor he will continue receiving therapy until another (successful) notice is served. The therapy might be ending because the patient has used the 100 maximum days of his therapy benefit, or it might be that the patient appears to have met his maximum level of functioning. If the patient's benefit has been exhausted, he will lose any appeal that he files. However, if the company that reviews the notice believes that the patient would continue to improve and still has therapy days left in his insurance benefit, the appeal will be successful.

There are three types of NOMNC notices; the first is a determination letter that informs the Medicare Part A beneficiary that the nursing home no longer believes that he is appropriate to continue receiving skilled services such as physical, occupational or speech therapies, or specialty nursing care in the facility. The NOMNC also advises the patient & family that the payment for his room & board will end when the 2-day notice expires. If the patient remains in the nursing home, he will have to make arrangements to pay for his room & board; otherwise he will have to leave.

The second type of NOMNC is targeted toward patients who are receiving supplemental therapies under the Part B benefit. The difference between the two notices is that Medicare Part A pays for the patient's room & board while he receives the therapies, while Part B is supplemental to his room & board in the nursing home and only pays for the therapy. For example, a patient can receive therapy under Part B while his room & board are paid by Medicaid. The notice that advises the patient/family that services will end doesn't address his continued stay in the nursing home because it's usually not an issue.

The third type of NOMNC is provided by the nursing home at the instruction of a Medicare Advantage plan. The main difference between this NOMNC and the one issued to Part A & Part B recipients is that in this case the insurance company – not the nursing home – determines that the patient has met his goals and requests that the nursing home issue a 2-day notice. Advantage plan members have the right to appeal this decision in the same manner as if they had traditional Medicare.

Regardless of the type of notice, it must contain the date that the services will end as well as a phone number the patient or family can call to appeal the decision. There is a place for the patient to sign; if the patient isn't competent to make decisions, the patient's responsible party should be notified in person, by fax, or via certified mail that the services will end; otherwise the nursing home will have no proof that the notice was served.

The nursing home is required to provide the patient with a telephone and even assist him in filing an appeal if he isn't able to do so on his own. It's easy to file an appeal; all that the patient must do is call a number on the form and request an appeal. This call takes about five minutes, and the nursing home can't retaliate against the patient if he chooses to make an appeal. Once the call has been made, a CMS contractor will notify the nursing home and request that certain medical records be faxed to them for review. The recipient is usually notified within 24 hours as to whether or not his appeal was successful and if he will continue to receive therapy under the Medicare benefit (unless there's a weekend or holiday that slows down the process). This decision often favors the patient, so if the family or patient believes that he would benefit from continued services it might be worthwhile to file an appeal. The patient will continue to receive his therapies during the appeal process, and if the Medicare Administrative Contractor rules in the patient's favor the nursing home will serve another NOMNC when it believes that therapy services have been completed.

In the event that the nursing home doesn't complete the NOMNC correctly, the patient will continue to receive the therapy free of charge until the nursing home correctly completes another form. Again, the nursing home can't retaliate against the patient if he appeals <u>any</u> notice he receives from the nursing home. I have seen many NOMNC's that were overturned by third party contractors, so if the patient or family believes that the patient would benefit from additional therapy, it's worth their while to file an appeal. For additional information about an appeal served to your family member, speak with the nursing home's social worker or a case manager. Feel free to call the number on the forms at any time to discuss your concerns.

Laundry Service

The nursing home offers laundry services at no cost to its residents, using huge commercial washers that intermix the laundry of many different patients. The clothing items don't receive personal attention and are often lost or ruined. There can be benefits to allowing the nursing home to do the laundry, especially if the family doesn't live nearby. The patient's clothing will be washed and returned to him at least twice a week, and the family doesn't have to worry about running to the nursing home to pick up his laundry.

The nursing home is required to replace any lost or ruined clothing. In many cases the nursing home will attempt to deny responsibility for the items, especially if they're not individually listed on the inventory form in the back of the nursing home chart. They will also ask for a receipt before any items are replaced. It's best to take a photograph of everything that is brought into the nursing home as well as to have the staff add each item individually to the inventory form; that way the nursing home will be forced to replace them with comparable items. However, the facility isn't responsible for replacing items ruined by everyday wear & tear.

Laundry is usually returned to patients within a couple of days as long as the clothing has been legibly marked with the patient's full name. It's important not to mark them with the patient's room number, because patients often change rooms as there are changes in their level of care. Chances are that the clothing will then be sent to the room number marked on the clothing and not the room in which the patient now resides. This is one way that clothing and other items are lost.

The found clothing items in a nursing home can take up quite a bit of space. There can be hundreds of items, and it's difficult to categorize them. Once an item of clothing is lost, chances are great that it will never be returned to its rightful owner. Many nursing homes throw away unclaimed clothing items after a month or two, or give them to other residents.

Patients aren't required to use the laundry service, though. It's possible for family members to bring a hamper and request that all of the patient's clothing be placed inside for the family to take home and wash. Not only do the items receive personal attention, but the family members also feel good about helping out the patient. The only time that it isn't possible for the family to do the laundry is when it is soiled with human waste; the nursing home will send these items to be cleaned and sanitized immediately regardless of the family's wishes. Many family members prefer to wash the patient's clothing at their home so that the clothing will last longer and retain its original color. Laundry that's been washed at home often smells better than the laundry that has been washed by the nursing home.

Room Transfers

Nursing homes often move patients to different rooms throughout the facility; this can happen for various reasons. It might be that the patient has completed his rehabilitation under Medicare Part A and will be moved to the facility's long-term wing, or it's possible that the bed he is currently using is needed by another patient. Many patients don't want to move – they like their current room and the thought of another change might be too much for them to handle.

Patients have the right to refuse a room transfer and must be served written notice in advance of the move. Even if the nursing home is attempting to transfer him from a private room to a shared room because he can't afford the private room rate, the patient has the right to refuse and the nursing home will have to legally evict him from that room to another in the nursing home. The nursing home can bill him for the difference between a private and shared room if he or his family refuses to allow the move, but if he doesn't have any money it's an empty threat. In most cases, patients are amenable to a room change if the nursing home can provide a valid explanation as to why it's necessary.

It's possible that an emergency room change will be required for the health and well-being of a patient – such as when he requires isolation for an infection – and in those cases patients can be moved against their wishes. Nursing homes aren't allowed to arbitrarily move patients from room to room, although the administrator might attempt to force the patient to move. In most states, the nursing home is required to give a patient a minimum of a 24-hour notice prior to moving him; the notice must be in writing, must be signed by the patient or his family, and must include the reason that the patient is being moved.

> One nursing home administrator bragged about her ability to maintain control over her residents, and that she was able to move them throughout the facility at her whim. A patient filed a formal complaint, and the facility was forced to develop a plan of corrections. The nursing home was required to provide written notice of every room change at least 24-hours in advance. This notice must be signed by the patient or family, and must be followed up after the move to ensure that the patient was satisfied after the transfer had occurred.
>
> This didn't slow down the administrator at all; her response was to have a staff member present a blank form to the patient for his signature and have it completed after the fact to give the appearance as though the patient had requested – or was at least in agreement with – the room changes.
>
> Unfortunately for the administrator, the blank (signed) forms were intercepted by a staff member who faxed them to the state licensing agency. These were compared with the ones that were found in the patients' charts. The state wasn't amused; this violated the patient's rights and the facility was penalized for these (and other) behaviors.

If a nursing home moves a patient without his permission, he has the right to complain to the long-term care ombudsman and also to file a formal complaint with the state regulatory agency. It can be a form of intimidation to move a patient from room to room as well as a manipulation on the nursing home's part to make the patient appear more disoriented than he really is. Confused patients will have a difficult time finding their room when they move constantly and will appear to be even worse off than they really are. This might possibly add to their "complex medical needs" and result in a higher Medicare reimbursement to the nursing home. If the patient is clearly confused, the nursing home should coordinate with his family regarding room changes.

Patients also have the right to request room changes, and the nursing home must do its best to accommodate their wishes. Patients who prefer the room colder can room together, as can those who like the same television shows. It's difficult to get along with someone in the bed next to you; it would be the same thing as staying in a motel room with someone you've never met. Sometimes it takes several moves before a patient is satisfied with his roommate, and each move can be difficult for the patient. Change is difficult, and the patient will need extra support making the room more "home-like" each time. Sometimes the nursing home staff is able to help with the transition, but it's helpful if the family is able to assist with moving the patient's personal items and hang his photos on the wall where he wants them to be. If at all possible, give the patient as much opportunity as possible to make choices about decorating his room.

Patient Abuse/Neglect/Exploitation

Some nursing homes provide excellent, patient-based care and there is no reason that the family will need to worry about the safety & well-being of the patient. Many nursing home staff members are top-notch and truly care about the patients in their charge. Nursing homes are required to have many checks and balances to ensure that patients aren't mistreated, which is great as long as they actually follow their policies.

But, then there are those nursing home staff members who treat their patients more like inmates than as people who are deserving of care, compassion and dignity. It is important to choose a facility carefully and to visit often, not just during visiting hours, but also at different times. It's possible that patients are being mistreated and are afraid to say anything for fear of retaliation. Listen to the patient; if she is constantly complaining about a specific staff member, it's possible that there is a problem that needs to be addressed.

If patients are truly being abused, it's possible that one staff member might be responsible for the mistreatment. It's also possible that the problem is systemic (with the full knowledge and permission of the administrative team). Don't trust that the nice social worker isn't part of the problem; there have been cases of social workers stealing money from patients or participating in neglect. You can always speak with the administrator, but you should also feel free to report your suspicions to the ombudsman and/or licensing agencies whose missions are to keep patients safe and well-cared for.

Patients are at the mercy of the nursing home staff because all of their needs must be met by the facility. If the problems are systemic, it might make things worse for those patients who complain about the way that they've been treated. Patients might not receive their pain medications on time or at all, their movements throughout the facility might be restricted or they might be forced to room with someone who screams constantly as a punishment for their complaints. The nursing staff can document that patients are confused or agitated, and in response the doctor might prescribe medications that further impair their thinking. Patients are understandably concerned about filing a complaint, because doing so can create problems far worse than those they complained about in the first place.

If a patient tells a family member that he is being abused or that he has witnessed abuse, it's vital that the incident be reported immediately. A family member should be able to report his concerns to any employee, as every member of the staff is a *mandated reporter* required by law to report any suspected abuse or neglect. Additionally, every nursing home is required to designate one staff member as the facility *Abuse Coordinator*. In most cases, the abuse coordinator is either the administrator or the director of social services; it's their job to immediately report the incident to the state and ensure that an internal investigation is begun

Be cautious when speaking to the staff; it's possible that the staff members or even the administrator himself is part of the problem and that a report of abuse will go no further. This is why it's vital that the family or patient also contact the ombudsman or state licensure agency with their concerns in addition to reporting it to the administrator. Nursing homes are required to post the phone numbers to make such complaints in public areas. I've also included the contact information for each state's ombudsman agency in the chapter "*Nursing Home Survey Agencies*." Don't be concerned that you are unnecessarily involving a state agency; the facility itself should already have done so as part of their protocol. I've seen administrators who were fired as a result of such investigations.

Remember that the complaints of patients diagnosed with dementia or paranoia might not be taken seriously, but their concerns might be valid. A formal investigation will provide insight into the issue. Elderly patients have tender skin, and it's possible that bruising isn't an indication of abuse, but it's also possible that the patient is being harmed. If you aren't satisfied with the nursing home's response, feel free to take a dated photo of a wound for proof (you should only take a photo of your family member; otherwise you could be invading another patient's privacy). If the nursing home staff treats the patient any differently after the complaint has been made, that also needs to be reported to the state. Any abusive or inappropriate behaviors that are observed while visiting a patient should be reported immediately, even if the victim isn't your family member.

If you've taken a photo or video of suspected abuse, the nursing home staff members might immediately demand that you give them the camera or camera-phone. Do not surrender the camera; leave the facility immediately and call the police if the staff attempts to impede your exit. Refer them to your family attorney if you have one. Even confused patients are aware of abuse: a patient once told me that other patients were being physically shaken by a facility LPN and the family believed the nurse when she told them that the patient was paranoid; a full investigation later found that the nurse was truly abusing patients and that the administrator had known of her behaviors for years.

I've known of family members who brought in tape recorders so that they could prove the patient was abused; it's a good idea to speak with an attorney before conducting a personal investigation to ensure that the investigator is acting legally. In some states it's illegal to record someone without their knowledge; also, the facility can accuse the person recording of violating patient confidentiality and threaten them will all sorts of legal action in an attempt to intimidate them. Patients already feel vulnerable, but when they've participated in a formal investigation the staff might attempt to change the patient's story through any means possible, including intimidation and threats.

Don't assume that every staff member is aware of an ongoing abuse investigation and that they are part of a vast conspiracy; each employee will only know what his supervisor tells him. Obviously, a staff member who is suspected of abusing patients isn't going to share this information with many people. If you report your concerns, keep notes of the date you reported, to whom and an overview of the conversation. Document their response, if any.

Remember that most elder protective agencies have up to 72 hours to respond; if you believe that the patient is in immediate danger call 911. You have the right to call 911 at any time; describe the situation and they will send out someone to investigate the matter. Ask for the event number, and provide it to elder protective services when you call to report.

When a staff member reports abuse, the nursing home can either help to investigate or attempt to cover it up. In those facilities with a history of abuse & neglect, it's common for the administration to retaliate against staff members suspected of participating in the reporting or subsequent investigation. This is because an investigation such as this can result in thousands of dollars in fines (and potentially millions of dollars in lawsuits). Even though the state attempts to keep confidential the names of those staff members who cooperated, it usually doesn't take a rocket scientist to figure out who they are. The rest of the staff will become immediately aware of their firings, and will probably refuse to cooperate with the complaint investigation in order to preserve their jobs. Once a worker has been branded as cooperative in a state investigation, it's possible that he or she will have a tough time obtaining a job in the industry again. These issues can get nasty real quick and an unscrupulous nursing home can ruin people in an attempt to defend itself against allegations of abuse & neglect.

Once allegations of abuse have been substantiated, the facility will hire a law firm that specializes in fighting nursing home inspection results and complaint investigations. They will use all sorts of tactics to fight charges on behalf of their clients. These appeals take time; if the process runs long enough those patients who were compromised are either too confused to cooperate or have died. This makes the charges much harder to prove. The nursing home will probably do everything possible to impugn the integrity of those employees who cooperated with the state in an attempt to shift the blame from the responsible parties. The system isn't set up to protect the employees and there's rarely a positive outcome for those workers strong enough to report abuse in a facility. Unless a staff member who is aware of abuse holds a professional license that requires he participate in such an investigation, it's doubtful that he will place his livelihood in jeopardy by cooperating. In today's economy, nursing home staff members are as afraid of losing their jobs as everyone else and unless they have direct knowledge of abuse, they will avoid any participation in a state investigation. It's doubtful that they will even call the company's compliance hotline due to the fear of retaliation.

Even those workers who hold professional licenses will do everything possible to avoid becoming entangled in an investigation of abuse and neglect in a nursing home. These workers are placed in a precarious position; they are mandated to report and to cooperate in a resulting investigation – and can lose their license if it can be proven that they were aware and didn't report – yet if they do report they might end up being forced to defend their professional license. A common method that the nursing home will use is to file complaints against the worker's professional license to retaliate against them for their cooperation (and to "encourage" them to stop cooperating). Families need to pay attention to the goings on and remain strong advocates for their loved ones in nursing homes and other medical facilities. Most of the time, unless the worker feels strongly about the abuse and is absolutely positive that it's occurring, he will avoid any participation with the investigation.

Do your homework; before a patient is admitted into a nursing home, it's best to contact the state licensing bureau and ask for the most current 2567 form and the outcome of any formal complaint investigations; it's also advisable to contact the state long-term care administrator's board to see if the administrator's license has ever been placed on probation for any reason. Even if the facility is the only one in town, it's much better to place a family member in a facility that's further away than to send them to a nursing home with a history of abuse. Unless the patient's choice is limited because of payment source, research all caregiving available options in the area.

Don't trust that the parent corporation of the nursing home is providing adequate oversight. All that the company knows is what the administrator reports to them, and the administrator might very well be part of the problem. The parent corporation is ultimately interested in the profits that the administrator brings in, and unless there is strong evidence of misconduct the company will stand firmly behind the administrative team. In most cases, the parent corporation will defend the facility rather than to investigate complaints. Don't be mistaken in thinking that a newer nursing home is better than an older one; just because they have a beautiful facility and haven't been in business very long doesn't mean that they're doing a great job. All that it takes is one bad employee, and patients can suffer.

In addition to physical abuse, patients can be neglected. Facilities that are understaffed might not have enough C.N.A.'s to toilet patients, meaning that an incontinent patient might lay in his own urine/feces for hours. This can cause skin breakdown resulting in life-threatening infections. If your family member appears to be in pain, check under the covers to see if his skin is intact and report it to the nurse immediately if there are open wounds. Another type of neglect is lack of feeding those patients who aren't able to feed themselves; they might be forced to sit in front of their food tray without the ability of eating it. If your family member isn't able to feed himself, visit the facility during meal times and ensure that he's eating. If he isn't being fed, speak with the administrative staff and call the ombudsman or state licensing agency.

Patients do have the right to refuse to shower; if your family member smells as if he isn't being bathed, speak with the administrative team and see if you can help to convince him to bathe. It's possible that he doesn't feel like showering, but it's also possible that the staff isn't caring in its approach to showering patients and they need to change their procedures or train their staff.

There are many types of neglect; patients should have access to water, be able to maneuver throughout the facility (within reason), to participate in activities and should be able to access snacks whether or not they are overweight. They have the right to be free from pain and should have the ability to complain about the way that they are being treated without the fear of retaliation by staff.

Nursing home residents can be also exploited financially – I've had patients and their families report to me that staff members complained to them about their home situation and how poor they are. One patient wrote a check for $10,000 to an employee, and when I reported it to the administrator she told the family that she didn't recognize the name on the check. The investigation went no further; but about a year later it was discovered that the billing office manager had embezzled well over a hundred thousand dollars from the nursing home by using aliases to cash checks. Had the $10,000 check been reported at the time, it's possible that she could have been caught much sooner – and it's also possible that the employee would have been prosecuted for exploitation of an elderly person, rather than the lesser theft charges she eventually faced. She was out of jail in less than a year, and will never truly be held accountable for her actions.

Nursing home residents should not "tip" staff members, nor should they offer Christmas bonuses or other financial incentives to employees. It's actually illegal for workers who are paid by federal monies to accept additional payments from patients and/or their families. Generally speaking, workers shouldn't accept anything with a value of more than $20 and it should never be cash. If you want to express your appreciation toward the staff or a specific staff member, buy them chocolate, but they aren't allowed to accept gifts. I've worked for facilities where the family members bought pizza for all of the workers on shift; before doing so, check with the administrator or the charge nurse to make sure it's okay.

Nursing homes can be wonderful, caring places or can be horrible, controlling environments. Patients who file multiple complaints with no resolution might be making up the whole thing, or their problems might just be the tip of the iceberg. Nursing homes are required to run federal background checks of their employees, but if an employee hasn't been convicted of a crime the facility might not be aware of the worker's history. If the accused employee is a close friend of the administrator, the complaints might not be investigated or will be covered up during an investigation.

It's also possible that patients are confused, and their allegations of abuse aren't true. The ombudsman can help to either substantiate or clear the nursing home's reputation. Patients who complain of neglect might be expecting personal service 24/7, which simply isn't possible; or they might be angry at a specific staff member. I've seen situations where patients and their families lie about abuse in an attempt to get a staff member fired, or in an attempt to get the facility to settle and make some quick money. One nursing home administrator told me that attorneys are taught that there's always money to be made when suing a nursing home. and that corporations will settle quickly rather than to suffer the publicity.

There are many situations that sound abusive on the surface, but when investigated they're found to have been baseless accusations. According to CMS, there are over 16,000 nursing homes in the United States providing patient care. The majority of these facilities provide excellent service and work hard to help their patients, but abuse does happen. Even though it is difficult to prove abuse, neglect or exploitation, if a family member believes that the patient is being mistreated they should do everything possible to ensure his safety. Simply reporting it to the nursing home staff might not be enough. Call the ombudsman, the licensing agency and if necessary, contact an attorney. It's important that patients be kept safe and are free from retaliation when reporting suspected abuse.

Leaving Against Medical Advice (AMA)

Patients who are sent to nursing homes – whether on a long-term or short-term basis – have the right to leave whenever they would like. As long as the patient has the capacity to make this decision, the nursing home can't keep him from leaving. Those patients who lack the capacity to make such a decision can leave with the help of a family member, the person designated as power of attorney or legal guardian, and the nursing home should do everything possible to assist with discharge planning. However, as discussed in the chapter **Methods Nursing Homes Use To Maximize Revenue**, nursing homes often do their best to delay patient discharges by several days or even weeks in order to maximize their Medicare payments.

Nursing homes, hospitals and other practitioners often tell patients that their insurance company won't pay their bills if they leave *AMA (against medical advice)*, but this isn't always true. The medical provider is usually paid because the services were provided; in fact, it's doubtful that the payment will be delayed at all. The insurance company might be hesitant to authorize another admission within 30 days for the same reason; however, in most cases the bill will be paid without a second thought.

This doesn't mean that the patient won't encounter some problems if he chooses to leave AMA. Nursing homes and other medical facilities aren't able to set up aftercare services if the patient leaves on his own due to liability issues. Basically it's either one of two scenarios: 1) the patient is being discharged as part of his treatment plan and the nursing home will set up aftercare services, or 2) he's leaving on his own and the nursing home isn't able to assist with any part of the arrangements. It can be difficult for patients who require transportation, medications, home healthcare, equipment, therapies, etc after they leave. If at all possible, it's best to work with the nursing home to ensure that the patient will be discharged according to their protocol so he will continue to recover at home. Most doctors will give a discharge order if they're advised that a patient will otherwise leave AMA in order to ensure that the patient receives services when he's discharged. The doctor also has a healthy fear of having to deal with a lengthy and uncomfortable state and/or federal investigation if the patient reports that a facility is delaying his discharge.

If the patient chooses to leave AMA, the social worker might be able to offer a list of agencies in the community, but she isn't able to assist with arranging for aftercare services. It's possible that the nursing home will make a referral to Elder Protective Services or another agency to check up on the patient after he's left the facility. The call might be made whether or not the facility staff believes that the discharge is unsafe; it's generally part of their protocol to cover their liability in case the patient encounters problems after discharge. The nursing home is not allowed to physically block a discharge unless they believe that the patient is in physical danger by leaving the facility – but in those cases they can only block the patient's discharge until the police arrive. In many instances, staff members threaten the patient and/or his family with referrals to Elder Protective Services in order to delay the discharge; during this time, the facility continues to bill Medicare hundreds of dollars each day.

One way to obtain services after a patient has left a facility against medical advice is to call his primary (home) physician and explain the situation. He will probably have the patient come into his office to be seen and will order all of the necessary equipment and/or home healthcare services from there. If the patient doesn't have a primary physician or the wait to be seen will be too long, it's possible to access care by calling a home health agency directly and having their medical director provide the orders to be seen.

While leaving AMA isn't the best choice, if a patient is ready to leave and the nursing home is delaying the discharge it might be the only viable option. Nursing homes must report AMA's to their parent corporation and defend them to the state, so they will often assist with a discharge if they feel that they have no other options. I actually witnessed an extreme case, where the nursing home administrator herself threatened a family with having them arrested when they attempted to remove a patient from the nursing home; the family backed down and the nursing home continued to bill Medicare for another week before the family wised up and brought the patient home. I reported this to the state bureau, and to the parent corporation. She no longer works for that company.

Discharge Planning Concerns

Planning for the patient's discharge starts the date that he arrives in the nursing home. The discharge plan can be anything from "transfer to home," to "long-term care." Federal requirements mandate that the patient must have a discharge plan written in the chart, and documentation that proves that the patient and nursing home are working to help him attain his goal. The discharge plan is developed with the patient and his family, and can't be the one that the nursing home decides is in his best interest.

Discharges are often delayed so that nursing homes can continue to bill Medicare at the very high rates that are paid for rehabilitation. Patients and their family members mistakenly believe that the nursing home has the right (and the power) to delay the discharge and that the facility is acting in the patient's best interest. However, patients have the right to leave, even if the nursing home believes that the patient is making a poor choice by leaving. Patients have the right to self-determination, meaning that they have the right to make choices no matter how poor the nursing home might consider them to be. And so, nursing homes utilize delaying tactics in the hopes that patients & families won't realize that's what they're doing.

It's possible for a facility to delay a patient's discharge without appearing to be blatantly unethical. It's common practice for a patient and family to be summoned for a "discharge planning meeting" prior to his leaving – and for the facility to delay this meeting for several weeks. These meetings aren't required and can't be used as a delaying tactic. All that a patient or family must do is refuse to attend this meeting and request an immediate discharge. If the facility refuses, call the ombudsman or state licensing agency. It's amazing how fast the meeting will be held (or dismissed) once the state has become involved.

Another method that facilities use to delay the discharge process is to use the excuse that the doctor won't discharge the patient, when in actuality he hasn't even been contacted. A way to address this is to call the doctor yourself and let his staff know that the facility is unnecessarily delaying the patient's discharge. If the doctor isn't responsive, feel free to call the ombudsman or state licensing agency – both the doctor and the nursing home usually want to avoid contact with these agencies if at all possible.

It's possible for the nursing home to delay the discharge by calling the doctor and telling him that the patient isn't ready to be discharged or that his home situation is "unsafe." It's important to remember that the treating physician probably won't know the patient well, with all of the information he knows about the patient having been provided by staff nurses who have been instructed by administration to delay the discharge. All that the nursing home staff must do is imply that the patient's home situation is unsafe, and the doctor probably won't be willing to discharge him until a "safe discharge" can be arranged. This could delay the discharge for weeks, during which the nursing home will continue to bill handsomely for his care. It's important to note that nursing homes can't block a discharge or dictate the environment to which the patient will be discharged; they can only call Elder Protective Services after the patient has left the building.

The facility might also attempt to delay a patient's discharge by telling him that he must have written prescriptions to take with him when he leaves, and that they're having difficulty obtaining them from his physician. However, they don't tell you that these prescriptions can be called into a pharmacy with no problem. The nursing home also must send the remainder of the patient's medications home with him when he leaves. Some facilities have policies that won't allow for patients to take controlled substances with them, even though in most states the medications are the property of the patient and he should be free to take them with him when he leaves. A quick call to the state licensing agency can resolve this issue (this tactic might not be helpful after hours or on weekends).

Physicians are independent contractors; they won't receive as many patients from the nursing home if they fall out of favor with administration. This is often why doctors tend to follow the nursing home's recommendations regarding patient care (including delaying discharges). However, if the family were to call his office and explain that there is a good caregiving plan in place and the patient has a safe place to go, the doctor will probably change his mind. Again, doctors who follow patients in nursing homes often only see their patients upon admission and sporadically thereafter; even though they are responsible for the patient's medical care they generally follow the nursing home's recommendations.

As mentioned earlier in this book, nursing homes can't dump patients out on the street because they don't have a payment source. However, it's different if the patient chooses to leave the facility and is capable of making that decision. The nursing home can't legally block a patient's discharge if he is competent, even if it's their opinion that the patient has unreasonable expectations. Sometimes nursing homes will call the ombudsman and ask them to speak with the patient in the hopes that he will agree to stay and allow the staff assist in developing a safer discharge plan. However, if the patient wants to leave, is able to make the decision and has the ability to follow through with his plans he has every right to do so.

For those patients without a payment source, it's a different story altogether. Nursing homes might make the decision easier by encouraging the patient to walk out the door. They can do this by telling him that every day he stays, he and his family will be billed hundreds (or thousands) of dollars – but if he leaves they'll discount the bill. They can also attempt to make his stay unbearable so that he'll want to leave, which solves the non-payment problem. Once he's been discharged, the facility is no longer responsible for his care. The facility can't be held responsible if a competent person makes informed choices as long as the staff members document their discussions with the patient.

Nursing homes can't place unreasonable demands on patients before they're "allowed" to leave. I knew of a nursing home administrator who told a patient with a history of alcoholism that she couldn't leave the facility until she went to AA meetings every day for a month before she left. There weren't daily AA meeting offered in the town where the facility was located. After a call to the ombudsman, the patient was discharged home where she remained until her death over two years later.

Nursing homes aren't prisons, and patients can't be forced to stay against their will. The administrator can't require that a patient have counseling or meet with a psychologist before he is discharged, and can't block the discharge in any other way. Patients have the right to discuss their discharge plans with an agency that is called a "Local Contact Agency" (as mandated by the Centers for Medicare & Medicaid Services); it's possible that these agencies will be able to assist with community referrals. Unfortunately, people aren't aware that the nursing home must provide a private area for patients to make telephone calls, which can be a barrier to patients being able to discuss their concerns with a state agency or complaint investigator. Most nursing homes are willing to assist patients in setting up a safe discharge plan, but if you believe that a nursing home is delaying a discharge you have the right to speak with the ombudsman or state licensing agency about this issue.

Patients in the process of being discharged from nursing homes must be provided with access to appropriate follow-up care from the provider of their choice; they must be provided with any medical equipment that they need such as oxygen, wheelchairs, walkers, referral to a medical equipment company and a home health agency as needed. They also must have the ability to obtain their medications. If the patient isn't able to afford these items, the nursing home must make every effort to obtain them for him and to refer him to any program that might help with payment. If the patient can't afford the equipment and has no reasonable chance of success in obtaining the items, the nursing home is required to discuss this with him as well. The patient has the right to refuse any follow-up care he chooses as long as he has the capacity to make these decisions.

Nursing homes can't limit the patient's choice of aftercare providers, such as home healthcare agencies or equipment providers, unless the patient's insurance plan limits these options to their contracted providers. If a nursing home refuses to refer to an agency you request, you have the right to call that agency yourself and to complain to the state licensing agency. It's highly illegal for agencies to provide kickbacks or incentives to nursing homes in order to obtain more referrals, but it happens all of the time.

Nursing home patients have the right to refuse to leave, and the nursing home must then go through a formal eviction process. If the patient requires placement, doesn't qualify for Medicaid and can't afford to pay, no judge will force him to leave and the nursing home might be stuck with him for years. If the non-paying patient is physically able to discharge but can't afford to go anywhere else, the nursing home might possibly make arrangements for him to go somewhere else and pay for him for awhile. Most facilities are too smart to accept such a patient because "once the head is in the bed," they become responsible to care for him. This is why the nursing home does its best to research the patient's history before he is admitted.

The patient who has nowhere to go might receive a discharge known in the industry as ***Greyhound Therapy***. This is where a patient is placed on a bus, with the facility paying for the cost of the ticket, and sent to another city or state. Their instructions to the patient are to find a shelter or go to a local hospital for assistance upon their arrival. The state of Nevada has recently been in the news for allegedly providing greyhound therapy to mentally ill people. Although patients have the right to leave the area and return to their home state, the facility is responsible to set up an aftercare plan. Medical providers are paid handsomely for the care that they provide while the patient is there and can't simply dump patients out with no assistance.

If the patient no longer requires the level of care that the nursing home provides – or even if the nursing home simply wants to get rid of him – it is the nursing home's responsibility to find him another place that he can afford and is able to meet his needs. For the non-funded patient, the social worker might have to get creative by finding placement in another city or even another state. Patients who have no income might need assistance with applying for financial assistance, including transportation to social service agencies. If the social worker finds an apartment that can meet his needs, she might have to assist with finding furniture and other household items. This is all part of the discharge plan

If he was homeless when he arrived, he has the right to go back to the streets if he chooses but the nursing home is required to find as many resources for him as possible and this must be documented in his patient chart. However, if he lost his home when he was admitted (for example, was evicted from his apartment), the nursing home has to help him find another apartment that he can afford and to ensure that he has furniture and food that meets his needs. The nursing home social worker can do this on her own, or can use local agencies to assist with this endeavor.

Local Contact Agencies

It used to be that patients who hoped to discharge from nursing homes were at the facility's mercy when it came to discharge planning. If the nursing home didn't want the patient to leave, they would do everything possible to block the discharge. A recent addition to the MDS assessment is the discharge planning area, where patients can ask to speak with a *Local Contact Agency*. This is an agency federally designated to accept referrals from nursing homes and to provide information and assistance in accessing community resources. Nursing homes are required to work with these agencies to ensure that the patients needs will be met upon discharge. Nursing homes don't have to wait for an MDS assessment to trigger a referral to an agency; they can refer to these agencies at any time. These agencies can be valuable tools in helping a patient to access community services.

Local contact agencies also link patients to agencies that can provide assistance under the *Olmstead decision (1999)*, a lawsuit that paved the way for patients who reside in nursing homes to be discharged to a lower level of care with the help of community programs. Each state has implemented a Medicaid-based program that helps these patients so that they can return to the community, although the programs and the method in which they provide services can vary from state-to-state. The rules are complicated; patients must be able to maintain their independence with the program's assistance; however, if their care needs are too great they probably won't qualify for the program.

Nursing homes that don't want to discharge their patients can instruct their staff members to check "No" in the box on the MDS that asks about whether the patient would like to speak with an outside agency. Unless the person completing the form holds a professional license (such as a social worker), there's no guarantee that the nursing home staff member will make a referral to the local contact agency. I worked for a nursing home administrator who refused to allow staff members to refer to local contact agencies; in an extremely uncomfortable meeting, she screamed at several staff members and threatened us with our jobs. This clearly violated Medicare policies, and we continued to refer to the local contact agencies anyway. When the agency workers came into the facility, she insisted that they check in with her first and monitored their interactions with the patients. She was later fired for such behaviors when I and several other staff members called both the company and the state regulatory agency to report her. She still works in the industry.

The nursing home is required to post notifications throughout the facility offering information about local contact agencies – but a patient in a wheelchair might not notice a sign that's posted at the average person's eye level. Family members might not even be aware that this assistance exists. It is federally mandated that nursing home social workers contact these agencies if the patient asks for assistance in discharging; if the nursing home refuses to give a patient the phone number and access to a phone to call the ombudsman, state licensing agency or Area Agency on Aging, have a family member help you call the local contact agency as well as to open an investigation into the nursing home's discharge practices. You can also report any licensed personnel to their licensing board, such as the social work board, nursing board, etc.

30-Day Notice to Evict

As mentioned previously, nursing homes do have the right to legally evict patients. According to the Code of Federal Regulations (CFR) 483.12 the only legitimate reasons that a patient can be discharged from a nursing home are as follows:

- The transfer or discharge is necessary to meet the resident's welfare; and the resident's welfare cannot be met in the facility; (i.e. resident requires hospitalization);
- Resident is physically well enough to be discharged to a lower level of care and no longer requires nursing home placement;
- The resident has become a danger to themselves or others in the facility;
- The resident's health status is a danger to others in the facility; (i.e. he has been diagnosed with an infectious disease)
- The resident has failed to pay their bill after a reasonable amount of time and appropriate notice (rules vary by state); or
- The facility ceases to operate.

The need for all discharges must be appropriately documented by physicians and clinical staff. It's up to the doctor as to whether he prefers to actually see the patient for a face-to-face interview for the purpose of documenting the need for a discharge; the term "physician's documentation" is open to interpretation. Whether the physician's documentation is written by a nurse on a telephone order or on a progress note during a face-to-face interview, in some manner the need for the patient's discharge must be written in the patient's chart by the MD (telephone orders are forwarded to doctors for their signatures at a later date).

The nursing home has to meet specific federal and state requirements by serving the patient or his responsible party with a minimum of a 30-day notice that must include the following information:

- The reason for transfer/ discharge.

- The date of the proposed transfer/ discharge.

- The location to which the nursing facility proposes the patient be transferred or discharged (the discharging facility must find a place that is able to meet the patient's needs).

- The patient's right to a hearing to appeal the transfer/discharge.

- The procedures the patient must follow to request a hearing.

- The date by which you must request a hearing in order to prevent the transfer/ discharge.

- Resident's right to representation at the hearing.

- If the resident is being transferred to a hospital (unless it's an emergency); information regarding the facility's bed hold policy and the facility's policies regarding readmission to the facility.

- Contact information for the Long-term Care Ombudsman.

If the 30-Day Notice doesn't meet every federal and state guideline, it must be reissued and the 30-day period starts all over again. However, even if the form is completed correctly the patient can refuse to leave and the process can drag on for years. Simply stated, if the patient wants to leave, it's his right to do so. On the other hand, if the nursing home wants to evict him, they'll have a difficult time making him leave. The laws are on the side of the patient in nearly every instance.

Regardless of the reason he's leaving, the facility is responsible to arrange for a safe and appropriate discharge if at all possible. It's important to remember that the patient is able to refuse to leave or to allow the facility to assist him in developing a discharge plan. There was a case in Florida of a patient residing in a hospital for over 1,000 days because the family refused to allow him to be discharged to the closest appropriate nursing home, about 50 miles away. This certainly isn't a typical situation, but most nursing homes or hospitals are afraid of the publicity and the possibility of state & federal sanctions that result from their attempts to force a patient to leave a nursing home or hospital.

There are those rare cases that patients have no payment source available to pay for placement elsewhere and there's simply no viable discharge plan. It's less expensive for a facility to continue to care for a patient in-house rather than to pay for him to go elsewhere, which helps to explain those patients who remain in acute hospitals for months on end.

Nursing Home-Based Hospice Care

Hospices provide care to patients in a nursing home in the same manner as if they lived in their own homes; they instruct the caregivers (nursing home staff) how to care for the patients and provide all of the same items as if the patient was living at home. Additionally, the hospice will send in staff members to supplement the care that their patients receive in the facility. Medicare will pay for hospice in a nursing home, even if the patient's room & board are paid by the institutional Medicaid benefit. In order to provide care in a nursing home, the hospice must have a contract with that facility that specifies the services each company will provide to its patients. Hospices sell their services to nursing homes by stating that the patients, their families, and the nursing home all benefit from the extra care that the hospice provides. Sometimes they do, but sometimes the additional care provided by the hospice doesn't appear to make a difference to the patient or family at all. Every situation is different.

Medicaid reduces its payments to the nursing home by 5% for those patients whose nursing home room & board are paid by the Medicaid benefit. This is because some of the services that the hospice provides are considered to be a duplication of the services Medicaid is paying the nursing home to provide (an example would be the personal care provided by the nursing home's aides). The federal government does allow the hospice to pay that 5% back to the nursing home without considering it to be a kickback. Not all hospices choose to pay the 5%; it's up to each hospice agency as to whether it wishes to do. If a hospice doesn't pay the difference it's possible that the nursing home won't renew its contract to provide service to its patients. Besides that 5%, the hospice isn't allowed to offer any additional money or services to the nursing home in return for referrals.

A nursing home is still able to benefit financially by its patients being on hospice by saving money on supplies that the hospice will provide. The nursing home is required to provide supplies and specialty equipment to Medicaid recipients at no extra cost to the patients, meaning that the nursing home "eats" the cost of these items. Hospice patients will receive these items from the hospice, saving the nursing home hundreds of dollars each month. As long as the patient benefits from the additional care the hospice provides and meets the clinical criteria to be considered terminal, it's a win-win situation. If the only benefit appears to be to the nursing home, however, this can be considered an abuse of the system.

The patient who is paying a nursing home privately for his room and board will also benefit financially from the hospice care by saving money on equipment, briefs, supplies, and other types of care for which he would normally pay out of his pocket. He will also save the cost of oxygen, which could be several hundred dollars per month. In many cases, Medicare pays thousands of dollars for hospice care in order to save the patient or nursing home hundreds of dollars in ancillary charges. Hopefully the patient will also benefit from the extra care that the hospice provides.

If a patient has significant pain issues, or has greater needs than the nursing home can address on its own, it might be beneficial to the nursing home and patient to have a hospice providing the additional oversight. Hospice nurses are trained in pain management and are able to use combinations of medications to alleviate a patient's discomfort; standard nursing home protocols often don't allow these medications unless the patient is receiving services from a palliative care team (hospice). This assumes that the nursing home is willing to work closely with the hospice and will administer the medications to the patient as directed, although some nursing home staff members won't follow the hospice protocol and their patients aren't able to benefit from the hospice intervention.

If the family requires emotional support beyond what the nursing home might offer, it might be in the patient's or family's best interest to utilize the hospice social worker or chaplain for counseling. The hospice social worker can also assist the family with making funeral arrangements, referrals for financial assistance, and provide emotional support that the nursing home staff simply doesn't have time to offer. Unfortunately, nursing home social workers are often buried in federally mandated paperwork and meetings, which significantly limits the amount of time and support they are able to provide to patients and their families.

The Medicare Part A program will pay a nursing home to provide rehabilitation and skilled nursing care, or will pay for hospice – but doesn't pay for both services at the same time (except in extreme cases). If a patient is receiving services under Medicare Part A, the nursing home will probably do everything possible to keep the patient from signing onto a hospice program. This is because nursing homes receive their greatest profits from billing under Medicare Part A, and allowing the patient to sign onto hospice means a potential loss of thousands of dollars in billed charges. The nursing home administrator who is looking at the financial bottom line might not care if the patient has pain or symptoms that could be better managed by the palliative care specialists of hospice. It's common for patients to wait to start to receive hospice care because the nursing home is billing every possible dime from Medicare. This can be hell for the patient who is in pain or distress, because they aren't told that they can elect the hospice benefit at any time.

I've personally witnessed therapists forcing physical therapy onto an actively dying patient for no other reason than to continue billing Medicare for aggressive treatment. Nursing home administrators will often do whatever they can to discourage hospice intervention, and might not allow family members to stop aggressive treatments by insisting that they don't have the right to make such a decision. There are tens of thousands of dollars on the line, and often the administrator has little corporate oversight and is free to act however he wishes.

Families often trust the nursing home staff recommendations and will allow therapies to continue because they don't know the difference. The doctor, who rarely visits nursing home patients (the usual minimum requirement is every other month), receives all of his information about the patient from the nursing home staff and often follows the nurse's recommendations. He might not realize how poorly the patient is doing, and will be met with resistance if he refers a patient to hospice while the nursing home wishes to continue billing for therapies. I once sat in on a meeting in a small-town nursing home where the family – who personally knew the Assistant Director of Nursing – accepted her recommendation to use medications to stimulate a dying woman's appetite in order for the nursing home to continue billing for additional therapies. The patient was in horrendous amounts of pain and it was difficult to watch her suffer through therapies, but the Medicare (patients receiving rehabilitation services) census was low and the administrator insisted that every patient receive the maximum amount of services. The patient died a week later, receiving therapy until the end.

Some nursing homes even offer special Medicare approved palliative care programs in an attempt to keep their patients from signing onto a hospice program, allowing the facility to receive a substantially higher rate of payment than if the patient were to choose to receive hospice care and pay the nursing home for room & board. In nearly every case, a palliative care program (or hospice referral) will be offered only after every attempt has been made to coerce a patient into receiving as much therapy as possible. Nursing home staff members refer to this as "rehabilitating the patient to death."

It's important to understand that families don't have to request services from a hospice program in order to accommodate for dying patients. Nursing homes are often able to make patients comfortable without the extra step of involving a hospice program. However, if a nursing home patient appears to be in pain or distress it's best to ask the doctor for a hospice referral (or call a hospice directly). You have the right to choose a hospice (nursing homes are required to contract with more than one provider). Regardless of what the nursing home might want, patients and families have the right to request a hospice evaluation – and an honest hospice will only sign the patient onto service if the patient is actually terminal.

Dying with Dignity

Patients are usually admitted to the nursing home for the final years of their lives. The nursing home is required to do everything possible to assist the patient to maintain his weight and good health, but eventually he'll die anyway. The nursing home might recommend medications that will to stimulate his appetite and therapy to help maintain his strength and balance, but the patient and his family have the right to refuse these treatments. If the nursing home provides good patient care, they'll order medications to keep the patient as comfortable as possible as he goes through the dying process. If they're not successful, the family should call the doctor to request hospice (or call their preferred hospice directly).

Patients die every day in nursing homes without utilizing the services of hospice care, and there's often no reason that they have to elect to use hospice services. Sometimes however, it's easier for the nursing home's staff to have him on hospice, because the federal regulations that require patients maintain their highest level of functioning don't apply to those patients being served by a hospice agency. In other words, they're not spending a lot of time completing paperwork that explains what they are doing to keep the patient from declining when a patient is referred to hospice. Of course, there are better reasons than saving the facility paperwork as to why a patient and family should choose to accept hospice care, including pain & symptom management, family support and saving the patient from unnecessary tests and treatments.

The patient who is paying privately for his room & board might face resistance from the nursing home if he or his family requests hospice care. This is because in most cases the nursing home is able to bill patients ancillary fees for items such as oxygen and incontinence supplies at a substantial mark-up (these are the same items for which Medicaid does not pay extra). Signing a private-pay patient onto hospice means that these items will be provided by the hospice, saving the family hundreds or possibly thousands of dollars in ancillary fees each month, depending upon the patient's needs. Facilities don't like losing the revenue and might do everything possible to impede the patient from receiving hospice care.

Hospices specialize in pain & symptom management, and they are able to supplement the care that the nursing home is providing. Hospices are able to use combinations of medications that nursing homes aren't able to provide – and can be beneficial to nursing home patients. It's truly up to the patient and family as to whether they would like to use the services of a hospice, and they have the right to choose which hospice they would prefer (as long as the hospice has a contract with the nursing home).

When the nursing home patient dies, the nurses will call the physician and he will usually allow the facility (or hospice) nurse to pronounce the patient's death. This allows patients to be picked up by the mortuary in a timely manner rather than to have to wait for the doctor to arrive and make the pronouncement. Most nursing homes don't have morgues or holding rooms; they will contact the mortuary and the patient will be picked up within an hour or two. It might be possible for the family to visit the patient before he is transported to the mortuary, but this depends upon how long it will take for the family to arrive at the nursing home. If the patient and/or family haven't designated a mortuary, the nursing home will usually assign the next one from a rotation list of all of the mortuaries in the area. There are often state and local agencies that assist patients in paying for burial, although they usually pay for the minimum service only after they've verified there is no family member who can pay for the services.

Before the mortuary arrives, the nurses and CNA's will clean the patient and possibly remove any jewelry if the family is able to retrieve it. The mortuary handles things from that point on. Whether or not the family has prearranged the services, the mortuary will set an appointment with the family to review the arrangements and complete necessary paperwork.

After the Death or Discharge

After a patient leaves the nursing home, the nursing home must follow its written policies regarding the patient's belongings. Generally speaking, most nursing homes will immediately pack up the patient's items so that the family can pick them up at a later time. They will deep-clean the patient's room to get it ready for a new patient.

If the patient owned a specialty mattress, motorized wheelchair or other piece of equipment, it's up to the family as to what they will do with the items. The staff might do their best to have the family donate the items to the nursing home, but if the nursing home is operated for-profit it isn't possible to take a tax write-off for any items that have been donated. It's also important to recognize that once the items have been donated, the nursing home will charge other patients to use them. There's nothing wrong with donating items to the nursing home as long as you understand these issues. It's worth it to take a little time to find a non-profit entity that could benefit from the donated items, while the patient's estate enjoys the associated tax breaks.

If at all possible, remove expensive items such as laptop computers, cellular phones, etc. from the facility at the time of the patient's death or discharge (or even before, if the patient isn't using them any longer). In most cases, the nursing home will attempt to deny responsibility for any missing items, especially if they weren't listed on the patient's inventory list. If the family pushes the issue, the nursing home will replace items for which the family presents receipts.

Unfortunately, the nursing home administrator might use your grief to its advantage in these situations. If you're not thinking straight, you might sign away your rights regarding replacement of items that have clearly been stolen or misplaced. Don't sign any forms that alleviate the nursing home from responsibility for your family member's missing items without first discussing the issue with the ombudsman or even your attorney.

Any money that was in the patient's trust account might possibly belong to the family; it depends upon the rules of the state in which the patient was located. If the patient was a Medicaid recipient, the Medicaid program might require that the monies be sent to the state. A patient who was the recipient of a Miller Trust will probably forfeit any leftover funds to the state. For additional information about asset recovery, refer to the Medicaid asset recovery program located in your state.

l.e. green

Methods Nursing Homes Use To Maximize Revenue

Nursing homes have experienced numerous cutbacks in their payments from the Medicare and Medicaid programs over the past few years, with many more anticipated in the future. The cutbacks in Medicaid payments have caused nursing homes to rely upon the higher revenue from their Medicare patients to offset their losses. Nursing homes hire consultants whose sole purpose is to maximize profits, which is fine as long as it's not at the expense of the patients. But more and more often these methods infringe upon the patient's rights and the family's plans; they don't realize that they have the upper hand in this matter. The nursing home can't force patients to accept treatments they don't want, nor can they delay a discharge in order to increase their Medicare billings.

Understanding the different tactics that nursing homes use to maximize their profits will help the patient & family to make decisions as to which type of care they will accept or reject. Remember that nursing homes can't mandate the type of service a patient receives, nor can the staff refuse to allow a patient to discharge if he wants to leave. The nursing home can make recommendations as to the patient's treatment plan, but can't force the patient to follow the plan of care.

A simple method of increasing profits is to use every possible diagnosis to describe a patient's condition (an example of "*up-coding*." Nursing homes receive a higher reimbursement for patients who are considered to be medically complex, so it only follows that the nursing homes will do their best to use as many medical diagnoses as possible to describe the patient in order to justify the need for skilled services. Using the information sent from the hospital, a nursing manager will scour the paperwork looking for every diagnosis possible, and will manipulate the information in order to use several diagnoses for one condition. For example, a patient whose physician has documented his diagnoses as "confusion due to Alzheimer's Dementia" can be up-coded as being diagnosed with Alzheimer's disease, Dementia, and Altered Level of Consciousness.

Using such tactics, patients are often diagnosed with conditions they never knew that they had in order for the nursing home to make more money. Nursing homes will say that they are simply transferring the information from the hospital onto their paperwork, but by doing so they're also increasing their revenue. Even though this is an obvious manipulation of the regulations, it's legal. It can be distressing for a patient or his family to find that he has several diagnoses he never knew he had.

CMS is now requiring that nursing homes only be allowed to utilize the codes that correspond to the patient's current treatment; if he isn't actively being treated for a particular condition the nursing home isn't supposed to utilize that diagnosis for billing purposes. An unscrupulous nursing home can report symptoms that the patient doesn't display (or embellish the patient's need for medication) in order to bill at a higher rate. For example, a nursing home can't utilize "High Blood Pressure" as a diagnosis unless the patient is currently being treated for the condition, so the nursing home might report that the patient has elevated blood pressure readings *whether or not they exist* and request the very lowest dose of blood pressure medication in order to use this diagnosis. If the condition was mentioned at all in the discharge paperwork that was sent from the hospital, the patient will probably be actively treated for it.

Another method nursing homes use to increase their Medicare reimbursement is to place a patient with a potentially contagious infection into an isolation room while he is receiving services under the Medicare A skilled benefit. This increases the rate that Medicare pays to the facility, as the patient will require a private room. It would only make sense if the nursing home were to place patients who have been diagnosed with the same infection into the same room, but if they're housed together, the facility can't bill Medicare for a private room.

The moment that same patient no longer qualifies for Medicare he'll be moved to a shared room *whether or not he still has the infection.* The decision to isolate a patient is often made by the administrator for financial reasons, not by the doctor for medical reasons. It's a manipulation of the system in order to bill Medicare at a higher rate, but the practice is legal as long as no patient's health has been placed at risk. Infections are common in facilities, and even if a patient is diagnosed with the same type of infection as his roommate it's difficult to prove cause & effect. It's simply not possible to provide isolation for every patient with an active infection, but it takes on a greater urgency if there's a financial incentive for the nursing home.

Most skilled nursing is provided in concert with therapy services, which greatly increases the amount that Medicare pays the nursing home. For example, a patient who is receiving wound care services and the maximum amount of therapy will provide the highest possible revenue. Patients might be "strongly encouraged" (forced) to participate in the maximum amount of therapy possible whether or not they are actually benefitting from the service. Those patients whose treatments are prohibitively expensive, such as radiation or chemotherapy, might be "strongly encouraged" to participate in physical or occupational therapy in order for the nursing home to turn a profit.

I worked for a nursing home where the administrator sent her staff members in to threaten a patient with being discharged home without services unless she agreed to work harder in the therapy room. She also called the family and told them that the patient would be discharged if she didn't work harder. The patient was participating at her highest level of participation, but that wasn't good enough for this administrator. Her phone calls and threats were illegal and unethical; unfortunately the administrator and her loyal staff members continue to work in the industry because such allegations are hard to prove. In this case, the patient died of cancer before the state was able to investigate.

It's common practice for nursing homes to continue providing therapy to patients up until the day – or nearly the moment – that that they die in order to squeeze every last penny out of them. I was present at a bedside family meeting when a speech therapist bragged to a patient's wife that he had consumed 60% of his lunch (while, as we spoke, the patient lay on the bed, obviously dying). He died about half an hour later; while the nursing home benefitted by being able to charge Medicare for the extra therapy he'd received, his wife hadn't been prepared for his death. It was most inhumane.

Of course, there's always the possibility that the nursing home is billing for therapy it doesn't actually provide. The Medicare program trusts that nursing homes are providing the services for which they bill, but this leaves the door open for fraud. It simply isn't possible to monitor every patient in every nursing home, especially since the agencies that provide oversight have also experienced cutbacks. A nursing home can lie about the amount of therapy provided to the patients or can continue to bill for therapy even though the patient isn't improving. Unless a complaint is filed, it's doubtful that the nursing home will ever be caught. Those nursing homes that have been able to get away with overbilling Medicare for years will continue to do so until someone is willing to come forward, but don't count on that happening; workers who report abuse are ostracized and their careers are irreparably damaged.

Nursing homes are often able to bill for the full 100 days of Medicare Part A services for long-term patients who are first sent to the hospital for three days; the goal for the nursing home is to find a reason to send a patient to the hospital in order to maximize their profits. I worked for a nursing home where the administrator wielded such power that she sent a long-term patient to a hospital to have a feeding tube inserted even though the family clearly stated that they didn't want the patient to have to endure an invasive procedure. The facility was able to bill the Medicare program at the very highest rate until the patient's death three weeks later.

Medical providers aren't supposed to force treatments upon patients; in the abovementioned scenario, the administrator told the family that they would have to go to court to stop the unwanted treatment. That simply wasn't true, but the family members were ignorant of the law and afraid they'd be stuck with thousands of dollars in legal bills, so they chose not to challenge the administrator. A call to the ombudsman would have ended the argument, and if the family had contacted an attorney they probably would have received a sizable settlement from the nursing home and its parent corporation. The problem is that families assume that the administrator is knowledgeable and is acting in the patient's best interest.

Employees are often terrified of losing their jobs, so they don't report such behaviors.

That particular administrator ran the nursing home unobstructed for over six years, with such behaviors as sending patients to a psychiatric ward for three days and billing Medicare for rehabilitation services upon their return (she bragged that she had an "arrangement" with the medical director of the psychiatric unit). She refused to allow the therapy department to stop providing services until she decided that patients had completed their therapy (usually when they had utilized all 100 days of their Medicare benefit). This administrator exhibited many behaviors, but no member of her staff reported her to the corporation due to the power she wielded over their jobs (and careers). She wasn't investigated until a report was filed at the same time that the nursing home failed the same annual inspection three times and was required to pay thousands of dollars in fees. It was only at that point, that the company investigated and fired her.

Other ways that nursing home are able to maximize payment includes cutting back on treatments and supplies. Buying cheaper supplies or cutting back on the number of treatments provided can save the nursing home money in the long run. Nursing homes can get away with providing non-working hospital beds, broken wheelchairs and other equipment as long as no one reports the practice. Nursing homes often use cloth bed pads rather than the more sanitary disposable ones, or use tab-sided briefs rather than the pull-up type.

It's possible for a nursing home to increase a private-pay patient's bill by claiming that he is using supplies and equipment, even if he isn't. The nursing home can make huge profits by applying substantial markups for these items. They can also apply markups to medications; recently a nursing home told one of my clients that the $400 she was billed for non-covered medications was actually $1,200 due to "facility markup."

If your family member is paying privately, buy your own supplies if at all possible and make sure that they are set aside only for the patient. Monitor the medications that the patient receives; if he is able to sign up for drug companies subsidized programs or have them supplied via the Veteran's Administration, he can save hundreds or thousands of dollars each month. Medications can also be ordered from mail order pharmacies in 90-day supplies in an effort to hold down costs. In most instances, it's substantially cheaper to obtain the medications from a private pharmacy and have the commercial pharmacy that serves the nursing home place them in a bubble-pack than to trust that the nursing home has your family member's best interest in mind. Nursing homes are huge profit-driven facilities, and you have the right to hold down costs in whichever way you can.

The latest trend is to delay the discharge for patients receiving services via the Medicare benefit as long as possible in order to maximize profits. The longer the patient remains in the nursing home, the greater the amount billed to Medicare. As mentioned previously, there are many delaying tactics that nursing homes are able to use to accomplish this:

- Requiring a discharge planning meeting before the patient is allowed to leave the nursing home. It's common to set these meetings at least a week in the future. This delaying tactic buys the facility at least seven days.

- Claiming that it takes extra time to set up home health care services, when in actuality this can be accomplished in one day. This delaying tactic can buy the facility several days or weeks.

- Delaying the coordination of home healthcare or equipment that the patient requires, and then refusing to discharge the patient because he has no aftercare services set up. This delaying tactic can buy the facility several days.

- Claiming that it takes time to arrange for medical equipment or specialty supplies to be delivered. In most cases, these deliveries can be arranged the same day the patient is discharged. This delaying tactic can buy the facility several days.

- Refusing to discharge patients on the weekend (or even Friday), claiming that the patient won't be able to receive home health care until the following Monday. This simply isn't true; home health evaluations are performed every day of the week. This delaying tactic buys the facility up to 4 days.

- Blocking or delaying a patient's transfer to another nursing home by refusing to cooperate with the new facility. They might not allow other nursing homes to review their patient charts, insist that the doctor won't allow the discharge, or use every other delaying tactic possible. Once the patient has been accepted by another nursing home, they might refuse to contact the doctor to request a discharge order and transfer summary. The nursing home can insist that the family attend a discharge planning meeting a week or so in the future; these delaying tactic can buy the facility at least a week, usually longer.

- Insisting that the doctor needs to physically see the patient before he is discharged. This is rarely necessary, and any prescriptions can always be called in to the pharmacy. The patient can always follow up with his own doctor when he leaves. This delaying tactic buys the facility up to seven days.

l.e. green

- Claiming that the patient isn't "safe" to return home, with no basis for this determination. Uninformed patients won't know that they have rights, and that the nursing home can't legally block a discharge. At most, the nursing home can call the police in an attempt to stop the patient from leaving. In most instances, the police will consider it to be a civil matter and won't stop a patient from leaving unless he truly appears to be a danger to himself or others – and then the patient is sent to the Emergency Room for a mental health evaluation. The facility can also call elder protective services to follow up if they truly believe that the patient isn't safe, and EPS will follow up within 72-hours.

If your family member is in a nursing home and the staff appears to be using such delaying tactics, you have the right to contact the nursing home ombudsman, state licensing agency, or even your attorney to assist with the discharge. Nursing homes don't like attorneys; if your family member is in a nursing home and they appear to be using delaying tactics (or refuse to discharge him altogether), feel free to call your attorney for assistance. In most cases, just the threat of having an attorney called is enough to encourage the administrator to work with you. The patient can always leave and follow up with his personal physician for referrals if necessary. It shouldn't have to come to this, but unfortunately some facilities will do whatever it takes to delay a discharge in order to bill Medicare for even one more day.

Remember that the nursing home's goal is to make as much money as possible, regardless of whether or not it's run for-profit. Unless a family member (or employee) reports overbilling, refusal to discharge patients or any number of profit-increasing tactics, nursing homes will continue to act in whatever manner they wish.

The cutbacks in programs designed to provide oversight need to be addressed. The funding should be reinstated; ombudsman programs should be staffed by professionals (not volunteers) and the current annual inspection system reviewed to allow for more stringent oversight. Other options, such as implementing a "secret shopper" type of program, might make a difference in the lives of all patients in nursing homes across the United States. If nursing homes were to be required to contribute toward the cost of additional oversight, the industry would change for the better.

Better protections need to be provided to those workers who are willing to report wrongdoing; at the present time, staff members who participate in an investigation are risking their jobs. It doesn't stop there; it's possible that a worker will be forced to defend his professional license and pay for any associated legal bills, whether or not he's working at the time. Additionally, he risks being black-balled in the local medical community and losing his ability to earn a living.

210

Nursing homes are able to retaliate against workers who report fraud and abuse. In the end, the staff members who were brave enough to file a report can end up losing everything while the facility pays a relatively small fine and moves on.

Most nursing homes operate in an above-board manner and are happy to assist their patients in having the best possible experience. Although many nursing homes utilize some of the above-mentioned methods to maximize their revenue, not all of them will do so at the expense of the patient. Most facilities recognize that patients and their families are in charge of their own healthcare decisions, and include them as part of the process. However, those that don't allow patients and their families to participate in developing their plan of care should be held accountable. If you aren't satisfied with the care your family member is receiving, feel free to discuss your concerns with the administrator, ombudsman or state regulatory agency.

At the present time, the odds are stacked in the nursing home's favor. Families must remain diligent in ensuring that patients receive the best care possible. There are ways to address many of these issues; in addition to discussing them with the administrator, feel free to report to the ombudsman, the state licensing agency and even the Medicare & Medicaid hotline for your state. You have the right to advocate for your family member. As the administrator of one facility liked to say, "This is WAR!"

l.e. green

The Nursing Home Bill of Rights

The Nursing Home Reform act of 1987 mandated that patients have certain rights in a facility – and that these rights must be posted in an area where they can be seen by patients and families. The full bill of rights can easily be found online or is hanging on the wall in any nursing home. A copy of the bill of rights is required to be provided in each patient's admissions packet. These resident rights include:

- The right to self-determination.
- The right to be free from abuse & neglect.
- The right to be informed in writing about any services and fees before the patient enters the nursing home.
- The right of a patient to manage his own money, or to choose who will manage his finances for him.
- The right to be free from physical restraints.
- The right to refuse medications and treatments.
- The right to privacy (including for married couples).
- The right to keep and use their belongings as long as they don't infringe upon anyone else's health, safety or well-being.
- The right to make private telephone calls.
- The right to be treated in a dignified and respectful manner.
- The right to voice complaints without fear of retaliation.
- The right to receive their medical records in full.
- The right to contact any state or federal agency without fear of retaliation.
- The right to discharge from the facility, free from intimidation.

l.e. green

Advanced Directives

Death isn't a subject that most people like to think or talk about; because of this, there is much confusion about the different documents available that convey a person's wishes about the care he'll receive at the end of his life. People often change the subject when the topic turns to end-of-life issues, as if they're somehow inviting death by discussing the subject. We're all going to die sometime – some of us sooner than others – and everyone should have the opportunity to provide their input about the care they do (or don't) want if and when they are considered to be terminal without any possible quality of life.

Advanced directives is the general term used to describe the many documents that contain a person's wishes concerning the medical treatment he would prefer if he were to become incapacitated and unable to make decisions. These forms should be completed long before one's health has deteriorated to the point that a decision needs to be made. Unfortunately, people usually deal with them when the forms are thrust upon them as they're being admitted to a hospital. At that point they are rarely of the mindset to consider all of the available options and make appropriate decisions.

If a person hasn't completed any advanced directives and decisions must be made on his behalf, it is up to the physician and the patient's family to guess what he might have wanted. The patient is in no shape to provide his input at the point that it's needed the most, which is unfortunate. What if the patient would want to have all treatments withheld, and the family member making the decisions doesn't feel the same? Or worse – what if the person considered to be his legal next of kin is the one person the patient wouldn't want to be involved? Unless they're documented, the patient's wishes probably won't even be considered.

A common misperception regarding advanced directives is that only old or very sick people need to complete them, but by that time it's often too late for the patient to make an informed decision. Every adult should have the opportunity to complete an advanced directive in order to ensure that his wishes will be known in the event of a life-threatening condition. Completing advanced directives can lead to an honest discussion between family members, a conversation which should also include such financial issues as whether there are any insurance policies or investments, where important papers are located, and the telephone numbers of people to contact in case of emergency.

No one is immune to tragedy, and it's helpful to have the information available for others to access. Many people keep this information on their home computer, but unless someone has the password and knows which file to access the information might be overlooked. Just as many police departments urge people to list their preferred telephone contact person under "ICE" (In Case of Emergency), you should have the information in a file that is easily identified and provide your password to someone who can actually access the computer. It might not be helpful if you send the information to someone who lives out of the area; without someone in the area who is able to retrieve the information, it might as well not exist.

There's a common misperception that there's a huge computer somewhere that contains everyone's personal and financial information that can be accessed in case of emergency. Nothing could be further from the truth; if the person completing the documents doesn't make the information readily available it might never be found. There is no way of knowing who to call in case of emergency unless the patient is able to provide the information himself; this is the reason that there are so many unclaimed accounts and other property listed in the newspapers every year.

Advanced directives are valuable documents, and it is important that someone know how to access them when they are needed. It's a good idea to have several photocopies made, and to give a copy to each person named in the documents. Although it might seem hard to believe, family members who disagree with the type of care a person has chosen might not present his doctor with a copy of the advanced directives, claiming that they aren't able to locate the forms. The possibility of this occurring will be greatly decreased by giving the forms to more than one person, including the patient's primary physician. Another option might be to check with your state government to see if they offer a registry (aka lockbox) where the information can be accessed in case of emergency.

You will probably need to provide a copy of your advanced directives every time you enter a hospital, nursing home or other medical facility. It's not necessary to complete new advanced directives each time the patient enters a health care facility as long as there haven't been any changes, but don't trust that they will hold your advanced directives "on file;" many facilities don't pull the information forward from past medical charts. Don't assume that they will request your advanced directives from your primary doctor, either; the hospital might not even know who your doctor is. Simply stated, if the documents can't be located, they don't exist in the eyes of the law.

It's a good idea to review your advanced directives every year or so, because the information might have changed. For example, you might have been divorced and remarried, yet your ex-spouse might still be listed as your power of attorney for healthcare. Even if the person designated as power of attorney is the same, their contact information might have changed and this information should be updated.

When advanced directives have not been completed and end-of-life decisions are forced upon patients in crisis, patients and their families often look to the person asking about the existence of such forms for answers. The guy providing the forms might be a marketer with no medical expertise at all whose job depends upon signing the patient onto his company's service (such as hospice care). This person might not understand end-of-life issues at all, especially as they relate specifically to the patient, and yet families will trust the information he provides. A marketer will do or say whatever is necessary to convince a patient to sign onto the service he represents, which is how people whose goal is to aggressively treat a serious healthcare condition end up signing onto hospice programs and discontinuing their treatments. This is a lot more common than most people realize, and the answer is simple: don't allow a marketing person to give you advice about your healthcare options.

It's important not to sign any documents that you don't understand completely, and to always make sure you receive a copy of the paperwork as soon as possible. If the person presenting the forms isn't qualified to explain them to your satisfaction, ask for a professional who is, such as a physician, nurse, or social worker (licensed professionals must adhere to certain ethical guidelines). If an agency worker isn't able to take the time to go over the forms with you, wait and find someone who is willing to take the time for this very important issue.

I've known patients who completed advanced directives because they didn't want to make the salesperson mad at them, so they just checked the boxes and signed the form. Medical care isn't about the health care provider; it's about the patient; only the patient's needs should be considered when completing advanced directives. If you need more time to consider your options, don't sign the forms. It doesn't matter whether the person asking you to sign is on a deadline, it's not *your* deadline, but it's your *life*. Take your time to consider your options, and remember that a healthcare provider can't refuse to serve you because you lack advanced directives.

In the event that a decision must be made and no advanced directives were ever completed, someone will probably need to make a decision on the patient's behalf. Although the patient's family members might get together and appoint someone to speak for them, it's possible that the hospital won't recognize their authority. Each state has a statute addressing the exact succession of people who are able to make the patient's end-of-life decisions. In many states, the people who can make decisions are as follows:

1. An attorney in fact (durable power of attorney), or
2. Any previously appointed legal guardian, or
3. The patient's spouse, or
4. The patient's adult children (over the age of 18), the majority of whom can reasonably be found, or
5. The patient's parents, or surviving parent, or
6. The patient's nearest reasonably available living relative 18 or older, or
7. A legal guardian appointed by the courts for this purpose.

Even the healthiest of families can break down under stress. When you factor in such issues as life-partners, patients who have had no contact with their family members for several years, and patients with substantial assets, it's a recipe for disaster if no one has been named to make decisions on a patient's behalf. By completing a durable power of attorney for health care, the patient can help to avoid family arguments and drama.

Powers of Attorney for Health Care

The best way that a patient can ensure that his wishes will be implemented when he isn't able to make his own decision is to complete a ***power of attorney for health care (POA)***, which is the form that designates the person he wants to make decisions on his behalf. The person named in the document as primary decision-maker is called a ***health care designee***, ***health care proxy***, or ***attorney-in-fact***. Although the health care designee might speak with other family members to gain their input, ultimately it is his decision as to the course of treatment that the patient will receive *when the patient is no longer able to make his own decisions.*

As long as the patient has the capacity to make his own decisions, he has the right to do so. Neither the family nor the health care designee is able to override his wishes, although they are able to provide their input if asked. This can be particularly frustrating to family members who aren't ready to "let go." As long as the patient understands the decisions he is making, he is free to choose the care the he wants. A power of attorney does allow the family to obtain and provide information on a patient's behalf, but it doesn't give them the authority to override the patient's decisions. He always has the right to direct his own care as long as he is able.

 If the family or other interested parties disagree with the choices made by the health care designee, the only way they can stop him is by court order. Hopefully it won't come to that; this is an expensive and emotionally draining process where no one wins. These situations can become nasty; I've seen families hire security guards to keep unwanted people away from the patient and spend thousands of dollars attempting to change the patient's treatment plan. Ultimately, the power of attorney or legal next-of-kin is able to make decision on a patient's behalf regardless of what the family might want.

If the patient completed a power of attorney in another state, it should still be valid as long as it was completed in accordance of the laws of the state in which the patient resides. I've heard stories about nurses who refused to honor powers of attorney because they weren't completed in the state in which the facility was located. In one case, a patient had a stroke while on vacation and her best friend – her legal power of attorney – arrived with a copy of the documents. The hospital charge nurse refused to allow the friend into the ICU, and wouldn't speak with her about the patient's condition. After the friend met with the hospital administrator, they were more than willing to accept her as the power of attorney. The commonly accepted rule is that a power of attorney form that was completed in accordance with state law is accepted across the United States. It's not realistic to expect that a patient will complete a power of attorney in every state he visits.

Most powers of attorney for healthcare include a *durable* provision, which is a paragraph on the form that specifically states that the power of attorney for health care remains in effect even after the patient no longer has the capacity to make informed decisions. Without a durable provision, the power of attorney ends when the patient is no longer competent to make his own decisions. In that case, either the legal next of kin will have to step in or a legal guardian might need to be appointed to make decisions on the patient's behalf, which can be expensive.

It's possible to have a power of attorney that is limited to a specific purpose; for example, a patient who has a lump in her breast might undergo exploratory surgery. Depending upon the results of the procedure, a decision will need to be made as to whether a lumpectomy is sufficient or a full mastectomy is warranted. Because she will be under the influence of general anesthesia at that time, the patient can designate a family member to make the decision on her behalf. This is an example of a limited healthcare power of attorney; this form ceases to be valid after than specific surgery has been conducted.

A person can only complete a power of attorney if he has the capacity to do so. Usually referred to as *alert & oriented times four (A&Ox4)*, a person must know who he is, where he is, the general date or day of the week and what he is signing (and why). If the patient lacks the capacity to make informed decisions, he certainly can't decide who should be named as his durable power of attorney for health care.

A person can only assign his own power of attorney; it's not possible for a third party to reassign someone else's power of attorney. The person named power of attorney was specifically chosen for that task, and if for any reason he isn't available or chooses not to make decisions, the patient's power of attorney reverts to the person listed as an alternate decision maker on the document. If there is none, the legal next-of-kin is designated as the decision-maker for that patient. Simply stated, the person who is named the health care designee can't appoint someone else to make decisions for the patient; he can only defer to the next person listed on the power of attorney document.

Many people don't consider that the person that they appoint as their power of attorney might not be available to make decisions. For example, if a married couple is in an auto accident and they had only named each other as their durable power of attorney for health care with no back-up designees, the hospital must follow the state statute and locate the next-of-kin. Unless advanced directives are in place, it's possible that the legal next of kin might be a family member with whom the patient hasn't spoken in several years.

When completing a durable power of attorney for health care, it's a good idea to name one person who can make decisions, and at least two alternates. If two people are named as primary ("John and Mary Doe" or "John or Mary Doe"), then the hospital must attempt to contact both parties, and hopefully the two people will agree on treatment choices. If they don't agree, most of the time the doctors will err on the side of whoever might sue them. This means that even though a patient has clearly stated his wishes not to be kept on life support, it's possible that he'll be kept alive until the attorneys-in-fact can agree on a course of treatment. Valuable time can be lost trying to determine who can legally make end-of-life decisions. Naming one person as the health care designee is the easiest way to make sure this doesn't happen.

A person who is alert & oriented can *revoke* (withdraw permission for the form to be valid) a durable power of attorney for health care at any time simply by stating *in front of witnesses* that he wants to revoke the document. The revocation needs to be done in front of witnesses because the person who was named as the health care proxy can take the matter to court, and without witnesses it will be difficult for the judge to verify what the patient's wishes were at the time. There is no requirement that the revocation be written, although it's helpful if the patient is able to put it in writing. The patient doesn't have to explain why he is revoking the power of attorney, nor is he required to physically speak with the person he had previously named as his durable power of attorney. Another way to revoke a power of attorney form is to complete another that contains a provision revoking all previous powers of attorney (most POA forms contain this provision).

When a patient informs a health care provider that he wishes to revoke his power of attorney, the best course of action would be to complete another as soon as possible; in fact, the easiest way to revoke a power of attorney is to complete a new one. Health care providers should do their best to encourage open communication between patients and their families, especially when it comes to revoking advanced directives. It can be quite distressing when a family member is "cut out" of the process, and can cause hurt feelings that last for years after the health care crisis is over. Powers of attorney should not be assigned lightly, and if family members are aware of the patient's wishes regarding end-of-life decisions long before the situation occurs it is possible to alleviate many of the issues that can tear families apart. However, if the patient states that he wants to revoke a power of attorney, he has the right to do so and the health care provider has no right to force the patient to discuss the issue with anyone.

The person designated as durable power of attorney for health care doesn't have to be a relative; it is completely up to the patient to decide who can direct his healthcare. The wishes of family members can't take precedence over the decisions made by the person named as health care proxy. This can be distressing to the family, especially when the durable power of attorney for health care is a life-partner of the patient and the family doesn't accept the relationship. When people live together without being legally married, family members might attempt to shut them out of the decision-making process. This can be addressed by naming the life-partner as the power of attorney for healthcare.

If the DPOA for health care doesn't address this issue, each state mandates the method used to deem a person incapable of making decisions. In most cases, two physicians must agree that the patient is not able to make decisions based on his cognitive or physical status. A patient's cognitive status can vary during the day, and various healthcare providers might have differing opinions about the patient's capacity to make informed decisions. I've seen incidences of three or more physicians, including psychiatrists, who were called in for consultations in order to make a determination about the patient's ability to make informed decisions. If at all possible, patients have the right to make decisions as to what treatments they will receive. Even if their capacity is in question, they are still able to refuse invasive treatments such as injections, IV's, surgeries, etc.

> Mrs. Smith is in the hospital and feels that her daughter (who was named DPOA) is interfering with her treatment. Mrs. Smith prefers to make her own healthcare decisions and states that she wants to revoke her DPOA. She also has decided that she no longer wants to allow her daughter access to her medical records. Although she intends to complete another DPOA, she doesn't want to be confronted by her daughter about the revocation and asks the medical staff to inform her daughter of the change. The social worker consults with the physician and reviews the medical chart to ensure that there is nothing that indicates that Mrs. Smith lacks the capacity to make decisions.
>
> The social worker meets with Mrs. Smith's daughter in another room, and explains that her mother revoked the power of attorney effective immediately. The daughter is upset and demands a copy of the medical chart, but the hospital staff refuses to give her the information. The daughter is told that unless she has a court order she will not be provided with a copy of the medical chart. If Mrs. Smith doesn't want to speak with her daughter about the issue, she isn't obligated to do so.

There are rarely court proceedings associated with powers of attorney, unless there is a question as to whether the durable power of attorney for health care is valid. However, if there is a question as to the patient's cognitive ability, it might be for a court to decide whether or not he is competent to make decisions. If a patient never wanted to be kept alive by artificial means yet has been placed on a ventilator while the hospital awaited for a decision from the courts, the issue then becomes whether to withdraw treatment that already been started rather than to withhold it in the first place. This can be distressing for everyone involved.

Until a patient meets the criteria to lack *Capacity*, the patient is legally able to make all of his own decisions. This is called the *right to self-determination*, meaning that people have the right to make choices no matter how poor they might appear to be as long as they are able to make informed decisions. I have discharged patients to situations that I felt to be unsafe, but they have the right to choose their living situation. One of my former hospice patients chose to live in an old camper so small that he had to place his feet in the oven when he stretched out (obviously it wasn't on at the time), but he was competent and able to decide where he wanted to live and die. I have seen family members who discover that their parents gave away some or all of their estate, even though there was a will that directed all assets be given to their family members upon their death. It's not uncommon for adult children who were counting on an inheritance to find that there is no money left over and that they are powerless to get the money back. Families can be torn apart when one particular family member appears to have exploited the patient, but if the patient is competent he has the right to do whatever he wants.

The powers of a DPOA end when a patient dies. It is common for healthcare facilities, banks and other entities to refuse to release the patient chart or account information to the person named on the document after the patient passes away. Providers often request a court order before providing the information; this is especially true if there is an issue where it's possible that a lawsuit might be filed. This is why a copy of the medical chart should be requested while the patient is still alive. Remember that the longer it takes for a chart to be provided, the greater the opportunity there is for the documents to be "scrubbed" and any incriminating information removed from the file. This isn't supposed to happen, and in a perfect world it wouldn't be an issue – but it does happen more often than you'd think.

General Powers of Attorney

A *general power of attorney* (also known as a *financial power of attorney)* is a form that designates the person to whom the patient gives his authority to make general decisions, including financial arrangements and completing contracts on his behalf. It can be limited, such as specific to the sale of a home, or unlimited in the scope of powers that it grants. A general power of attorney can also contain a health care clause allowing the designee to make the patient's health care decisions, although most don't address the person's health care. Even though these forms can be obtained at almost any store or on-line, if you have any questions at all it's worth the cost of paying for legal advice because they give such a broad authority to the designee. It is important to name someone that you can absolutely trust as your general power of attorney.

Many banks and other institutions won't honor a general power of attorney unless it has been completed on an approved form at that institution, and some entities such as banks or investment firms won't honor anything short of a court order. Many banks will only allow a person access to the patient's bank accounts if they've actually been added to the account as a co-owner. Each place of business must decide what it will and won't honor, and it's becoming increasingly common for a bank to refuse to allow a third person access to a patient's accounts even if they have a power of attorney in-hand.

> Mrs. Smith is recuperating from surgery in a skilled nursing facility. She has signed a financial power of attorney allowing her daughter access to her account. The bank teller alerts her manager when the daughter presents a check signed by Mrs. Smith, but the rest of the check is in the daughter's handwriting and is made out for over twice the amount Mrs. Smith usually spends each month. The account is frozen and the bank manager contacts **adult protective services (APS)** to investigate. APS determines that there is no exploitation and informs the bank of their findings. The bank refuses to allow the family access to the accounts, requesting that Mrs. Smith either add her daughter to the account or that the daughter be appointed as legal guardian of her mother's estate.

The policies and procedures that banks impose can be a problem for a family member who is attempting to assist a patient. As in the above example, it's fairly common for a family member to alert the bank that the patient is in the hospital only to find that the patient's bank account is immediately frozen. The family thought they were doing the right thing, but by doing so they made it difficult to access the patient's monies to pay his ongoing bills. The bank is only trying to protect an elderly customer; this type of action protects the patient from possible exploitation, but can also slow down the process of placing a patient in a nursing home or with paying his monthly household bills.

This doesn't necessarily mean that without a financial power of attorney a patient's needs can't be met; much of the time a patient's income is automatically deposited into his bank account and his bills can be paid online. It's possible to set up such a system if the patient is able to provide his password and login information, but if he never set up online banking there might be problems accessing his account. It is also possible to have the patient sign several checks before going into the hospital, or to give a trusted family member access to the account with an ATM card. As long as it can be shown that the patient's money is being used for his benefit, there shouldn't be any legal problems associated with accessing his account.

It is important to remember that having general power of attorney means that the designee is responsible for paying the patient's bills out of the patient's finances; the designee is not personally liable for the patient's bills or the decisions that he makes unless it can be proven that the patient's finances were used for the designee's own personal gain.

Some patients allow a family member to become a co-owner on their accounts so that the money can be accessed in case of emergency, but it might not be in the best interest of the patient to share a bank account with another family member unless the money in the account is only used for the patient. When applying for Medicaid or other assistance, the entire balance in the account will probably be considered to be the property of the patient. This is the case even if it can be proven that some of the money belongs to the family member; if at all possible, never *co-mingle* the patient's funds with anyone else's. Patients are often denied public assistance as a result of co-mingled funds.

Being added as a co-owner of a bank account won't help with any other accounts that the patient may own. For example, if a patient adds her daughter as co-owner of a checking account, that won't automatically grant her access to the savings or investment accounts even if they're at the same institution. When adding a person as co-owner, make sure that you include all of the accounts or there can be problems later on.

Whether or not a family member is listed as co-owner of the patient's bank accounts, it's possible that a financial decision will be required at some point. Without a power of attorney it will be ambiguous as to whether anyone can legally make such a decision for the patient. Again, there are so many issues regarding powers of attorney that can affect a person's finances, it is best to obtain legal advice before allowing a person full access to yours or your family member's finances.

Legal Guardianship

Family members often mistakenly believe themselves to be the *legal guardian* of a patient because they live closest in proximity to the patient, or because they are named as the patient's power of attorney. This simply isn't the case.

A guardian is a person or entity appointed by the courts to make decisions on a person's behalf, involving a legal process that usually includes hiring attorneys, paying fees, appearing in court, etc. The court may appoint a legal guardian for the person, but the term for guardianship over his estate is called a *conservator*. There is no guarantee that the person who is petitioning to become guardian or conservator will appointed by the courts as the person to act on the patient's behalf; if for any reason there is a question as to who should be named as conservator it's possible that the judge can appoint an unrelated party such as an attorney or accounting firm.

If the patient has the assets to pay the costs, the court will approve a schedule of fees to be paid to the conservator from his estate. However, if the patient can't afford to pay for all of the costs associated with the guardianship process, the person filing the petition will be responsible for all associated court fees. A legal guardian/conservator of the estate will be required to provide the courts with an accounting of all transactions, and must be able to prove that each expenditure was made for the patient's benefit. The process can be quite expensive, especially if there are several people petitioning to be appointed and there is a protracted battle over control of a person or his estate.

An emergency (temporary) guardianship generally takes at least a week, while the process of appointing a permanent guardian/conservator can take months or even years. There are many factors that can cause a guardianship application to be delayed, such as those situations when there are multiple family members involved and they all wish to be heard. For those patients who have been referred for a public guardian, the length of time that they'll have to wait depends upon whether they're in danger of losing their housing or if an immediate healthcare decision must be made on their behalf. It also depends upon how many other referrals for guardianship that the agency might have pending as to how quickly the agency might act. Those patients who have substantial assets are often served immediately, because they will probably require financial decisions made on their behalf – and it doesn't hurt that the agency will be paid for its intervention.

The appointed guardian must be a resident of the state in which the patient lives, although out-of-state relatives are able to act as co-guardian with a party that lives locally. This person can be a family friend, an attorney, a private guardianship agency or a public agency. In most cases, the courts won't grant guardianship to a person who has been convicted of a felony, financial crimes, or any crime against a person.

Most courts require at least one physician (often a psychiatrist) to certify that the patient lacks the capacity to make decisions. If there is any question as to whether a guardian should be appointed, the judge might designate a *guardian ad litem* to conduct an independent investigation and make recommendations as to how the courts should proceed. The patient himself has the right to attend the hearing to defend his right to self-determination, and it's possible that the judge might not deem him to be incompetent even though two physicians have certified that he lacks the capacity to make decisions.

The decision as to whether a family member should apply for guardianship on behalf of a patient can be difficult. The only reason that an application should be submitted is to protect the patient and/or his estate because he isn't able to do so himself. In most instances, as long as a patient is able to make informed choices, he isn't a candidate for guardianship (unless he is physically unable to sign his name and requires a co-guardian to act on his behalf). Some communities offer information about the guardianship process; if none are available in your area, consult with an attorney.

Last Will and Testament

People are often confused about their status as the *executor* of a patient's *will*. An executor is the person appointed to be responsible for distributing a person's property after they die. The will comes into effect only when the patient is no longer living; an executor does not have any legal authority to make decisions for a patient before he dies.

As was previously discussed, the authority granted by a durable power of attorney for health care ends when the patient dies. After the patient's death, the executor of the patient's will is the representative of the patient's estate (in accordance with the terms of his will). Any demand for his medical records in anticipation of a lawsuit must be requested by the executor, or by his attorney.

Wills must be prepared according to the laws of the state in which the patient resides; otherwise, they might not be valid. There are many websites that offer assistance in completing a will, and in many circumstances they work just fine. However, if there are any questions (or if there are substantial assets) it's usually best to discuss them with an attorney.

Living Wills

A *living will* is a document that specifically addresses what treatment the patient might wish to have at the point that he is no longer expected to recover with any reasonable quality of life. This document includes such information as whether the patient wishes to have intravenous fluids and feeding tubes placed to keep him alive, whether he wishes to have CPR (cardio-pulmonary resuscitation), and whether or not he would want to be placed on a ventilator.

A living will can be a separate document, although it doesn't have to be; it is often included as a provision in a durable power of attorney for healthcare. A patient with a terminal disease might wish to be made comfortable and allow nature to run its course, or might want to extend his life as long as possible without regard as to the quality of life he will experience during the time that he has left. He has the right to make this choice, even though the cost of providing life-saving measures for a terminally ill person can easily run into the hundreds of thousands of dollars. This decision is emotionally taxing for family members to make on their own; by completing a living will the wishes of the patient can be honored without the family feeling responsible for the decision that has been made.

There is much discussion about whether withholding artificial nutrition and hydration is uncomfortable for the patient; at the point that a patient refuses to eat and drink it's a personal decision as to whether he would want to receive an invasive treatment such as the placement of a feeding tube or the administration of IV fluids. There are arguments supporting both views of the issue, but in most cases the doctor or a hospice provider can make the patient as comfortable as possible during this very difficult time.

Medical Treatment Plans

Medical treatment plans are documents developed by the patient's physician, either with the patient or his health care proxy, which details the course of treatment that the patient would prefer to receive. These documents usually include much of the information contained in the living will. The main difference between a living will and a medical treatment plan is that a living will provides direction as to which treatments that the patient would prefer, while the medical treatment plan is the actual plan of care that the physician will follow for the patient.

Developing a medical treatment plan provides the patient with an excellent opportunity to discuss his treatment options with his physician, and to direct his own care. Treatment plans can be changed according to the patient's physical status; a healthy patient's plan will be vastly different than that of a person who has been diagnosed with a terminal disease.

Do Not Resuscitate Orders

A *Do Not Resuscitate Order* (*DNR*) is an order from a physician that directs the medical staff to allow the patient to expire without performing heroic measures such as CPR. A DNR can be a verbal order, a written order in the patient's chart, or a separate form that is approved by the state in which the patient is receiving treatment.

Many states require that a DNR be completed on a state approved form and signed by the physician in order for it to be considered legally valid. Without the specific form being present, *Emergency Medical Technicians (EMTs)* are required to perform resuscitation procedures and to transport the patient to the emergency room. The original of the form is designed to follow the patient from the hospital to another facility or to his home, so in theory it won't need to be completed more than one time. However, since these forms can be easily misplaced or a care provider might file the original away, it's possible that more than one will need to be completed during a patient's sickness. The main objective of the form is to provide direction to EMTs so that they will have a doctor's order to provide or withhold treatment.

Some states require that a patient register their DNR with a designated agency such as the health department; the form is signed by the doctor and mailed in for registration. Without the official registration form, EMT's are required to act as though the patient has no DNR and do everything possible to resuscitate the patient. If registration is required in your area, make sure to complete the forms and mail them in or hand-carry them to the agency if necessary. It's distressing when a terminal patient awaiting the return of the official DNR form is sent to the hospital and placed on a ventilator. This registration often costs a few dollars, which can be difficult for a low-income patient to come up with; in most cases, the state or local agency will waive the fee if the patient can't afford to pay.

Home hospice patients who haven't received the official state-approved form back after sending it in for registration probably won't have any problems, as long as no one calls 911. In most cases, the patient or caregiver will call the hospice provider in case of emergency and the hospice will send a nurse to the house. However, if *anyone* calls 911, it's probable that the patient will be resuscitated and transported to the hospital without the official form being present. Even though the family might be instructed not to call 911, there might be a problem if a concerned neighbor calls 911. This is why it's always best to complete all forms in accordance with state laws.

Organ Donation

Another type of advanced directive is the issue of ***organ donation***. A patient might have an organ donor card or the option is marked on his state issued driver's license, but it is still a requirement for the next-of-kin or the person designated as power of attorney to provide written permission for a loved-one's organs to be harvested for transplant. The family members might have different religious beliefs than those of the patient and can refuse to allow the patient's organs to be donated. In most cases, the removal of the organs is not a painful process because care is taken to ensure that the patient has sufficient pain medication, even though he is non-responsive and unable to make his needs known. The patient's vital signs are monitored for any indication of a pain response such as elevated heart rate or blood pressure. The only time that organ donation is an option is when the patient has no reasonable chance of recovering and has no measurable brain function.

Due to modern mortuary practices, the family who allows for organ donation won't notice a difference in their deceased family member even if there is an open casket. Unless the disease process has rendered his organs unusable, the patient's organs can give other people the opportunity to resume a semi-normal lifestyle. It's important to understand that sometimes organ donation is not possible, such as the death occurring in a rural area where harvesting and transporting the organs might not be a viable option, or the disease process or treatments the patient received caused damage to the organs. If the organs aren't in a healthy condition, transplant might not be possible; in this case, the patient's body might still be valuable for research or other purposes such as teaching.

Elder Law Attorney Intervention

While it's not necessary to hire an attorney to complete advance directives, if there is any question as to whether the forms will be contested, it's best to access the services of an attorney who specializes in elder law. An attorney can also answer questions about whether the advanced directives completed in one state will be accepted in another state, as well as whether they will remain in effect if the patient travels out of the country. This could solve many future headaches.

Hiring an elder law attorney to complete a patient's advanced directives also allows for the attorney to take a "snapshot" of the patient's financial situation and review his eligibility for Medicaid, Veteran's benefits, or other programs that might help with caregiving.

Medicaid eligibility is a confusing process; any financial decisions can affect a patient's ability to qualify for the program. When a person is appointed guardian, they are able to act on the patient's behalf to apply for any benefits for which he might be eligible. Utilizing the services of an elder law attorney to complete advanced directives will ensure that the patient will receive the best advice possible. I've known people who were positive that they didn't qualify for Medicaid find that, after meeting with an elder law attorney, Medicaid began pay for the patient's room & board immediately.

l.e. green

Institutional Medicaid Eligibility

Back in the good old days, pretty much anyone could qualify for **Institutional Medicaid** to pay for room & board in a nursing home. All it took to qualify was that a patient give away **(gift)** his assets to someone else or somehow hide them from the prying eyes of the eligibility worker, and Medicaid would pick up the tab for the nursing home stay. With a little creative accounting, everyone from the very wealthy to the poorest of people qualified for Medicaid to pick up the tab for nursing home placement. It wasn't necessary to hire an elder law attorney in order to become eligible, the process was simple and nearly everyone qualified.

It wasn't long before the nice folks at the **Department of _H_ealth & _H_uman _S_ervices (HHS)** realized that the government was spending a lot of money to help people who didn't really need the assistance. They began to tighten the eligibility guidelines so that hopefully Medicaid would only be awarded to people who actually needed the help. Between those changes and the technological advances of the computer age, it became much harder to qualify for assistance to help pay for nursing home placement. It wasn't as easy to hide assets because Medicaid workers were able to access public records over the internet. Patients were still able to gift money away; the Medicaid program required that patients wait a couple of years or so to be eligible but eventually they qualified. It was still possible to apply for Medicaid without the assistance of an elder law attorney, but there was a pretty good chance that the patient would be denied. Although it was a little harder to become eligible, a good elder law attorney was still able to get just about anyone approved at that point.

HHS eventually realized that people were still able to hide their assets and eventually qualify for Medicaid. The **Deficit Reduction Act (DRA) of 2006** took care of that, drastically changing the eligibility guidelines to the point that it is now much more difficult to qualify for Medicaid. The most significant difference was that the attitude of the Medicaid program seemed to change; instead of helping patients to become eligible for assistance, the goal for Medicaid eligibility workers appeared to be looking for reasons to deny benefits. It's still possible to become eligible for Medicaid, but more often than not it requires hiring a professional to assist with the application and there are no guarantees the patient will be approved.

Unfortunately, many people still aren't aware that the Medicaid eligibility criteria has changed, and choose to accept information about Medicaid from family or friends (or people they meet in line in the grocery store), rather than to pay for professional advice. Hiring an attorney doesn't always guarantee that a Medicaid application will be approved, but it might very well give the patient a fighting chance. Consulting an elder law attorney can help to decrease the amount of time he'll have to wait before his Medicaid is approved, potentially saving the patient or his family tens of thousands of dollars.

Thanks to the **DRA**, many people are now paying thousands of dollars per month out of their pocket for the exact same care that Medicaid patients receive at about half the cost. But the dirty little secret that no one seems to want the public to know is that it's still possible to plan ahead and qualify for **institutional Medicaid,** which is the formal name for the type of Medicaid that pays for nursing home placement. Institutional Medicaid is also the payment source for programs called nursing home waivers, which provide limited assistance to patients so that they can remain out in the community rather than to be forced to live in a nursing home. Each state offers several versions of nursing home waiver programs; for additional information about programs in your state call your local Medicaid office or Area Agency on Aging.

People often tell me that they don't want to apply for Medicaid because they can afford to help their family member pay for his placement and they don't want to accept "welfare." I've been told that the family wants to "do the right thing" and pay for the patient's room & board, or that they're concerned that the federal Medicaid program will go broke. I do understand their reasoning, but there are strict eligibility guidelines for Medicaid and if a patient fits into the criteria, he's not taking anything away from anyone else by accepting assistance. Most people aren't able to afford the $6,000 (minimum) that it costs for nursing home placement, and end broke. Patients often are sent to board & care homes with the family bearing the costs of upwards of $2,000 each month (these homes offer less staff and offer substantially less supervision than nursing home patients receive). These costs will continue to go up; why not allow Medicaid to help out if the patient is at all eligible?

The Medicaid program contributes as much, if not more, to local communities than it costs the taxpayers. Medicaid pays for real people to be cared for in their old age, which in turn pays the salaries of nursing home employees who pay income taxes, property taxes and sales taxes that benefit the community. They shop at local businesses and pay for goods & services that benefit others in the community. Medicaid funding also pays the salary of the employees who administer the program, office space to house them, and the dollars continue to trickle down to the community in many other ways. In other words, the money associated with Medicaid not only helps real people with their caregiving needs, it also benefits the entire community in many, many ways. As long as the patient is eligible, there's no reason that he shouldn't benefit from the program.

There are two opposing ways to view a patient's assets: 1) the patient worked hard his whole life to save for his old age, and now that he's old he should spend every dime of his money to pay for his long-term care needs; or 2) as long as there are ways to legally qualify for Medicaid, why not allow the program to work for the patient?

Many people are under the (mistaken) impression that all they need to do to make their elderly parents eligible for Medicaid is to deed the house out of their parent's name. However, by doing so it's probable that Medicaid will be denied for at least five years after the home was gifted. In those cases where the family sells the home and splits the proceeds, Medicaid will not only be denied, but those family members who spent their share will have to figure out a way to come up with the money to pay for their parent's ongoing placement or in-home care needs. Even when the family is acting in what they believe to be the patient's best interest by meeting with an attorney to develop an estate plan, it might not help them at all when it comes to Medicaid. This is because there's a huge difference between estate planning and elder law. Estate planning is focused on arranging for the disposal of an estate and reducing taxes, while elder law has an estate planning component that focuses on benefits (including Medicaid) eligibility and advanced directives.

People often pay thousands of dollars to create revocable living trusts in an attempt to protect their estates, only to find that the trust didn't protect the assets in accordance with the Medicaid process. A revocable trust can be changed (revoked) at any time, and in most cases the Medicaid program will view the trust as an asset that is available to the patient. A primary residence (home) that is placed into a trust can be considered an asset, even if a *community spouse* (the wife or husband of a patient in a nursing home) lives there. The home might not have been an issue if it hadn't been placed into a trust in the first place. Depending on the rules of the state in which the patient lives, he might not ever be eligible for Medicaid; at the very least the family will have to pay an elder law attorney thousands of dollars to fix the problem that they paid an estate planner thousands of dollars to create.

I have witnessed family members who filed a declaration of homestead on a parent's home; there's a misconception that by doing so they can protect the home and make the patient eligible for Medicaid. Filing a homestead and applying for Medicaid require completely different legal strategies; before doing so, it's best to speak with an elder law attorney. Otherwise, it's possible that such a move will guarantee that the patient will never be eligible for Medicaid to pay for his nursing home placement.

Patients who have been paying privately to remain in a nursing home might not be aware they're actually be eligible for Medicaid; family members of private-pay patients often assume that the nursing home staff will tell them if and when the patient appears to be eligible for financial assistance. The nursing home staff doesn't know anything at all about the patient's finances unless the family shares the patient's financial information with them, and in many instances the nursing home staff members don't understand Medicaid well enough themselves to advise the patient and his family as to when they might be eligible. Nursing homes are required to post the telephone numbers of Medicaid and Medicare program offices, but many don't offer assistance with the actual applications nor do they understand the intricacies of the ever-changing program eligibility criteria.

Lack of knowledge about the program isn't the only reason that nursing homes often discourage families from applying for Medicaid on a patient's behalf; the amount that Medicaid pays is often substantially less than the amount that the facility can charge the private-pay patient. There's no financial incentive for the nursing home to refer the patient to the Medicaid program, so it depends upon the administrator's attitude as to whether patients and their families are informed about eligibility. Family members can quickly go broke attempting to "do the right thing" and pay for mom & dad's nursing home placement, never having been told that they're not legally obligated to pay these costs. The nursing home business office will continue to accept the payments unless the patient or family meets with them to discuss the patient's finances. In most instances they'll pay out-of-pocket until the family hires a professional to assist with Medicaid eligibility.

Many nursing homes provide excellent care in a home-like environment for their patients at the end of their lives; they recognize that patients can quickly run out of money when paying $6,000+ a month for their care and some even employ eligibility workers to help with the Medicaid application process. These workers are able to help guide patients and their families through the system, saving them the cost of having to hire a professional to complete the process. It's to your benefit to meet with the eligibility worker to discuss Medicaid, as long as the nursing home where your family member resides offers this service. If there is no eligibility worker, it's usually in your best interest to seek private advice about Medicaid eligibility.

For the patient who hasn't yet been admitted to the nursing home, don't trust that a state Medicaid worker will be of assistance with your application. Most state agencies don't provide any direction in the pre-eligibility process and will only evaluate a patient's Medicaid eligibility after the application has actually been submitted. To make matters more confusing, an application that's submitted while the patient is at home will be automatically denied because he's not physically located in a facility, and there will be no further assessment of the patient's eligibility for Medicaid. At best, the family might be told *if* the patient qualifies according to the broad eligibility requirements, but usually won't be informed as to what steps they can take to *become* eligible. Some states are easier to work with than others when it comes to the Medicaid eligibility process. With state Medicaid budget cuts, there are fewer workers with huge caseloads and they simply don't have the time to help a patient/family with the Medicaid process. Additionally, the focus has changed from assisting a patient become eligible to looking for a reason to deny as many applications as possible.

Medicaid programs are always on the chopping block when it comes to program cuts, meaning fewer workers available to provide personal attention to increasing numbers of applications. Accessing an elder law attorney or other professional to assist with the Medicaid application might save the patient or his family thousands, or tens of thousands, of dollars in out-of-pocket costs as well as to expedite the admission process. Nursing homes often give priority to accepting patients whose Medicaid applications are prepared by professionals over those who the facility will have to help. It's less work for the facility if the patient has a professional in his corner.

Seeking Professional Advice

The many changes to the Medicaid eligibility criteria that have occurred over the years has spawned a whole new generation of attorneys called *elder law attorneys* whose mission is to help their clients navigate through the system and become eligible for Medicaid if at all possible. These attorneys are worth their weight in gold; as changes have been made over the years they have had to remain knowledgeable as to how each state interprets the federal rules. They are often able to assist patients to become eligible and might possibly be able to fix problems that existed before they became involved with the application. Elder law attorneys can also help with applications for veteran's programs if the patient is eligible for that type of assistance.

Many people are clearly eligible; if they are considered to be low-income and have no assets or fall below the asset limit for their state (a nursing home can tell you the asset limits, which vary from the norm of $2,000 to about $14,000 in New York State), it's possible for the family to complete the application themselves. However, most people don't plan their lives in anticipation of applying for Medicaid, and their finances include miscellaneous deposits and withdrawals. If there is *any* question as to the patient's Medicaid eligibility, it's worth meeting with an elder law attorney to see if they can assist you in the application process. It's a lot easier to be proactive and present the patient's personal and financial information in a favorable light in the first place than it is to wait until the application has been denied and try to "fix" it. Once the application has been processed and Medicaid has been denied, it's much more difficult to win an appeal.

When looking for an attorney to help with Medicaid eligibility, ask how long he has been specializing in Medicaid and what his success rate has been. Ask for references, and feel free to interview a couple of attorneys before you make a decision. Bring an adult child or friend who can help understand (and remember) what the attorney says. New attorneys aren't necessarily a bad option: elder law attorneys all have to start somewhere. Many attorneys who specialize in elder law start out working closely with an experienced elder law attorney for the first few years, which is a good idea considering that the intricacies of Medicaid law takes a while to learn. Don't choose an attorney based upon how much he will charge for his services because you could end up saving hundreds in legal fees while spending thousands on the patient's medical care. Be wary of attorneys who are willing to discount their rate if you purchase an annuity from them; they might be trying to help you, but they also might receive a huge commission from the purchase of the annuity. Attorneys are required to disclose any potential conflicts to their clients, such as commissions from outside vendors.

Many elder law attorneys provide free informational seminars about Medicaid or related issues. These seminars are a way to attract customers, but if they require that you sign in and provide contact information they might not be providing a public service as much as they are attempting to trick people into using their services. Many elder law attorneys offer a free initial consultation to potential customers, but others charge for this service. One elder law attorney explained to me that he provides an introduction to the services that he can provide through his seminars, and that if clients choose to meet with him he charges a consultation fee. Remember that elder law attorneys are businessmen and women, and that they have overhead costs including the salaries of support staff. Simply stated, they can't give away their services for free or they'll be out of business.

Even if a patient doesn't require assistance from an attorney, families often feel overwhelmed by the application process. It's possible to save some of the cost of attorney fees by hiring companies or individuals who are knowledgeable about Medicaid to assist with applications. These companies are often staffed with retired state eligibility workers, and can assist a patient in almost the same manner as an elder law attorney would. They are usually able to push an application through at a lesser cost than the amount charged by an attorney. Some attorneys perform the legal work necessary for a patient to become eligible for Medicaid, but contract with these companies to assist with the actual application.

Many hospitals hire companies that apply for Medicaid on behalf of their patients, but remember that their goal is to get the hospital bill paid. They probably have little interest in obtaining ongoing benefits for the patients, and often aren't available to answer questions. They probably aren't applying for institutional Medicaid, and the patient will be no closer to being admitted to a nursing home when the hospital's application has been approved. If at all possible, work with a professional of your own choosing when it comes to the Medicaid application.

Again, not every patient requires legal representation; many people are approved for Medicaid without ever having consulted an attorney. Each state has its own eligibility process, and it depends upon the attitude of the worker and the amount of leeway that she has in the assessment process as to whether or not a patient is eligible for Medicaid. Unless the patient is clearly eligible and there are no other issues to be addressed (such as joint bank accounts and extra assets), it's probably worth the money to pay for a professional to assist with the application.

Medicaid in Simple Terms

Although Medicaid is never really simple, there are some basic guidelines for Medicaid:

- Income limits – patients are eligible for Medicaid if they are below the maximum allowable income limit, which varies according to the rules of the state in which the patient resides. Your local Medicaid office or any nursing home eligibility worker can provide you with the amounts specific to your state. Don't panic if your family member is over the limit, because there may be legal strategies to help maneuver around this rule.

  Some states allow a "spend-down," which allows the patient to pay the amount he's over the income limit to the state and still receive Medicaid assistance. For example, if the patient's income is $3,130 and the Medicaid income limit is $2,130, the patient is able to pay that extra $1,000 toward his placement in addition to the amount he would already be paying for his share-of-cost. Please note that this is a simple explanation; eligibility is further explained in this section.

  If a person's income is too great to qualify for Medicaid – and he doesn't live in a spend-down state – yet he doesn't have the assets to pay the full cost of placement out-of-pocket, it might be possible for him to assign his income to a special trust account that reduces his monthly income to an amount that fits into the Medicaid guidelines. These trusts are known as **Miller Trusts**, although they're also referred to as **Qualified Income Trusts** or **Income Cap Trusts**. Essentially, the patient's income is assigned to the trust, and the trust pays the patient a monthly amount that is just under the Medicaid limit (when the patient dies, the proceeds of the trust belong to Medicaid). Obviously, it's more complicated than that, but it is possible to be over the income limit and still qualify for Medicaid as long as the patient meets all of the other Medicaid criteria. It will probably be necessary to hire an elder law attorney to set up one of these trusts.

- Allowable assets for unmarried (single) applicants – in most cases, single applicants are allowed to have a home, one car that is available to be used for the applicant's transportation, a pre-paid burial plan, and up to $2,000 in liquid assets (this amount can vary according to the state, with New York allowing about $14,000 in assets). The term **liquid assets** refers to any asset that is easily converted to cash, such as the cash value of a life insurance policy, non-residential property, coin collections, artwork, etc.

  Since most of the unmarried applicant's income will be paid to the nursing home as his **patient liability** (also referred to as his **share of cost**), there will be no money available to maintain the home & car that he's allowed to keep. In most cases, family members can pay for the upkeep without jeopardizing the patient's Medicaid eligibility. Generally speaking, the resident's home must be located in the state where the nursing home is located because his primary home establishes his state of residency. Patients who live in another state must either put their homes up for sale or prove that the property can't be sold due to market conditions (there are a very few exceptions, including family farms and other income-producing properties). Medicaid might be approved while the home is for sale, and once the home has been sold the patient will need to pay privately out of the funds until he has spent down to the state's maximum asset limit. At that point, Medicaid will again pick up the cost of the patient's room & board.

- Allowable assets for married couples – a married couple can keep the home, one car, burial plans, and some (or all) of the household income to help offset expenses. The name of the program that allows for the patient's income to be available to the community spouse is **Spousal Impoverishment**. The community-based spouse is also allowed to keep approximately the first $20,000 in liquid assets (these amounts can vary according to the state). Any assets above that amount are split between the patient and his spouse, although an elder law attorney can advise as to how to legally split the assets and spend the patient's portion so that he can become eligible for Medicaid. The patient can continue to keep up to $2,000 in his name if he wishes, but the spouse who remains at home will be able to maintain the household and keep at least some of the assets. Unmarried patients who cohabitate (live together), even for long periods of time, might not be viewed as married no matter whether the state recognizes common law marriages. This can be financially devastating for the partner who remains at home, but if the patient has the capacity of entering into a marriage it's possible for the couple to marry in order to become eligible for Medicaid. An elder law attorney can provide information about this strategy.

- Medical need (level of care) – in order to be admitted into a nursing home, an applicant has to present a physical need for nursing care and will be assigned a *level of care*. He must require assistance with several of the *activities of daily living (ADL's)*, which include walking, dressing, toileting, eating, & personal care. If a patient doesn't require the services provided by a nursing home, he won't be allowed to remain there regardless of what his payment source might be. People who require some oversight but are able to complete most activities of daily living might not meet the medical criteria for nursing home placement.

  The patient's level of care must be justified to *The Centers for Medicare & Medicaid Services* on an ongoing basis. The nursing home does this by transmitting an MDS assessment of the patient at regular intervals. If at any point the patient no longer meets the criteria to remain in the nursing home, he must be discharged to a less restrictive setting.

How Assets Affect an Application

Before the Deficit Reduction Act took effect in 2006, it was possible for a patient to transfer assets to a family member or into a trust a few years before he needed to go into a nursing home. As long as the date of transfer occurred more than three years before the patient entered the nursing home, his assets weren't considered at all when determining his Medicaid eligibility.

At that time, the patient who transferred assets out of his name could become eligible for Medicaid to pay for the placement by utilizing a formula that took into account how much that the patient *would have paid* if he had been in a nursing home from the date of the transfer. For example, if the state allowed $4,000 for this calculation, a patient could give away $40,000 in December and become eligible for Medicaid to pay for his placement ten months later, in October of the next year. People who planned ahead simply transferred their assets into other people's names and by the time they were ready to move into a nursing home, Medicaid would foot the bill.

The DRA changed this rule; now the ineligibility period begins when the patient applies for (and is otherwise eligible) for Medicaid, not when the assets were transferred (with a five year **look back period**). In the same scenario, a patient who entered the nursing home and applied for Medicaid in October wouldn't be eligible for assistance for ten months from the date of his application (October), regardless of when the money was transferred out of his name. The end result is that a patient might have to remain at home (with or without caregivers) regardless of how desperately he requires nursing home care. It doesn't matter where the patient is physically located; even if he has already been admitted into the nursing home, Medicaid won't pay the patient's room & board.

Unfortunately, even the dates of transfer can be open to interpretation. A very real example is an application I once submitted on behalf of a patient. Her home was quit-claimed to her daughter in 2000, but due to an oversight at the title company the deed wasn't recorded until 2007. The state in which I worked considered the date of the transfer to have been when the document was recorded rather than the date of intent. Even though the patient appealed the determination, the Medicaid office wouldn't budge and the patient wasn't eligible for Medicaid. Decisions such as this vary from state to state.

Proceeds from Reverse Mortgages

Reverse mortgages are United States Government-backed loans that allow seniors to cash out their equity to help them get by while they continue to live in their homes. The money that is paid out from reverse mortgages isn't taxable and doesn't have to be paid back until the senior sells the home, leaves it permanently (such as being placed in a nursing home), or dies. It's a way for seniors who are "house poor" to increase their income for whatever purpose they choose.

The proceeds of a reverse mortgage can be structured in any number of ways, such as monthly payments, annual payments or a lump sum payment. The proceeds of a reverse mortgage can be used for any purpose: to pay off an existing loan, take a vacation, make improvements on a home, or as an additional source of income. It can be an excellent financial tool to allow a senior to remain in his home as he ages. This is called **Aging-In-Place**; it allows a senior to remain in a familiar environment and provides him with an income by allowing him to tap into the equity he's built over the years.

One of the requirements of reverse mortgages is that the home will be sold at fair market value and the mortgage paid back from the proceeds as soon as the patient leaves the home on a permanent basis. If the loan amount exceeds the proceeds from the sale (i.e. the house is "underwater"), the balance due is written off. If there is still equity after the loan is paid off, the proceeds are assigned to the patient's estate or whomever was named in the Will.

Should the family decide they want to keep the home after the patient dies, they can always pay off the mortgage themselves. They will be required to pay off the full cost of the mortgage in order to satisfy the loan whether or not the home is underwater. For example, if the loan amount is $100,000 and the home is worth $50,000, the family will have to pay off the entire $100,000 or the home will be sold to a non-related party for $50,000 and the bank will essentially write-off the loss. Oftentimes families don't want seniors to apply for reverse mortgages because they will lose their claim to the family home, although these same family members might not be willing to contribute to the senior's income in order to help them out.

The US Government guarantees reverse mortgages, which is why there are higher up-front for this type of mortgage. The fees are typically $6,000 to $10,000 for your average reverse mortgage, and the amount borrowed is typically 50% to 75% of the home's value depending upon a formula developed by the US Department of Housing and Urban Development. This formula takes many things into account, including the anticipated life span of the borrower – and the terms don't change once the mortgage has been issued. Many reverse mortgages that were taken during the real estate boom are now severely underwater, but the government guaranteed them and the lenders lost nothing on the deal. The federal government, on the other hand, experienced huge losses.

Even though the proceeds from reverse mortgages aren't considered taxable income, they're countable income for Medicaid purposes. A lump sum can render the patient ineligible for Medicaid for several years (or forever), and monies paid out on a monthly basis can increase the senior's income to the point that he might not be eligible for Medicaid. This can be a catch-22; a patient might be over-income for Medicaid due to the proceeds of the reverse mortgage, but the income will stop soon after he is admitted to the nursing home. An elder law attorney can assist with this situation, because it could keep a patient from being approved for Medicaid.

Because most mortgage brokers don't consider (or even have knowledge of) Medicaid eligibility, these issues are rarely addressed when assisting a senior with a reverse mortgage. Even if the mortgage broker is aware of how reverse mortgages and Medicaid affect each other, it's doubtful that he will turn away the business. Mortgage brokers are sales people and their goal is to make as much money as possible, regardless as to how it might affect the patient in the long run.

Reverse mortgages can be valuable tools to allow seniors to improve their lifestyle, but if the possibility exists that a senior will be entering a nursing home within the next five years it would best serve the senior to consult with an elder law attorney before taking out a reverse mortgage. By seeking legal advice, the proceeds can be structured so that the patient's future Medicaid eligibility isn't affected.

Even fairly healthy seniors should consider how a reverse mortgage might affect their future Medicaid; it's possible that a senior who enters a nursing home for short-term therapy services might need assistance with copayments and deductibles. In this case, they might apply for Medicaid and find that they aren't eligible due a lump-sum payment they received. Even if they spent the entire amount, they might not be eligible for Medicaid. A little planning goes a long way in these instances.

Asset Recovery Programs

The urban legends being passed around about someone losing their home to Medicaid might be *partially* based in truth, but they're always embellished to make the program seem as though seniors are torn from their home and left destitute because of a vindictive Medicaid worker. This simply isn't the case; a Medicaid worker doesn't remove you from your home. However, the Deficit Reduction Act implemented *asset recovery* programs that allow states to place liens on properties in an attempt to recoup some of the monies paid by Medicaid. The idea is that the state will be paid back the amounts they shelled out for the patient's medical care after his death.

The Medicaid program itself doesn't take possession of the house, nor does the program become involved in the sale of the home, but it does require that the home be sold at the time of the patient's death or that (in some way) the program be paid back for the monies it paid out. Any leftover equity will be applied to the patient's estate, but if amounts paid out by Medicaid are greater than the home's value the family won't be held responsible for the difference. The thought of losing the family home can be upsetting for family members who were counting on an inheritance. With asset recovery, the family has the option of satisfying the loans and keeping the home. Depending upon the state, it's possible that the Medicaid program will accept a negotiated amount rather than the full amount owed if the home is underwater. States have more discretion with Medicaid asset recovery programs than they do with reverse mortgages.

I've known many families who don't want to get embroiled in a "Medicaid situation," preferring instead to sell the patient's home outright and pay for his care until he's broke, then placing an application for Medicaid. Something to consider when placing an unmarried patient in a nursing home is that having Medicaid pay for his care can be viewed as an interest-free loan with additional built-in savings.

Medicaid often pays for a patient's room & board in the nursing home at a lesser rate than if the patient paid privately (both rates are set by the state). The private-pay rate doesn't take into consideration the cost of ancillary items such as incontinence supplies, oxygen, wheelchair rental, medication costs, wound supplies, etc which are provided to Medicaid recipients at no additional cost. These necessary items can cost hundreds, if not thousands of dollars each month – so even if the base Medicaid & private-pay daily rates are close to the same amount, the patient will save the cost of paying for ancillary items simply by using Medicaid to pay for his placement.

As illustrated in the table below, the asset recovery amount is further reduced by the amount he paid each month toward his share of cost. In this example I used $1,000 as the amount that the patient contributed toward his care each month; depending upon the actual amount of his *patient liability* as set by the Medicaid program, a patient's estate can be responsible to pay back more (or less) from the proceeds of the sale of his home after he dies.

Estimated Private Pay Rate $275.00 per day		
Estimated Ancillary Charges of $500.00 per month*		
Cost Per Month	$8,250.00	
Cost Per Year	$99,000.00	
Estimated Medicaid Rate $200.00 per day	**Billed Charges**	**Medicaid Share**
(Less patient's income of $1,000/mo)		
Cost Per Month	$6,000.00	$5,000.00
Cost Per Year	$72,000	$60,000.00
Potential Savings (before ancillary charges)	**$39,000.00**	
Potential Savings (after ancillary charges)	**$45,000.00**	

*Ancillary charges include supplies, equipment and medication costs.**

Once the patient passes away, the home will be sold and the Medicaid program will be reimbursed. Using the illustration above, the patient can sell his home for

$100,000 and spend all or most of the proceeds paying for his room & board plus ancillary charges, or he can utilize Medicaid to pay for his care and his estate will receive half of that back after he passes away. It's perfectly legal to allow Medicaid to pay a patient's room and board in order to help protect a patient's estate.

There can be some drawbacks to this plan; while the Medicaid program will allow the patient to keep the house, it won't allow any of his ongoing income to be used for home maintenance. As long as the patient is alive, the family will be responsible for the paying the taxes, insurance and maintenance on the home out of their pockets. These amounts can be negligible compared to the thousands of dollars it costs for a private-pay patient in a nursing home. If the patient outlives his equity, the family will have paid for these costs without being reimbursed.

It might be possible to rent out the patient's house in order to help cover these costs, although it's important that the rental income not be paid *to the patient*. Any money paid directly to the patient will probably be considered his income, and the Medicaid program will either increase his share of cost to the nursing home or deny him assistance altogether. As with other financial issues, any questions you have should be discussed with an attorney and/or accountant to ensure it doesn't create a tax problem for the patient or family.

There are exceptions to Medicaid's asset recovery rules; they might not apply to homes occupied by spouses. They also might not apply in cases where patients have handicapped adult children who reside in the home, income-producing properties (such as family farms), and in numerous other instances. Most states offer heirs the opportunity to request a waiver if the sale of the home would cause a hardship for the surviving family members who live there. It can be difficult to get these waivers to be approved without attorney representation.

It's always a good idea to hire an elder law attorney to help with complicated asset recovery issues, because if one form is missing or completed incorrectly the request for a waiver will be denied. Some towns offer a list of attorneys who will work pro-bono; call your Area Agency on Aging for additional information.

Completing the Medicaid Application

An application for Institutional Medicaid can be picked up at any Medicaid office, in most nursing homes, or might be accessed online depending on the state in which you are applying. The nursing home might have a copy on-hand and be willing to help you apply; many employ eligibility workers who will do everything possible to get your application approved. If the application is beyond their capabilities, they'll refer you to an attorney or other professional who can assist you with the process.

It's important to fully answer each question, and if one doesn't apply to the patient either cross it out or write N/A next to it. Anything left blank will be questioned. The application is only about ten pages long (several pages are disclosures, releases of information, etc), but the applicant must attach proof of everything that the applicant claims in the form of bank statements, marriage licenses, insurance policy binders, birth certificates, etc. The Medicaid eligibility worker might also independently verify the information by looking it up on the internet or sending a request for information. The process has changed over the years; it used to be that the eligibility worker looked for ways to approve the application, but now the attitude appears to be that the agency is looking for ways to deny benefits when at all possible.

Verifications

Most people are under the impression that there is a computer somewhere that holds all of their personal information, and that any government worker can look it all up at the press of a computer key. That simply isn't true; the applicant must present supporting documentation *(verifications)* for everything they've stated in the application when it is submitted to the Medicaid office. When the verifications are submitted, they will be carefully reviewed for additional clues about the patient's financial situation. It's the patient or family's obligation to prove that the patient needs the assistance; if this isn't accomplished the application will be denied.

People often go to great lengths to attempt to hide assets so that the patient will appear eligible for Medicaid, but assets are rarely successfully hidden from a Medicaid worker. There's generally a paper trail that leads back to the patient, such as miscellaneous deposits to bank accounts and transfers that are referenced in the verifications that patients present. If an asset is later discovered, the patient will be immediately denied assistance and it's possible that the applicant and/or family member will be required to pay back any money that Medicaid paid on the applicant's behalf. It's also possible that they will be prosecuted if the omission is serious and has the appearance of fraud.

The Medicaid application usually includes a general list of verifications that will be required, although they're not specific to everyone's situation. Please note that all of the verifications need to be provided for both the patient and his/her spouse, whether or not the spouse is applying for assistance as well. Even if the two parties are separated, it's possible that the Medicaid program will view them as a couple (another example of when to consult with an elder law attorney). As a general rule, Medicaid will require *at least* the following verifications:

• Proof of Citizenship status, such as birth certificate, naturalization certificate, or in some cases a baptismal certificate. These can be ordered from the county of the patient's birth.

- Picture ID for the patient and all members of his household (spouse/dependent children). They must be recent but don't have to be current – and roommates or other people who live in the home such as adult children aren't considered to be part of his household.

- Medicare card or other primary insurance card.

- Front & back of secondary insurance (Medigap) card, if any.

- Social Security Card – if none, it might be necessary to apply for a new card online at www.SSA.gov, or go to the local Social Security office.

- Proof of Social Security Income – most SSA income is deposited directly into the patient's bank account, and many states will allow the worker to use the bank statement as proof of income. Social Security sends out annual statements that can be used for this purpose. Verification of Social Security income can also be obtained by calling the Social Security Administration at (800) 772-1213.

- Proof of Supplemental Security Income (SSI) – this is a type of income that helps to supplement the income of seniors whose income is very low.

- Proof of income from the Veteran's Administration, if any – if the patient is a veteran or the spouse of a deceased veteran, it will be necessary to apply for Aid & Attendance from the V.A. and include a copy of the application with the Medicaid application.

- Proof of retirement or other income – this can be in the form of check stubs, annual statements, a verification of income from the company written on its letterhead, or any other correspondence from the company. Medicaid rarely allows a bank statement to verify non-SSA/SSI income; this is because the amount that is being deposited into the account might be only a portion of the actual income, with the rest being sent to another account or directly to the patient.

- If the patient has been maintaining his lifestyle by borrowing money, it might be necessary to have the person who loaned the money to him write a statement that explains how much the patient has received and whether or not the loans can continue. If the family member is able and willing to continue contributing to the senior's housing costs, Medicaid can reduce its payments to the nursing home by that amount. It's important to remember that if the patient's expenses are greater than his income, he will need to explain how he has been able to make ends meet.

- Proof of home ownership – if the patient owns a home, include the closing statements if the home was purchased within the past five years. If anyone else's name is on the home, it will be necessary to prove that the other party contributed to the down payment and monthly payments. Medicaid might view the home as belonging only to the patient, which could be a problem for estate recovery purposes after the patient passes away.

- Proof of home owner's insurance and property taxes – if they are part of the house payment this will show on the monthly statement.

- Rental or lease agreement if no home is owned.

- Household bills – including utilities, cable/satellite, internet fees, home security systems, credit cards, etc.

- Bank statements – generally they'll request monthly statements for the past year and the statements for January of each of the previous five years. This applies to all accounts that the patient has in his name. The number of bank statements requested varies according to each state's rules.

- Explanation of any large payments or deposits – you must prove anything that is listed on the bank statement. It might be necessary to provide receipts for large purchases.

- Explanation of any transfers into or out of the account that are reflected on the bank statement – if the bank statement references any other accounts, it will be necessary to provide a statement from that account (it doesn't matter whether or not the patient is listed as owner on that account).

- Explanation of any automatic payments or withdrawals – this includes payments for insurance and burial policies. If something is being automatically withdrawn and the patient/family has no idea what the item is about, it's possible that the bank can help research this issue.

- Life insurance policy information – you must provide the cover sheet and statement of cash value of any life insurance policies that the patient owns or is paying out of his bank statement. If there is a cash value, the amount will probably be viewed as an asset that the patient can use to pay for his placement. In the event that the patient isn't the owner of the policy, it probably won't be considered an asset, although Medicaid will do its best to assign the patient ownership. An elder law attorney might have to help with this issue.

- Proof of ownership of burial plots – if a patient is listed as the owner of several plots it might be necessary for him to sell them unless he can prove that they have little or no resale value.   This information can be accessed from either a mortuary or the city in which the cemetery exists.

- Cover sheet and statement of cash value for burial plan or policy – in some states, it is acceptable to Medicaid for a patient to irrevocably assign the cash value of a burial insurance policy to the mortuary; in other states this would still be considered an asset available to the patient. If that is the case, the Medicaid office or an elder law attorney can advise as to how to remove this as an asset to the patient.

- Certificate of registration and/or title for all automobiles – if there is more than one car it's still possible to qualify for Medicaid as long as the autos have negligible value. It's best to either pull up the information from the Kelly blue book online, or obtain a statement from an auto dealer. If the car has a loan against it, it will be necessary to provide a copy of the payment coupon and it will have to be affordable within the confines of the patient's income, or this will raise the question as to how the patient has been making the payment.

- Proof of insurance for all autos.

- Proof of ownership of all other assets, including ATV's, motor homes, etc.

- If the patient has a personal trust or is part of a family trust, it will be necessary to provide information about the ownership, successor trustees, whether the trust is revocable, and "Schedule A" which usually lists all of the items that have been deeded into the trust. The eligibility worker will have many questions and will probably forward the information to another department to review. They can and will request additional documentation regarding the assets owned by the trust.

The above list isn't all-inclusive. Each state has different requirements in order for the Medicaid application to be approved. It's important to understand that the patient is essentially asking for the state and federal governments to pay thousands of dollars each month on his behalf, and the Medicaid office wants to make sure that the patient is eligible for the program. Applying for Medicaid has been compared to applying for a home loan.

Remember that it's the patient's responsibility to prove eligibility, and the Medicaid worker will deny or delay assistance to anyone who appears to be hiding assets. When completing a Medicaid application, you are attempting to paint a complete picture of the patient's & spouse's finances so that there won't be any unnecessary delays. The more questions there are, the longer the wait for approval will be. A simple application can be approved immediately, while a complicated one can take six or more months for approval. During that time, the nursing home might be providing the care free of charge or it might be collecting from the patients' family members while waiting for the application to be approved.

Organizing the Application

The application itself is usually around ten pages (varies according to state requirements) and doesn't appear to be daunting. The verifications that must accompany the application are the most important component, and it's vital that they are easily understood. Unless the patient's finances are so simple that only a few verifications are needed, it's best to organize the application in a manner that makes it easier for the worker to quickly access the information.

I've found that a cover letter explaining the patient's situation can be quite helpful by filling in the gaps that aren't otherwise explained in the application. For example, if the patient was living alone since his wife died a few months ago but recently moved in with his children, there's no place on the application to explain the reason for his change in residence and circumstance. A cover letter will also personalize the application, which might help the eligibility worker remember that she's dealing with a person and not just a file. A letter of explanation such as this can decrease the amount of time it takes to become approved for Medicaid, because it answers many of the questions the worker has when she reviews the application and verifications. The letter should be simple and concise; if it's too lengthy, the worker might not even read it.

It also doesn't hurt to group multiple verifications into sections, such as income, assets, bank accounts, insurance policies, identifications, etc. and to provide a cover sheet for each section that explains what is being provided. For those applications that require many different categories of verifications, organizing them in a three ring binder might be a good idea. I also recommend highlighting items that have an explanation, so that they won't be missed. Remember that many states now require the application to be scanned into a computer system, so it's best to make it easy to scan (no staples, binding, etc). Don't provide information that isn't needed; if you include extra information it can make the eligibility worker angry and it's possible she won't want to work as hard to get the patient eligible for Medicaid. It happens.

Keep a copy of the application in the exact same order as the one that was submitted to the Medicaid office. If the worker calls with a question, she can reference the section and specific page and you can easily find it.

What to Expect After the Application Has Been Submitted

After the application is completed and as much supporting documentation as possible has been attached, it will need to be submitted. Depending upon where you live, you might be able to hand deliver it, or the nursing home might be able to help you deliver the application. If it needs to be mailed in, send it certified return receipt. Another option might be to Federal Express the application. Don't send it regular mail unless it can be easily tracked.

Once the Medicaid office receives the application, it can take anywhere from two weeks to several months for a decision to be made; each state has specific guidelines it must follow. An eligibility worker will be assigned, and she has about two weeks to review the application and all of the verifications. Her job is to identify anything that might disqualify the patient; if something is obvious, the eligibility worker will immediately request additional information or process a denial. The patient/family then has a couple of weeks to obtain the additional items. It's important to deliver them by the requested date or the Medicaid will be denied. Because these additional verifications are time sensitive, keep a copy of any fax confirmation sheet and also call to confirm that the Medicaid office has it in their possession. Document the name of the person with whom you spoke, as well as the date & time. If you deliver the documents in person, ask for a time-stamped receipt. Remember that items are lost everyday, and that the burden of proof is on the patient. I've known of workers who were so disorganized they had huge piles of paper on their desk – and yet, patients were denied Medicaid because the paperwork hadn't been placed in their files.

There are many issues that patients will need to resolve and the verifications are supposed to do just that. However, the verifications might raise more questions than answers. The Medicaid worker will review the application and address the following issues:

Home Ownership Issues

- *Date of the loan and the original amount* – if a large down payment was made to the mortgage company, the worker might question where the money came from. If it resulted from the sale of another home or piece of property, the worker will need the closing statements from that transaction as well.

- *Monthly loan payment* – if the home's monthly payment is a higher amount than the patient is able to pay with his stated income, the worker will question how the patient has been making the payment.

- *The home owner of record* – the worker can access the property assessor's records and find out when the home was purchased, how much it sold for, and who legally owns the property. This web page reflects whether there were any recent transfers of the home's ownership and verifies that the patient doesn't own other properties he hasn't reported.

- *If the patient is a renter* – the worker can search the property records to ensure the patient isn't trying to hide an asset by transferring the home to a family member and pretending to rent. They will also request a copy of the lease, and verify the origin of the security and cleaning deposit monies if they don't show as originating from the bank account.

- *Online searches of assessor sites* – if the patient recently moved to the area, the worker might review the property records from the past addresses he listed on the application, as well as to access property records for his family members. It's important to note that any out-of-state property owned by the patient is considered to be non-residential (not the patient's primary residence) and *at the very least* Medicaid will be denied unless the home is put up for sale.

- *If the patient recently sold/bought a home* – the worker will ask for the closing statements and will track where the money went. If the patient sold a home for $200,000 that had been paid-off and took out a loan to buy another $200,000 home, the worker will probably deny the Medicaid until it can be verified where the excess monies went.

- *Indicators of fraud* – house payments that aren't affordable based on the patient's stated income, and patients who are vague about property information.

Automobiles

- *The worker might be able to access DMV records* – and will probably find out how many autos are registered in the patient's name. If it's more than one, the patient probably isn't eligible for Medicaid. This depends upon whether the cars are in operating condition.

- *Auto purchase contracts* – the worker can review the contract from a recent car purchase and will question where the car that was replaced went (was it sold and the money hidden, or given to a grandchild?). The payment on the contract must match the amount that the patient is paying out of his account each month; otherwise the worker will question the transactions.

- *The worker can request insurance information* – the worker can ask for the insurance information and will verify how many cars are insured; since most people bundle their insurance they can also verify home ownership issues.

- *Indicators of Fraud* – car payments that the patient can't afford with his stated income, payments that are directly withdrawn from the patient's bank accounts when he claims that he doesn't own any autos.

Burial Plans

- *Prepaid burial plans* – the plan must be reasonable; if an applicant buys a policy with a value of $20,000, then immediately applies for Medicaid, the assistance could be denied. The burial plan allowable amount doesn't include the cost of the funeral plot, and if one was recently purchased the eligibility worker will need to see a copy of that paperwork as well.

- *Cash value* – most people don't realize that often a burial plan is an insurance policy rather than a prepayment for the funeral expenses to the mortuary. Buying a policy assures that the price for the funeral will be covered, but it also accrues a cash value that helps to offset the cost of inflation to the mortuary. The cash value also counts toward the patient's $2,000 maximum assets.

- *Transfers and changes to the burial plan* – any transfers of the ownership to remove the cash value from the list of the patient's assets might be considered gifting and can result in a Medicaid denial. It also might be allowed; each state is different.

- *Burial plots* – the worker will need proof of ownership of all burial plots. If the patient owns more than one, he will need a statement showing the value and whether or not it can be resold.

- *Other issues* – many state Medicaid programs will allow a burial policy if the cash value is irrevocably assigned to someone else or to the mortuary, while other states won't recognize that the cash value has been assigned to another party. It's important to check with the Medicaid program of the state where the nursing home is located because the rules vary.

- *Indicators of fraud* – burial plans for multiple family members paid out of the applicant's funds (they'll probably be in numerical order in the mortuary's records and can be verified by withdrawals from the patient's back account).

Bank Accounts

- *Social Security deposits* – direct deposits are noted on the statement and must match the amounts verified by Social Security. For couples, both deposits must be verified.

- *Automatic deposits* – if there are other automatic deposits, the patient's bank statement will show tracking information. The patient will need to provide a statement from each company of origin.

- *Miscellaneous deposits* – the worker will question where the money is coming from and might ask for proof. For example, if the spouse has been selling personal items on EBay for extra money, the worker will probably request a printout from EBay or a statement from Pay-pal.

- *Automatic payments* – every automatic payment is noted on the bank statement and can be tracked. I've known people who denied they owned a life insurance policy, yet there was an automatic withdrawal listed on their bank statement each month.

- *Miscellaneous payments* – the worker can question any transactions to/from the account.

- *Account transfers* – money that is transferred between accounts will have been noted on both account statements; the worker might request copies of statements from both accounts whether or not the patient is listed as the owner of both accounts.

- *Money that "magically" appears* – the worker will need to know where it came from. If an applicant is claiming that they borrowed from a family member, the worker will more than likely ask for a copy of the repayment agreement. It's best to have such an agreement notarized. At the very least, the worker will request a statement from whoever gifted the money.

- *Money that "magically" disappears* – sometimes the worker will ask for random statements from the past 2 years rather than to ask for every bank statement. If there is a high balance one year and the money is gone the next year, the worker will need to know where the money went.

- *Account owners* – for jointly owned accounts, the worker will need proof that half of the money belongs to the other person and that the account is used for the benefit of both parties. If the account appears to be used only for the patient's needs, the full value belongs to the applicant for Medicaid purposes regardless of the listed owners.

- *Indicators of fraud* – unexplained items, photocopies that appear to have been altered and accounts where family members were added as co-owners but there's nothing to show that the money ever belonged to them.

Loans & Other Debts

- *Home loans* – loan documents will verify amounts. As mentioned before, bank statements must match the amounts paid from or to the patient.

- *Auto loans* – loan documents will verify amounts.

- *Personal loans, or loans from family members* – the worker will need verification of where the money came from as well as written documentation of payment arrangements. Proof of any loans between family members should be notarized so that there won't be any questions later on. If the patient makes a large payment to a family member without supporting documentation, it might be viewed as gifting to become eligible for Medicaid.

- *Indicators of fraud* – unexplained items, photocopies that appear to have been altered and loans or debts that simply don't make sense.

Income Tax Forms

- *Income verification* – this information must match the bank account information provided by the applicant.

- *Interest income* – the tax return will show if there are investments, even if the information wasn't provided on the Medicaid application.

- *Real estate information* – if the applicant doesn't own a home yet claims to be paying real estate taxes, the eligibility worker will deny the application until the information can be verified.

- *Direct deposit of a refund* – the worker can compare the account numbers into which any refund was directly deposited, and will ask for statements from that account.

- *Indicators of fraud* – information that contradicts the financial situation presented in the application.

Life Insurance Policies

- *Cash value* – the worker will need statement of the cash value, if any.

- *Loans against cash value* – the worker will need to track the proceeds of any loans against the cash value of a policy to make sure the money wasn't hidden away to make the patient appear eligible.

- *Indicators of fraud* – if the policy was recently changed in or out of the applicant's name, it might be viewed as a divestiture of assets in order to become eligible for Medicaid. Any extra money paid on the policy can affect eligibility.

Additional Information about Medicaid

- The worker isn't there to pass judgment on the patient's or family's lifestyle. The only objective is to determine whether or not the patient is eligible for the program. Medicaid workers have probably seen finances that are much more jumbled than what you are presenting.

- Don't volunteer extra information. The worker doesn't need to know that the patient and spouse took an extravagant vacation several years ago. The worker might question where the money for the vacation came from. The law allows her to ask for information about the patient's finances, not about his lifestyle.

- Expenses and income should match. If the income is much greater than the expenses, the worker might question where the money went. If expenses are greater than income, how is the applicant paying his ongoing bills? Wherever the money is coming from, and why can't it continue?

- If the patient is already in a nursing home, work with a designated nursing home staff member for help with Medicaid applications if they have one. If the patient is at home and a social worker is assisting, allow them to help with the application if they're able.

- Always be honest and helpful. Just like everyone else, eligibility workers tend to respond better to people who are cooperative and friendly. The more difficult a person is to work with, the greater the chance that the application will be denied. Make sure that the applications and verifications are submitted on time and that all deadlines are met. If an application is denied make sure that the appeal is completed in the format and time frame that the application requires.

- Make sure that an application is in place the entire time the patient is attempting to apply for Medicaid. In most cases, an application that has been successfully appealed will pay retroactively to the date the Medicaid application was first submitted. However, if the application was denied and never appealed, but later another application was submitted, the period of time that no application was on file probably won't be covered.

- It's important to let the nursing home know as soon as you are applying for Medicaid; in addition to the Medicaid application you've submitted, the nursing home is required to submit certain forms to the Medicaid office. Without these forms, the nursing home won't be able to bill Medicaid retroactive to the date the application is approved. This means that the patient or his family will be responsible for the bill *even if the Medicaid is approved.* Don't worry about the nursing home attempting to discharge the patient because he's applying for Medicaid because they're not legally allowed to discriminate on the basis of payment source. If you have any problems, call the state regulatory agency or the ombudsman to discuss your concerns.

Appealing a Denial of Medicaid

A Medicaid application can be denied for any number of reasons. It's possible that a paperwork error might have occurred, or that the patient simply isn't eligible at all, even if he hires an elder law attorney. The official denial will include the reason that the program believes that the patient isn't eligible; if the patient has too many assets the Medicaid program will include the future date that the patient will be eligible for assistance.

Once the Medicaid has been denied, there is an appeal process included on the denial form. It's important that the appeal process be followed exactly (including submitting the appeal by the required date), or the patient will have to start the application process all over again. In most cases, when the application is finally accepted, Medicaid will pay retroactively for all of the months that an application was awaiting determination. In most cases, Medicaid won't pay for any lapses in time when there wasn't an active application pending.

The nursing home might be able to help with the appeals process; if so, take their advice. If they recommend that you consult with an attorney or other professional, it's probably a good idea to do so. Don't just accept that the patient isn't eligible for assistance because it's possible that the Medicaid office made a mistake with their determination. Don't call up and verbally abuse the eligibility worker, or chances are you'll never be approved for Medicaid. If you believe that you have a case for overturning a Medicaid determination, you should do so and follow the appeal process.

Other Medicaid Programs (non-nursing home based)

There are Medicaid-based programs for the aged that vary in the services for which they pay. Medicaid can pay for extra assistance in the home, or might simply act as secondary insurances to Medicare. None of these programs are available to patients who reside in nursing homes because they're not necessary; Institutional Medicaid generally covers all necessary costs that Medicare doesn't.

Traditional Medicaid

In order to qualify for traditional Medicaid as a Medicare supplement, the patient must be eligible for Medicare and receive **Supplemental Security Income (SSI)**. The income and asset limits for SSI vary by state, but the client must be over the age of 65 to be eligible for "aged" SSI. Supplemental Security Income is a financial program that raises the income of seniors to just over $721.00 per month (2014 amounts), although some states pay a higher amount to their residents – and if the senior is married and the partner is blind or disabled it is possible that the amounts will even be higher. Like nursing home Medicaid, the senior may have a home (it must be occupied by the senior and there can't be any extra income to the senior from renting out rooms), a car, a burial plan, and less than $2,000 in assets

l.e. green

(varies according to state). Call Social Security at (800) 772-1213 to see if a person qualifies for SSI or visit each state's website for more information.

Medicare beneficiaries who also have Medicaid are considered to have **Dual Eligibility**. Medicaid pays the patient's portion of the billing amounts that Medicare approves but doesn't pay. Medicaid programs usually pay a contracted rate that is less than the private rates paid by a Medigap policy; because of the lower reimbursement rate some providers won't accept Medicaid at all.

Dual eligible patients often qualify for special Medicare Part C Advantage plans that cover more than the regular HMO/PPO coverage offered to Medicare beneficiaries; they'll often include dental care, hearing aids and prescription glasses and will have little or no out of pocket costs with these plans. Some states offer only one provider for this plan, while other states allow insurance companies to compete for patients. Other than the name of the provider on the insurance card, it generally doesn't make a difference to the patient as to which company he chooses. Even though these plans provide extra benefits, they also severely limit the patient's choices as to providers and services they'll receive.

Nursing home-based patients are able to select dual eligibility Part C Advantage plans, but it can be difficult for the nursing home to coordinate the insurance company's plan patient's care with that of the nursing home. Things become even more complicated if the patient requires physical therapy and the third-party therapy company contracted with the nursing home isn't a plan provider. It's always best to discuss enrollment – or disenrollment – of a Part C Advantage plan with a nursing home administrator or billing office manager before you make any changes on the patient's behalf. Don't trust that telling the charge nurse is enough to address this issue. Floor nurses don't understand insurance and billing issues and you might make a change that you regret.

Depending upon the state in which the beneficiary lives, even without enrolling in a Part C Advantage plan the patient might also receive dental care, hearing aids and prescription glasses. There are usually limits on the types of services and amounts that Medicaid will pay. Medicare beneficiaries who receive Medicaid also might also receive additional items such as incontinence supplies, home bathing assistance, additional equipment and services such as blood draws that Medicare doesn't pay for. For additional information about these extra services, it's best to contact Medicaid, a local Senior Center or your local Area Agency on Aging. It is also possible that a medical equipment provider or home health agency might have information as to how to access these services.

Qualified Medicare Beneficiaries

Qualified Medicare Beneficiaries (QMB) is another program offered by Medicaid that acts as a supplement policy to Medicare. Like Medicaid, there is no charge to the client for the program, which is designed to assist beneficiaries who

256

can't afford to pay for a supplemental policy. QMB pays for the Part B premium, meaning that the patient's income will increase by $104.90 each month (2014 amounts), and the beneficiary must present a Medicaid card to each medical provider at the time of service.

QMB doesn't offer the extra services for which full Medicaid pays, such as the incontinence supplies, home bathing assistance, additional equipment and services such as blood draws. QMB also doesn't pay for prescription eyeglasses, hearing aids and dental care. To qualify for QMB, clients must have less than $6,940 in assets (single person) and $10,410 (married couple), and no more than a burial plan, a car & a home; there are also income limits that start at $951 (single person) and $1,137 (married couple) although income limits vary according to state. For additional information on QMB, contact your local Medicaid office.

Again, Medicaid program eligibility varies from state-to-state and there are often ways to become eligible for assistance even though the patient or family believes that the patient doesn't qualify. Contact your Area Agency on Aging for additional information about your state or research the specific eligibility criteria for your state on the internet.

Specified Low Income Beneficiaries

Specified Low Income beneficiaries (SLMB) is a program for seniors who are over the income limit for QMB, but are still considered to be lower-income. SLMB pays the monthly Medicare Part B premium for the senior, effectively raising his income by $104.90 each month (2014 amounts). While SLMB isn't a supplement to Medicare, it does save the client a little over a hundred dollars per month. Just like the other Medicaid programs, the Part B premium is not deducted from his monthly income but unlike the other programs SLMB does not cover any other services for the client. The income and asset limits for SLMB varies by state; for further information on SLMB, contact your local Medicaid office.

Aging Waiver Programs

Medicaid Aging Waiver programs are designed to provide assistance in patient's homes or wherever the patient resides, including the homes of family members or in assisted living facilities. The goal of waiver programs is to assist patients who meet the criteria for nursing home level of care, but are able to maintain elsewhere with the help of agencies and/or family members. Aging waivers are wonderful programs, but there are often waiting lists that result in long delays before the patient is even assessed for the program, much less approved to receive the actual care.

Waiver programs are often difficult to understand. In order for the patient to qualify for the program he must meet the nursing home level of care but must still not require 24-hour care. If the patient is too independent, he won't qualify – but if his level of care is too high, he also might not qualify. The program will send in staff from a home-care agency to bathe the patient, provide him with a homemaker, shopping assistance, senior companions to sit with the patient, pay for specialty equipment and food supplements, and also might provide up to a couple of weeks of *respite care* in a facility so that the patient's caregiver can take a break. Some waiver programs pay for adult day care so that a patient can live with a family member who holds a full-time job. It's best to speak with the actual agency that administers waiver programs, because the more people that you ask about them the greater the opportunity to receive incorrect information.

Depending upon the rules of the state in which the patient resides, it's possible that a family member can be paid to help care for the patient. Some states offer programs that pay the family members directly, while others pay agencies that are able to add the family members to their payroll. In most cases, the amount that's paid is substantially less than full-time wages.

There are also waiver programs designed to help a nursing home patient to be discharged to a lower level of care such as an assisted living facility or group home. These waiver programs may pick up part of the cost of the assisted living facility or group home, although the amount that the Medicaid program pays is considered to be payment for the services while the patient pays for his room & board. Like most waiver programs, these programs vary from state to state and might have long waiting lists. In order to receive more information about such a program that might offered in your area, contact your Area Agency on Aging or the assisted living facility itself.

Because each state must offer waiver programs – and each state has the opportunity to tailor the waiver programs to their perceived needs of their patients – waiver programs are complicated. There truly is no "clearing house" that offers concise information about programs that are available in each state. I run across situations on a daily basis where a patient has been misinformed about the availability of assistance and the financial eligibility requirements. The information that the patient/family receives depends upon the experience and training of the person answering the question. Asking a community social worker might not be helpful; even though each state has an education requirement regarding ongoing social work licensure, it's possible that the information they received during an in-service two years ago is no longer valid. There are always new programs being introduced while others are being shuttered, so it's best to call your area agency on aging for information about waiver programs.

Like all Medicaid programs, aging waiver programs have income and asset eligibility guidelines that vary from state to state, but they usually mirror the criteria for institutional Medicaid. The client is allowed to keep some or all of his income to maintain the household; if the senior is over income it's possible that he will be able to "spend-down" (pay the amount of overage to the Medicaid program) in order to qualify. Concessions are often made for medical-related expenses in order to ensure that the patient's needs are met.

Patients with traditional Medicaid who apply for a waiver program might not be eligible because they must first utilize the services of the program for which they are eligible. They will only be able to access waiver programs if traditional Medicaid isn't able to meet their needs. To apply for waiver programs, it's necessary to contact the agency managing the specific program for your area and follow their instructions. In most cases, applicants are screened for eligibility and then placed on a waiting list. It's possible that the patient will be contacted every few months to ensure that he wants to continue waiting for services, although in many cases he won't hear from the program until his turn comes up on the list.

Once the patient's name comes up, he will be contacted by a worker who will assist him in completing an institutional Medicaid application. It is not possible to speed up the process by applying for institutional Medicaid on your own, because patients aren't eligible for this type of Medicaid if they're not in a nursing home *unless they're working with a waiver program.* After the application has been approved, the services will generally start within a month or two. The length of time that it takes to begin services might be too long for the patient to wait, and it's common for patient to end up in nursing homes long before they are accepted into a Medicaid waiver program.

Jim's mother (Mary) lives in an Assisted Living Center. She becomes increasingly dizzy, and suffers a fall in the dining room. Mary is sent to the Emergency Room and subsequently admitted to the hospital for complications due to a hip fracture. From there, she is sent to an Acute Rehabilitation Facility for comprehensive therapy. Two weeks later, she isn't quite ready to return home and is discharged to a Skilled Nursing Facility.

In each facility, Jim speaks with a social worker or case manager about Mary's need for additional in-home care when she returns to the ALF. Each social worker/case manager provides him with different criteria for programs that might be able to assist his mother in her home on a long-term basis. However, none of them are able to provide any written information, until his mother is discharged home and the home health company's social worker assists with a referral to a Medicaid waiver program.

Although the appearance is that waiver programs save the Medicaid program more money than if it were to pay for 24-hour care in a nursing home, they can cost the state and federal governments substantially more than those programs that pay for nursing home placement. Waiver programs are federally funded and loaded with requirements; the monies are first sent to the state, then funneled through multiple oversight agencies. Each agency takes their cut before the money finally trickles down to the agencies providing the actual patient care. Sometimes the oversight is necessary, but other times it appears that the only role each agency plays is to add to the layers of bureaucracy of which the Medicaid program is so fond. The only benefit to these programs is that patients are able to remain in a less restrictive environment rather than to be forced to reside in a nursing home.

Because eligibility guidelines vary from state to state, it's best to contact the Area Agency on Aging in the senior's community to find out if these programs exist and whether the senior might be eligible. These programs provide services to patients whether they are married or single, as long as they meet the eligibility requirements.

Medicare

Medicare is the federally funded health insurance program for people who are 65 or older, diagnosed with End Stage Renal Disease or Amyotrophic Lateral Sclerosis (ALS), or those whom the Social Security Administration has deemed to have been disabled for at least 24 months. People who are enrolled in the Medicare program are called *Medicare beneficiaries* or *Medicare recipients.*

The part of the United States Government that governs the Medicare program is the *Department of Health and Human Services (HHS);* the government agency within HHS that administers both the Medicare and the Medicaid programs is the *Centers for Medicare and Medicaid Services (CMS)*. The Centers for Medicare and Medicaid Services contracts with private companies to either provide a health insurance plan or to process billings for beneficiaries and tell the government how much to pay on the claim. CMS also contracts with various public and private agencies to provide oversight and hopefully ensure that the Medicare benefits are being administered in an ethical and ceffective manner. In other words, there are many different providers, both public agost encies and private companies, being paid to make the program work. It's difficult to navigate through this system, especially since you'll receive different answers to the same questions depending upon whom you ask.

The Medicare Program is complicated and difficult to understand, so to help explain it better, CMS sends out an annual booklet to Medicare beneficiaries entitled **Medicare & You**. This booklet is over one hundred pages long and is chock full of information that can be confusing even to professionals who deal with it on a daily basis. Imagine how confusing it might be to a senior who needs to make an immediate decision about which plan will provide the most coverage for his specific medical needs. A copy can be requested by calling 1-800-MEDICARE (1-800-633-4227), can be found at local senior centers, and social service agencies might possibly have extras that they can give out. The booklet can also be easily downloaded from the Medicare website at www.medicare.gov:

How to Order or Download a Medicare Publication Online*

- Go to www.Medicare.gov
- Across the top of the page are blue boxes; look for the one entitled **Forms, Help & Resources**. Hold your mouse over the box – it will give a drop-down menu.
- Click on **Publications**. Medicare & You will be on the first page, but there are other publications that can be found as well.

---

*Medicare changes its website often, there might be a different search for the information you want.

Medicare & You provides an overview of the program, information about client's *Medicare rights* and also explains how to *appeal a determination*, which is a decision made about payment for an existing medical bill. All of the information about Medicare is explained in detail, so it's a good idea to keep the booklet in a place where it can be easily found. **Medicare & You** is available in both English & Spanish, large print (both languages), audiotape (both languages), and in Braille. This isn't the only publication about Medicare; the website offers over 80 different publications that describe every component of the Medicare program in detail.

Medicare Eligibility

Approximately three months before a person meets his retirement age or becomes eligible for Medicare, the *Social Security Administration (SSA)* sends out information advising as to the health insurance options available to him. The SSA determines the client's eligibility for Medicare and calculates how much the client will pay for his monthly premium for both the A & B benefits; this amount varies according to the number of quarters that the client paid into the Medicare program over his lifetime, his annual income, and his retirement age. Most people are eligible to receive part A for "free" (after paying into the system for many years), but there is a monthly premium to participate in the part B program. Part A covers hospitalization, while part B covers outpatient services. Both are explained later in this section.

After determining that a client is indeed eligible for Medicare, the SSA collects the premiums from the retiree's monthly Social Security income beginning the month that he's eligible. Premiums are collected by deducting the amount due before the monies are deposited into the client's bank account each month (or applied to a debit card, if the recipient doesn't have a bank account).

People who choose to take an early retirement any time after they turn 62 years old won't be eligible for Medicare until they are 65 years old, although they will receive a monthly Social Security payment. The age that a retiree qualifies to collect a full retirement check is slowly adjusting upward, but according to current rules the age for Medicare eligibility will continue to remain 65 years old.

Year of Birth	Full Retirement Age
1937 or earlier	65 years old
1938 – 1959	65 years + 2 months to 65 years + 10months
1960 or later	67 years old

Retired members of the military and their civilian family members will receive *TRICARE Insurance* instead of the Medicare Part A benefit. TRICARE enrollees are required to apply for Medicare Part B, which compliments the TRICARE insurance coverage. It's possible that their medications will be provided by the Veteran's Administration; if not, the TRICARE enrollees will need to apply for Medicare Part D prescription drug coverage as well. TRICARE will notify the beneficiary about their available coverage for prescriptions.

Most retired railroad workers are automatically enrolled in the Medicare Part A program by the *Railroad Retirement Board* instead of them having to make an application for Medicare Part A; however, the railroad retirement program requires that their beneficiaries enroll in and pay for Medicare Part B for medical coverage and Medicare Part D for prescription drug coverage. The Railroad Retirement Board will send out information to their retirees advising them of the changes in their insurance benefits when they retire, and what they must do to continue receiving healthcare benefits.

People who have been diagnosed with End Stage Renal Disease, Amyotrophic Lateral Sclerosis (ALS – also known as Lou Gehrig's disease), or who are legally blind qualify for Medicare regardless of their age or the length of their disability. It's important that people with these diagnoses apply for Medicare immediately, because they will need the benefit in order to be able to pay for the medical care necessary to treat their illness. All other people who are receiving Social Security disability benefits are eligible for Medicare two years after they have been deemed disabled or when they reach 65 years of age, whichever comes first.

Applying for Social Security Disability

The application process for social security disability benefits is a long, drawn-out process. The majority of applications are immediately denied, and the client is required to follow through with a rather confusing appeal process for the next year or two. If the client misses a filing date, the application will probably have to be filed all over again.

When an applicant is fortunate enough to be deemed disabled and has been awarded disability income (often a two year process), his date of disability will be determined by the Social Security Administration. For example, a person who for all practical purposes was disabled in January might be "deemed" disabled as of June; that client will receive disability payments retroactive to June and will be eligible for Medicare two years from that date. The date that the SSA chooses often doesn't make sense, and it's not possible to appeal a positive determination in order to become eligible for Medicare at an earlier date.

When applying for disability benefits, the burden of proof is the applicant's responsibility. It's important to see a doctor as soon as possible to ensure that there is supporting documentation that can be provided to Social Security. The more information that can be presented to support an applicant's disability claim, the earlier in the process that he *might* be deemed disabled. This can be a difficult endeavor for the person who can't afford to pay for their medical care.

Unless a client has a private insurance policy (for which he is responsible to pay the premiums), he probably won't have any healthcare coverage during the time he is waiting for his disability to be awarded. There might be a Medicaid program that will pay the patient's bills retroactively once Social Security deems he is disabled, but the medical provider must be willing to wait a couple of years to be paid. Most doctors, therapists and pharmacies aren't willing to do so. Sometimes state or local agencies will provide medical care, or at least guarantee that they'll pay the bills if Medicaid is never awarded. In order to qualify for these programs, the applicant must be extremely low-income and can't have more than $2,000 in assets (this amount varies by state). Unfortunately, this is a confusing process for someone who desperately needs medical care and financial assistance. The Affordable Healthcare Act (ACA) might change this situation, although it's unclear as to how disabled people will be affected if they missed the open enrollment period. Several states are still quibbling over the Medicaid expansion at the present time.

A person who is filing for disability is claiming that he is no longer able to perform work duties *of any kind*, not just the type of work he was doing before. During the entire time period he awaits a determination, he *can't* work because, if he holds a job of any type, he's not really disabled. Although sometimes there are state and local programs available to help out financially while an applicant awaits a decision, the benefit amount is rarely sufficient to sustain a person or household. Some applicants will continue to try to work in order to make ends meet, but this alone will render them ineligible for disability even if they only last one day on the job. The system is difficult and demeaning, to say the least. It's helpful if the applicant has a supportive family to provide emotional and financial support as he awaits a determination.

Social Security and Medicare help out only when people are fully disabled, not partially disabled. Unfortunately Social Security doesn't help out if a person can't make as much money as before he was injured, or if there are no jobs available in his chosen field; the benefit is only awarded to people who are fully disabled and aren't able to hold a job.

As if attempting to qualify for Medicare isn't hard enough, the financial aspects of Social Security Disability are confusing: the first five months a client has been deemed disabled by Social Security he will only be eligible for Supplemental Security Income (SSI) as long as he meets the financial criteria. The 2014 federal SSI amount is approximately $721.00 per month; an applicant won't qualify for assistance unless he makes less than $721.00 and has less than $2,000 in assets. The $721.00 amount differs according to the state in which the applicant resides;

some states such as California pay an additional amount to SSI recipients. SSI will be paid retroactively if and when the patient is awarded Social Security Disability benefits as long as he meets the financial eligibility criteria (above).

After those first five months, the client's ongoing Social Security Disability payments will be a different amount that's based on his employment history and the amounts that he paid into the Social Security system. Simply stated, when the disability is finally awarded the patient might receive two retroactive checks: one for SSI and one for Social Security Disability. However, if they had savings that helped them to make it through those first months, they're probably not eligible for SSI.

Many people have no other source of income and can't afford to wait a couple of years to receive any income. While they're waiting, they might be able to receive assistance from a program called *General Assistance (GA)*, which is a federal program administered by state or local agencies that provides a minimal amount to clients who don't have any other finances available to help them out. The GA eligibility limits for income and assets are quite stringent and hard to meet, and those people who qualify for GA usually must pay it back out of their retroactive lump-sum checks from Social Security.

Before receiving any help from General Assistance programs, clients are first required to sign a form that allows their SSA award checks to be sent to the agency that provided the General Assistance. The amount of GA that was paid out will be deducted, and then the client will receive his money. I've heard it described as "dangling a carrot" in front of the clients; their lump-sum checks are sent out from Social Security but they must wait another month or two while the repayment is processed before they actually have their money in-hand. The worst part is that, during this period of time, the clients won't have *any* income to get them through. It's a catch-22; the client has already received his SSA award so he doesn't qualify for General Assistance, even though he doesn't actually hold it in-hand. It can be very frustrating, and can render the applicant homeless.

Some applicants hire an attorney to represent them during the Social Security application process, usually because the SSA has notified the client that he "may wish to have an attorney present" during a particular hearing. Those people who hire an attorney are often charged 25% of the total retroactive lump-sum payment the client receives from Social Security and SSI (not the amount left over after any General Assistance payments have been deducted). Although an attorney might be instrumental in helping with the process, it's also possible that the client would have been awarded disability without him or her.

It's a personal decision as to whether an attorney should be hired to assist with Social Security Disability applications, but applicants who plan on hiring an attorney should do so from the start. It's much easier for an attorney to be actively involved throughout the application process than it is for him to come in at the end of it and attempt to make sense of the situation. Hopefully his intervention will make a difference and he will be instrumental in the application becoming approved. Even if you decide to wait until the last moment, it's doubtful that an attorney will turn away the business. Regardless as to whether the application would have been approved without his intervention, he'll collect a fee. In the 25 years that I've been a social worker, I've only met one attorney who turned away a client because his application was solid.

Navigating Through the Sea of Information

People are bombarded with information about the various options available in their community at the time that they become eligible for Medicare. The plan choices differ according to geographical area of the country, but one thing is certain: participating in the Medicare program offers a huge financial payoff to its providers and the competition for patients is fierce. Insurers place expensive glossy brochures in every conceivable place that a senior might frequent, such as doctor's offices, hospitals, pharmacies, medical equipment companies, restaurants, and bowling alleys. I've even seen brochures in casinos and public restrooms.

Since the federal government doesn't have guidelines about the location and manner in which information about Medicare products is displayed, it's a marketing free-for-all. Medical providers (such as hospitals, doctor's offices, medical equipment companies, etc.) often prominently display the information for the insurance company with which they are affiliated, while relegating information about other providers to the back (if they display them at all). Questions about non-affiliated plans might be answered incorrectly in an attempt to steer customers away from the competition.

Companies that offer Medicare options often use trusted actors to help sell their products, pay for half-hour infomercials, or offer free "informational seminars" for the community that are thinly veiled sales pitches for their products. They participate in community health fairs, offering blood pressure checks or other services. Their goal is to get the customer to call their toll-free number so that they can subject them to their sales tactics. Each company represents their plan as superior to all of the others, and what they don't want potential customers to discover is that each plan follows the same guidelines and provides pretty much the same service as all the others.

Many pharmacies are affiliated with a national chain, and will often have a customer service representative available on-site to answer Medicare questions. The salesperson providing the information is usually a paid employee of the particular insurance company or health plan affiliated with the pharmacy and he receives a commission for each client he signs up. There's no guarantee that the plan he recommends is the best one available for the senior, but it surely will be the best one for the salesman. In most cases the sales staffs of insurance companies have little or no knowledge beyond the products their company offers, so the information that they provide won't include comparable plans from other companies – yet they will claim that their product is superior to the others.

Those seniors who were covered by private health insurance before they were eligible for Medicare (such as through a retirement plan) usually have the option of converting their coverage to a Medicare supplemental plan offered by their current provider. No matter the types of plans offered, the insurance company will do its best to keep a paying customer. The insurance company is banking that the patient's resistance to change will be a more important factor than whether the plan they offer is best suited to the patient's needs. It's possible that Medicare beneficiaries can receive the healthcare coverage that best suits their needs, but they'll have to sort through an awful lot of information to get there.

Because there's so much information to sort through when decisions about healthcare need to be made, seniors often turn to local senior centers or *AAA's (Area Agencies on Aging)* for help understanding the Medicare system. These agencies often provide trained volunteers that are usually seniors who are paid a *stipend* (a small non-taxable amount to supplement their income) to help others with these issues. Although they are able to answer some basic questions, these volunteers probably received only a couple of hours of training themselves. It's easy to see why there is much confusion when it comes to Medicare and other health insurances.

There are federal, state and local programs available that might help to offset the healthcare costs for low-income Medicare beneficiaries, although a lot of the time the beneficiary won't find out about these programs. There are hundreds of brochures explaining the different programs that exist, but they can be hard to find and even harder to understand. Many of these booklets can be requested from the Medicare website, but in most cases the beneficiary needs to know what to ask for – and that's assuming that the beneficiary is computer literate. It's also possible to get information by calling 1-800-Medicare and working your way through the automated voice jail.

I don't mean to imply that companies that offer Medicare insurance plans aren't providing adequate products; in most cases, the services provided to patients are well within accepted standards of practice. For the most part, the Medicare insurance provider supplies the payment and not the actual medical care; the only time the treatment becomes an issue is when an insurance company makes it difficult for a provider to obtain pre-authorizations for treatments.

It's difficult for people to understand that "necessary" doesn't mean "emergent" (life-threatening), and that many life-saving procedures are actually considered to be *elective*. An example might be surgery to remove a gallbladder; if the patient is admitted through the emergency room and the doctors believe that he will die without immediate surgery, the patient has an emergent condition. If that same patient goes to his doctor's office and the doctor makes arrangements for surgery at a future date, it's considered to be elective. The insurance company can refuse to pay for the surgery by requiring that certain medical tests be conducted beforehand, but it's much more difficult for them to deny payment for emergency surgery.

When choosing an insurance company or medical provider, remember that non-profit health insurance providers, including hospitals, hospices, home health providers and insurance parent corporations, still have to pay their expenses and that a non-profit status doesn't necessarily translate into better care for the patients. They operate under the same general rules as the for-profit plans and charge the same amounts as those that are run on a for-profit basis.

Every one will have to choose the Medicare plan that will best suit his needs when be becomes eligible for Medicare, but there are many things to take into consideration. In addition to the patient's out-of-pocket costs, it's important to verify that his physician accepts his insurance, and that there are local medical facilities that can provide the type of care that he requires. It won't be helpful to sign up with a company that provides dialysis if their closest contracted clinic is located 20 miles away; any financial savings can be wiped out by the cost of transportation or the amount of time the patient spends riding in a transport van. Determining whether or not a company is a contracted provider can be easily accomplished by calling them directly rather than to rely on an insurance sales person who is trying to meet his monthly quota. There's no guarantee that the provider list the salesperson holds is the most current one available; it's best to call the provider's bookkeeper or office manager to verify the information yourself.

If the insurance plan that the beneficiary is using doesn't meet his needs, it can be a difficult process to change plans, and that's assuming the beneficiary is aware that there are other plans that *can* meet his needs. It's human nature to avoid change, and many people stay with their current insurance plan even if it doesn't provide exactly what they need or if it costs more than other plans. People seem to have the idea that changing health insurance plans will create more problems than it would be worth, and are afraid to "rock the boat." The truth is that in many cases a patient who changes insurance companies can change back to traditional Medicare if they don't like their new plan. There are limitations on changing plans; this might need to be done during *open enrollment* periods, which is a set time period that beneficiaries can change insurance plan providers. To find out information about the open enrollment period for the healthcare plan you'd like to change, call Medicare at 1-800-Medicare or you are also able to search for the information online at www.medicare.gov.

Researching plan providers and benefits is important: I once worked in a rural area where a Medicare Advantage plan health maintenance organization came to the area and signed up several hundred clients. Unfortunately, the closest hospital just over the state line wasn't a plan provider. Customers were required to travel over 90 miles (one way) to a contracted hospital, which rarely occurred since ambulances transport patients to the closest hospital regardless of their insurance provider. Patients paid thousands of dollars in out-of-pocket charges as a result. There was only one local doctor who accepted the insurance and she wasn't accepting new patients, and the only nursing home/rehabilitation unit wasn't a contracted plan provider. Patients were assigned plan physicians near the hospital over 90 miles away, making it difficult to access proper medical care. One appointment was an all-day event (as long as the patient was able to find transportation to/from the appointment). The "winner" in that scenario were the marketing representatives who made thousands of dollars in commissions; they received $500 for each patient they signed on, as well as $500 for every year that the patient continued with that insurance plan. The sales people also received a $2,500 bonus if the patient remained on service for five years. This is precisely why it's vital that before a senior signs up with an insurance plan, he investigates exactly how he will be affected and asks the right questions.

Choosing the Right Medicare Plan

Knowledge is power, so it's vital that Medicare beneficiaries understand their choices and make informed decisions about which plan will best suit their needs. Some plans might save patients a substantial amount of money but remove their provider choices, or won't cover the beneficiary if he travels (other than for emergency care, but at a higher out-of-pocket amount). Others are expensive and yet might not provide the level of coverage the patient needs. In order to make a decision about which plan might be in the patient's best interest, it's important to understand how the original plans A&B work in concert with a *medigap* policy (Medicare supplement), and also to determine whether a Medicare Advantage plan that is able to manage that patient's care is available in the area. That way, a patient is able to make informed choices.

Choosing the correct Medicare plan is instrumental in ensuring a patient's continued health and well being, and it's always best to ask family members or trusted friends to help research your options and provide helpful insight. Patients who trust the advice of an insurance salesman without considering other plans available might be encouraged to choose a plan that provides the highest commission to the salesman. While that plan might be exactly what the client needs, it's better to make an informed choice based on patient need rather than to have regrets later on. In certain circumstances a Medicare recipient might not have a choice of Medicare plan. Recipients who are working full-time and are currently covered under an employer's healthcare plan (or are covered under a spouse or parent's plan) must sign up for Medicare. In most cases their current plan will remain primary and Medicare will be the secondary insurance.

Traditional Medicare Plan – Part A Hospitalization

Medicare Part A is provided to most Social Security recipients at no cost because they or their spouses paid Medicare taxes while they worked. If the beneficiary or spouse didn't pay enough to be fully vested into the system, SSA will calculate the premium amount that will be withheld from his Social Security check every month. The amount varies according to the number of quarters the person paid into the system, with the current (2014) maximum premium amount set at about $426.00 per month. Retirees are notified by mail about their eligibility and costs, and are also able to call the Social Security Administration (800) 772-1213 to find out exactly how much it will cost for them to enroll in the Medicare Program. Those beneficiaries who choose not to sign up for Part A when they are first eligible will have to wait for an open enrollment period before they are able to elect to use it – usually at the end of the calendar year.

Choosing Medicare Part A allows a patient to go to any hospital or provider that accepts Medicare, no matter where the facility is located. A patient who lives in one state but prefers to have a surgery in another state can do so without having to worry about whether the insurance will pay for the services. Even while on vacation, beneficiaries can be assured that they'll receive medical care, no matter whether the healthcare concern is routine or an emergency; this is true of all services provided under the Part A benefit. Traditional Medicare allows beneficiaries to choose all of their own providers without worrying about whether or not they're part of a provider network.

The copayments are calculated according to each *benefit period*, which starts the day the patient is admitted to a hospital or other facility. The benefit period continues until there is a break of 60 consecutive days that Medicare hasn't been used as the payment source for inpatient services.

Under Part A, the hospital or other provider sends the bills to a third party company, called a *Medicare Administrative Contractor (MAC)*. Essentially, the MAC is paid for each piece of paper processed; workers review invoices and determine how much is covered by Medicare as well as the amount the patient will be required to pay out of pocket (or the amount that the supplemental insurance will pay, if the beneficiary has coverage).

The MAC sends a *Determination Letter (also known as a Medicare Summary Notice, an Explanation of Benefits or EOB)* explaining billed charges and approved charges for both Medicare A&B. Until recently, these forms were referred to as EOB's, and many professionals still refer to them as such, so I will refer to them as EOB/MSN. The EOB/MSN states across the top "THIS IS NOT A BILL," and should be compared with the medical bills the beneficiary has received. The form explains how to file an *Appeal* if the patient disagrees with the decision that has been made. These forms can be confusing; they are printed in a regular sized type, and often cover several bills on one statement. Some people hire specialists to help them keep their Medicare bills straight due to the multiple charges, duplicate billings, and huge statements that result from even a simple hospital stay.

When using the Medicare Part A hospitalization benefit, there is a copayment that can either be paid out of pocket or can be paid by a Medicare supplemental policy. Under Medicare Part A, the patient's share of cost (also known as out-of-pocket costs, or deductibles) for 2014 are as follows:

Days 1-60	$1,216.00	Total
Days 61-90	$304.00	per day
Days 91-150	$608.00*	per day
Days 150 – ongoing	All Costs	
Skilled Nursing First 20 days	No Cost to Patient	
Skilled Nursing days 21-100	$152.00 per day	

These are "lifetime" days – once used they cannot be replaced. There is also a lifetime limit of 190 days for inpatient Mental Health Services.

Most medical providers accept **assignment,** which means that they will follow Medicare's billing guidelines. They agree to send the bills to the MAC, to accept the determination and to charge the patient or medigap provider only the amount that Medicare approves but doesn't pay. Many people are confused about assignment, mistakenly thinking that they won't have to pay anything out-of-pocket. When a provider accepts assignment, they are agreeing to collect a copayment from the patient or Medigap policy. If the MAC determines that Medicare isn't responsible for payment of a hospital bill and that the patient had no way of knowing the bill wouldn't be covered, it's likely that the patient won't be responsible for any part of the bill as well. This is because the provider accepts assignment.

Medical providers that choose not to accept assignment can require that the patient pay the charges in full at the time of service. The patient will have to follow up with the MAC in order to be reimbursed for the visit; this can be a time-consuming and intimidating process. Depending upon the state in which the patient was treated, providers that don't accept assignment can bill only up to 15% above the Medicare approved charges. Because this can be such a confusing process and patients don't usually have hundreds of dollars to pay out-of-pocket for all of the services provided, most doctors work with the Medicare program for patient billing. Requiring that patients pay up front in cash would also limit the potential patient base for the doctor.

Regarding the costs of hospitalization, it's important to remember that ancillary costs such as x-rays, laboratory fees, and physician charges are not covered under Medicare Part A; those charges will be covered under Medicare Part B and will be subject to different copayments and deductibles. The hospital billing might include both A&B items, or they might be billed separately. Because in most cases the physician is an independent contractor, each consulting specialist will bill separately as well.

Patients used to go to the hospital for treatment and stay until they had fully recovered, but things have changed over the years. Patients are now discharged to facilities that offer the necessary care in a much more cost effective manner such as **Long-_Term _Acute _Care Facilities (LTAC)** and **_Acute _Rehabilitation _Facilities (ARF)**. Patients are often able to remain in these facilities for several weeks, and will receive a separate bill for this admission as well as separate billings for lab fees, physician visits, etc. When they no longer require such comprehensive care, they will either be discharged home or to a skilled nursing facility for additional therapy.

Traditional Medicare Plan – Part A Skilled Nursing Benefit

People are often confused about the Medicare Part A skilled nursing and/or rehabilitation benefit. The rehabilitation services are usually offered in traditional nursing homes; some do not accept long-term patients – although they are staffed and licensed the same as every other nursing home – while others have a mix of both short and long-term patients. Some facilities offer private rooms, while others do not. Medicare doesn't pay for a private room unless the patient requires isolation for a healthcare condition; most facilities that offer private rooms are doing so to remain competitive with the other nursing homes in the area.

There are two basic types of care provided in skilled nursing facilities; custodial care and skilled nursing care. Patients who aren't able to live alone and require assistance with their activities of daily living are admitted into a nursing home for **custodial care**. This type of service provides 24-hour care to meet the client's basic needs, such as bathing, medication management, transferring assistance, meal preparation and/or assistance with eating. Medicare does not pay for custodial care, no matter whether the patient was recently discharged from the hospital or was admitted directly from his home. Please refer to the section entitled _Determining The Payment Source_ for additional information about the various types of payment for custodial care.

The Medicare program does pay for skilled nursing care; under Medicare guidelines a patient who has been discharged from an **acute hospital** following a qualifying three-day admission (over three midnights) within the past 30 days can enter a skilled nursing facility (SNF) using the Part A benefit as long as he presents a medical need. The services for which Medicare pays include specialized nursing services, physical, occupational and speech therapies provided at a higher level than can be delivered in the home.

Medicare pays the full charges for the first 20 days for skilled care in the nursing home, and as the patient continues to progress toward recovery Medicare will pay a portion of the charges for the next 80 days. The 2014 copayment amount is $152.00 per day. Please note that some medigap policies cover some or all of the cost of the facility copayments. The nursing home will have verified the amount that a medigap policy pays before the patient is admitted for therapies, and is required to notify the patient and/or family in writing about the potential out-of-pocket costs. Just like other providers, most SNF's accept assignment and bill the Medicare approved amounts in order to remain competitive with other local nursing homes.

Patients are eligible to continue receiving services in a SNF under the Medicare Part A benefit up to a maximum of 100 days *as long as the patient is showing progress*. A patient is considered to have a **custodial** need when he **plateaus** and isn't likely to progress further, unless he is receiving another skilled service such as wound care, IV's, etc. Without a need for skilled services or therapy, Medicare will not pay for the patient to stay in the nursing home *even if he isn't ready to go home*. Medicare is a health insurance, not a payment for long-term care.

Mrs. Smith, who lives alone and has Medicare A & B, falls and breaks her hip. She is admitted to the hospital for surgery, and afterward is discharged to a skilled nursing facility. The first three weeks after she has her surgery she is considered to be "non-weight bearing," meaning that she needs time to allow the bones to heal before she begins therapy. The nursing home is able to provide a limited amount of therapy for a week and attend to the wounds from her surgery.

After that first week, Mrs. Smith is totally dependent for all activities of daily living but has no skilled need. Medicare will not pay for her room & board and if she remains in the nursing home during this time period, she'll have to pay privately or apply for Medicaid.

When she is ready to start therapies, Medicare will again pay for her to receive therapy in the nursing home (including room & board) as long as it has been less than 30 days since she used the Medicare SNF benefit. If she has no money, isn't eligible for Medicaid and can't go home, the nursing home has an unpaid customer.

If the patient isn't able to go home and has no way to pay the room & board, the SNF will have to figure out a way for him to pay for his placement such as Medicaid (if he's eligible). Nursing homes aren't able to force him to leave without going through a formal eviction process, and even if they win in court they aren't able to discharge a patient to an unsafe environment. SNF's should do their homework before the patient is admitted, but many do not and are stuck with a non-paying patient.

Medicare doesn't provide care for those patients who have been discharged from the hospital after surgery and can't immediately begin therapies. Sometimes patients have to wait a few weeks as they recover sufficiently in order to begin physical therapy; an example would be the patient who has had hip surgery and is non-weight bearing for 2-3 weeks while his bones heal. If the patient doesn't require wound care and has no other skilled need, Medicare will not pay for him to remain in the nursing home during this recovery period whether or not he can receive adequate care at home. The patient will have to pay privately or find another payment source to remain in the nursing home because Medicare doesn't pay for custodial care.

When a patient is sent to the emergency room, it's best to tell the doctor that the plan is for the patient to go to a nursing home when he is discharged. If the doctor is at all able to justify making the patient's status a full admission from the start, this will expedite the Medicare SNF admission. However, the patient must present a medical need in order to remain in the hospital; it doesn't matter that the patient would benefit from the therapy offered in a nursing home, or even that the doctor is willing to write an order for him to be admitted directly into the nursing home. Medicare will not pay for a patient to be in the hospital for three days without a medical need, and without that three day qualifying stay Medicare won't pay for skilled nursing and therapy in a nursing home

Patients who are discharged from the nursing home before they use up the full 100 days might be eligible to return to the nursing home within 30 days of their discharge and receive additional therapies, but only for the remainder of the 100 days. After 30 days have passed, they'll have to be readmitted to the hospital for three days in order to use the rest of the 100 days they have left. Whether or not a patient uses the full 100 days, his Medicare skilled nursing benefit will regenerate back to the full 100 days once he hasn't used the Part A skilled benefit for 60 days.

Traditional Medicare Plan – Part A Hospice & Home Healthcare
Medicare Part A pays for the patient to receive home healthcare or hospice at virtually no out-of-pocket cost to the customer. Both of these programs are explained in more detail earlier in this book.

Home healthcare is a short-term service provided with no copayment to the patient; it is designed to rehabilitate the patient back to his former level of functioning. The benefit provides skilled nursing services, physical therapy, occupational therapy, and speech therapies to patients who are considered to be homebound.

Hospice is a type of palliative care designed to provide comfort to people who have been diagnosed with a terminal condition. Hospices can charge a co-payment for medications and inpatient respite care, but most don't charge their patients for these services in order to remain competitive with other hospice providers in the community.

Items Covered by the Medicare Part A Benefit

Part A Service	Amount of Medicare Approved Costs to be paid by beneficiary
Part A – Blood transfusions	100% of costs for first 3 pints, 20% of costs thereafter.
Part A – Hospice Care	$0 to the patient. Hospices can charge up to 5% of prescription drug costs and up to 5% for inpatient respite care.
Part A – Home Health Care	$0 to the Patient.
Part A – Hospitalization (costs per each benefit period)	$1,260 for days 1-60 $304 per day for days 61-90 $608* per day for days 91-150 *These are 60 "lifetime reserve days."
Part A – Skilled Nursing Facility (costs per each benefit period)	$0 for first 20 days, $152.00 per day for days 21-100

Traditional Medicare Plan – Part B Medical Services

Medicare Part B works in concert with Part A. It covers the rest of the medical bills that Medicare Part A doesn't. For most seniors, the Part B premium of $104.90 (2014 amount) is automatically deducted from their Social Security income before it's directly deposited into the beneficiary's account. The premium amount is waived (via the Medicaid program) for patients who are considered to be low-income, and is billed at higher amounts for recipients in the higher-income brackets. Higher-income recipients also pay a surcharge for the Part D plan of their choice, which covers medications. This charge is in addition to the plan premium.

Medicare Part B Premiums for Higher Income Beneficiaries

Income – Individual Return	Income – Joint Return	Premium Amount	Part D Surcharge
Up to $85,000	Up to $170,000	$104.90	No additional charge
$85,001 to $107,000	$170,001 to $214,000	$146.90	$12.10 + premium
$107,001 to $160,000	$214,001 to $320,000	$209.80	$31.10 + premium
$160,001 to $214,000	$320,001 to $428,000	$272.70	$50.20 + premium
More than $214,000	More than $428,000	$335.70	$69.30 + premium

Part B is a voluntary program; beneficiaries who are eligible for Part B but don't elect to use the benefit will be penalized an additional 10% of the premium for every year they were eligible but didn't sign up for it, and can only elect the benefit during open enrollment. There are annual deductibles and copayments for services received under Part B; medigap policies cover some or all of the copayments and deductibles (but not premiums). There are Medicaid programs that act as Medigap policies, covering Part B deductibles, copayments and premiums.

Although Part B is a voluntary plan, those beneficiaries who have coverage through TRICARE (military benefits), or Railroad Retirement benefits are usually required to pay for Medicare Part B in concert with their other benefits. Although Part B isn't a requirement for most Medicare recipients, it really doesn't make sense not to sign up because Part B pays for many services that would otherwise be out-of-pocket.

As mentioned above, Medicare Part B pays for the medical care that Medicare Part A doesn't cover, including visits to the doctor's office, durable medical equipment (*DME*), outpatient surgeries, transportation by ambulance, tests, and prosthetic devices. The only time that prescription medications are provided under Part B is when they are administered to the patient in a hospital or skilled nursing facility.

Like Part A, Medicare Part B claims are submitted directly to the Medicare Administrative Contractor (MAC) by the medical providers, and the beneficiary receives an EOB/MSN that says, "THIS IS NOT A BILL." It's important to read these determination letters, because sometimes the service is denied but the patient isn't responsible for the bill. The medical provider will be more than willing to help the patient with an appeal in such an instance because otherwise they won't be paid. This is because when a provider agrees to accept assignment, they are agreeing to accept the amount that Medicare approves. If Medicare denies the claim, the provider has agreed to accept the decision and only bill the client for the amount that Medicare has determined to be his responsibility, which would be nothing (no out-of-pocket cost) to the client.

When payment for an ongoing service is denied, such as for an item of specialty medical equipment, the provider has every right to retrieve the item from the patient's home. The provider can't legally bill for past charges denied by Medicare, but if the client wishes to continue receiving the service he will have to pay future costs out-of-pocket. This is true whether or not the doctor has written a prescription or has stated that the item is medically necessary. If payment is denied for equipment that is life sustaining, such as home oxygen, the provider can't remove it from the house unless other arrangements have been made to ensure the patient's needs will be met. It's important to remember that patients must medically qualify in order to receive oxygen; if they don't meet certain hallmarks (an oxygen saturation rate of less than 89%) to qualify for their oxygen, the provider may remove it from the house without making arrangements for another provider to help out the patient.

Items Covered by the Medicare Part B Benefit

Part B Service	Amount of Medicare-approved Costs to be paid by beneficiary
Part B – Deductible	$147 per year
Part B – Blood costs	20% of Medicare-approved amount after first 3 pints given outpatient.
Part B – Laboratory Services	0%
Part B – Home Health Care	0%
Part B – General Medical Care	20% of Medicare approved amount
Part B – Mental Health Care	50% of costs
Part B – Preventive Medical Care	$0 deductible or copayment
Part B – Durable Medical Equipment	20% of Medicare approved amount
Part B – Outpatient services	Copayments apply depending on service provided.

It is possible to win an appeal for a denial that has been issued under both Parts A & B. In most instances, the medical provider will help with the appeal because they want to receive payment. Patients can also hire private billing companies to assist with appeals as well as to help keep all of the patient's healthcare billings straight so that the beneficiary isn't overpaying providers.

Medicare Supplemental Insurance Policies (Medigaps)

As mentioned previously, the original Medicare parts A and B don't cover 100% of the billed charges; like many insurance plans there are annual deductibles and copayments for most services. In most cases, there are plans that pay the amounts that Medicare approves but doesn't pay. These are known as *Medicare Supplements*, or *Medigap Policies*. Both federal and state laws carefully regulate these insurance policies, which are provided by private companies. There are twelve standardized options for medigap policies, unless the beneficiary lives in Wisconsin, Massachusetts, or Minnesota (these three states have added their own requirements in addition to the federal regulations). It is important to understand that, while the coverage provided under the policies is standardized, the cost of premiums is not. It's a good idea to shop around for the best price for the policy that meets the specific needs of the beneficiary.

Medigap plans don't always allow you to choose any provider; there are plans called *Medicare Select plans* that are often a less expensive option than a regular Medigap policy. They are basically managed care plans, and they require that you only use providers with which they have developed contracts. Medicare Select Plans do allow more freedom than Part C plans, but they still limit the beneficiary's choices when it comes to providers and treatments.

Most health insurance companies provide some type of medigap policy in order to retain their customers who have private insurance as they transition into Medicare. If the beneficiary had healthcare coverage through a retirement plan, his policy was probably converted to a supplement at the time that he became eligible for Medicare. Supplemental policies can be confusing, and the high pressure sales tactics used on seniors can result in their accidentally purchasing several policies at once. This doesn't make sense, nor is it ethical for a medigap policy provider to knowingly sign up a client who already has a policy unless the beneficiary is willing to drop the coverage under the first plan. However, as mentioned previously, the sales person might not know, understand, or even care that the customer already has coverage and will sell him a policy anyway. Hopefully the computerized Medicare system will catch it, but I've found several clients to have more than one medigap policy. One patient wasn't able to get back the money that she paid until her family contacted their attorney; since the cost of a medigap policy is around $200 per month it's usually not worth the cost of hiring an attorney specifically for this purpose. I advised the others to contact the consumer advocate at their local television station to help with a refund.

Medigap policies make sense for beneficiaries who have chronic conditions, but they might not appear to make good financial sense for someone who is fairly healthy and has the ability to pay privately for the deductibles and copayments for a short period of time. Problems arise when a person with no supplemental policy suddenly becomes sick and is faced with huge out-of-pocket expenses. Unless the senior is very low income and qualifies for Medicaid, a Medigap policy that covers some or all of the copayments is a good idea. One serious healthcare crisis can wipe out a person financially, even if they have Medicare parts A&B. Although it's possible to wait until you need the coverage, it's only possible to elect a Medigap policy during open enrollment in order to keep from having limitations for pre-existing conditions. Medigap policies won't pay retroactively for bills that were incurred before the policy was in place.

Open enrollment for Medigap policies is the first six months after you are eligible for Medicare; otherwise you're subject to underwriting and will pay more if you have pre-existing conditions. This is called *Guaranteed Issue Rights*, or *Medigap Protections*. After the six month period has passed, the companies are able to exclude coverage for pre-existing conditions and are also able to charge higher premiums for their policies. There are certain exclusions to this rule, however. If a Medigap provider goes bankrupt or stops providing service in your area, your Medicare Advantage plan provider stops servicing your area, or you move out of the service area of your Medicare Advantage plan provider, you will be protected by the Guaranteed Issue Rights. You won't be subject to underwriting and will have your choice of any policy you wish. Additional information can be found at www.medicare.gov.

How to Choose a Medigap Policy using www.Medicare.gov

- On the top of the screen, click on **Supplements and Other Insurance.**

- In the drop-down box, click on **Find a Medigap Policy**

- On the next screen, fill in the requested information (**Zip Code & Health Status**); click **Continue.**

- Follow the prompts.

Insurance agents often encourage a client to buy the policy that pays the highest commission to the agent. Agents aren't required to provide information about state or federal programs that might help cover medical costs, and most agents aren't even aware that such programs exist. I've found that in most cases, agents are only knowledgeable about the products that their company sells. When an agent tells you that a certain policy is the best one available, he probably means that it's the best one his company offers (or the one that will pay him the highest commission). Once they've sold a policy, insurance agents count on the ongoing income from the commission they will receive due to the customer retaining that same policy year after year.

It's a good idea to review your coverage every year; I know of a couple where the husband's retirement-related supplemental policy costs him $360 per month and covers 100% of his out-of-pocket expenses. He has been very sick, and the policy has saved them around $25,000 in out-of-pocket expenses even after deducting the cost of the monthly premiums. His wife's supplemental policy (also retirement-related) costs $300 per month, and the only benefit it offers pays $1,000 per hospital admission after a $500 annual deductible. Since she hasn't been hospitalized even once, the more than $18,000 in premiums she's paid over the past five years has been wasted. During an insurance check-up, she was surprised to find that she has been eligible all along for the Medicaid-based program called QMB, which provides much better coverage at no out-of-pocket cost to her. When she called her insurance company, they weren't even aware that QMB exists.

In most cases, Medicare beneficiaries who have Medigap coverage through a previous employer aren't able to make any changes without dropping their entire policy. A patient who selects a different Medigap policy could lose his Part D prescription coverage, and if he's under the age of 65 it probably won't be easy to find another company to insure him. This isn't to say that Medigap policies provided by former employers shouldn't be dropped, but it's important to carefully consider your options and make the best choice possible.

It's possible to change policies to one that better suits your needs; make sure that you don't first carefully research the risks and benefits of dropping your current plan. The Medicare site can be helpful when comparing plans, and it's always best to check with your Area Agency on Aging to find out if you are eligible for a government-sponsored plan that better suits your needs.

Medicare Part C Advantage Plans

Part C Advantage plans are also known as *Managed Care* plans; in most instances they combine Parts A & B with the Part D Prescription Drug program into one healthcare plan. These healthcare plans are offered by private companies, such as *Health Maintenance Organizations (HMOs)* and *Preferred Provider Organizations (PPOs)*.

There are also Medicare *Private Fee-for-Service (PFFS) plans*, *Special Needs plans*, and *Medicare Medical Savings Account plans (MSA)*. It's necessary to do a little research about what is available in your service area in order to choose a plan that will meet your specific needs. Don't trust that a private insurance agent will provide you with the best plan for you – there are many publications available for order or download on the Medicare website that fully explain the different types of plans.

- **HMO's** are companies that contract with providers of all types in a specific service area to provide medical care to its members. Costs are reduced by using a primary physician and requiring pre-authorization for many services.

- **PPO's** are companies that contract with providers to provide service to members; unlike HMO's, these plans also offer the opportunity to see non-contracted providers, only at a higher out-of-pocket cost to beneficiaries.

- **PFFS's** are companies that offer private insurance to beneficiaries. They do have to offer a certain level of service required by Medicare, but they can also offer extra services beyond what traditional Medicare offers.

- *Special Needs plans* provide extra services for beneficiaries with certain chronic diseases and other specialized health needs and who have both Medicare and Medicaid.

- *MSA's* are insurance plans that offer coverage with a higher deductible; Medicare deposits money into a medical savings account that can be used for health care costs. These plans operate pretty much like most privately operated health care savings accounts.

When a beneficiary chooses to participate in an Advantage plan, his Part B premium will continue to be withheld from his monthly social security payments. In most cases, the Advantage plan provider will charge an additional monthly premium that can be paid out of the patient's pocket or might possibly be withheld from his social security income before it's deposited into his account. The cost of the premium depends upon the plan the senior chooses; each company generally offers several different plans. The most expensive plans usually offer the most services, but in most cases a traditional Medicare plan combined with a good Medigap policy will provide comparable prices with the added benefit of being able to choose your providers.

Medicare Advantage providers are able to offer coverage that is often less expensive to the consumer because the federal government heavily subsidizes these private insurance plans. The amount that's paid varies according to the geographical area of the country in which the plan operates. The government saves money by not having to pay a Medicare Administrative Contractor to process the patient's claims, nor does it have to pay the additional costs of a separate Part D prescription drug plan because most Part C plans include coverage for medications. The senior essentially "surrenders" his red, white, & blue Medicare card when he enrolls into an Advantage plan, and will present an ID card supplied by the insurance company. All charges are billed to the Advantage plan.

Advantage plan providers are able to raise their rates every year if they want; it's possible that a beneficiary will choose a plan because it is significantly cheaper than other plans, only to have the company substantially raise their rates the following year. The provider counts on retaining most of its patients because people become comfortable and don't like change regardless of the cost. However, it's always possible to change to a less expensive provider or to revert to traditional Medicare during annual open enrollment.

The greatest benefit of choosing a Medicare Advantage plan is the potential cost savings to the consumer. In exchange for the savings, beneficiaries who sign up with Advantage plans give up their ability to choose any provider they want. This might not be a bad thing; Advantage plans employ *case managers* whose sole responsibility is to coordinate the care their customers receive and ensure that all services are provided through contracted providers. For many plans, patients don't have to find their own doctors or set up their own services because the case manager does that for them.

The greatest disadvantage of signing up with a Medicare Advantage plan is that beneficiaries must almost exclusively use plan providers. Those beneficiaries who have had the same doctor for years might no longer be able access his services. In most cases members will only be able to access emergency services while traveling, meaning that a routine visit to the doctor while on vacation (such as to renew a prescription) probably won't be covered. Even a new condition is considered to be routine unless the situation requires a trip to the emergency room – but if the patient accesses the ER at a non-contracted hospital, it's possible that the bill won't be covered at all. At the very least, the senior might have to pay cash for the visit and request reimbursement from his insurance company, with no guarantee that any part of the bill will be covered.

At the very least, advantage plan members who are admitted to a hospital while traveling will experience substantially higher out-of-pocket costs, and non-emergent procedures won't be covered. In a variation of the above example, consider the beneficiary who, while traveling, is diagnosed with a painful hernia that needs to be repaired quickly although the condition isn't life-threatening. It will be the patient's responsibility to return to his service area, which can be a difficult process. If the patient is too sickly, he might not be allowed onto a commercial flight and will have to rent a car, ride a train or a bus, or make other transportation to return home. People traveling in a recreational vehicle might have an easier time, because the patient can lie down on a bed and remain comfortable during the trip home while someone else drives him back to his plan's service area.

Mrs. Smith, who is signed up with a Medicare HMO, is visiting her daughter in another state and hurts her shoulder. Her daughter takes her to the hospital, where the ER doctor recommends surgery. Her Medicare Advantage plan will only pay for her surgery in a contracted hospital. Both Mrs. Smith and her daughter would prefer that she have the surgery in the town where her daughter lives, but the Medicare Advantage plan is not willing to approve payment for surgery at an out-of-plan hospital.

Mrs. Smith has two options: Her daughter can take a week off of work, pay for both hers and her mother's airfare, and accompany her mother home to have the surgery; or

Mrs. Smith has the option of disenrolling from the plan, stating her intention to permanently move out of her plan's service area. It's possible that the insurance company will refer her to a plan in her daughter's area, and they might have to fight off agents who insist that they can enroll her in a comparable plan. She does have the option of enrolling in an Advantage plan in that area or reverting to Original Medicare A&B and selecting a Medigap policy. It will take a month or so in order to sort it all out.

All of this is frustrating for a woman who simply wanted to receive treatment while staying with her daughter – and later on, when Mrs. Smith receives her EOB/MSN, she finds that the plan paid very little of the ER bill and associated costs. In addition to the stress that she has endured, she owes the hospital hundreds of dollars.

The system isn't always kind when it comes to insurance issues.

Beneficiaries who require inpatient physical therapy after emergency surgery will probably receive the services in the geographical area of the hospital rather than for the insurance company to pay for his transportation back home. This can make it difficult for family members to visit the patient; the only other option would be for the patient or his family member to arrange and pay for the substantial costs of transporting him home in order for the patient to receive rehabilitation services near his support system. If the patient chooses to remain near the hospital where he had his surgery, he will experience a higher out-of-pocket cost than if he were to receive the rehabilitation services at home.

Even when a patient is at home, if he would like to use the services of a non-contracted provider he'll have to pay for some or all of it out of his pocket depending on the type of Advantage plan he has chosen. It's fairly common for a salesman to convince a senior that the plan he sells is the best one available and that most local physicians are plan providers, only for him to find out after they've signed on that his preferred physician is no longer a contracted provider (or never was). Some physicians won't work with certain insurance plans because they're too difficult to work with.

Most Advantage plans require that patients be assigned a ***Primary Care Provider (PCP)***, which is a physician who is paid a monthly amount to manage the care of all of his assigned patients. This means that the physician and his staff must complete paperwork and obtain authorizations for many, many patients, and that the physician will probably see his patients less often in order to dedicate time processing the necessary paperwork. Even if the patient is given the opportunity to choose his doctor, it's possible that he'll be assigned a different physician than the one who has provided him care in the past. This could be for one of many reasons, such as that his doctor has already been assigned the maximum number of patients under that particular HMO/PPO plan, or even that his doctor isn't a plan provider. It can be stressful to change to another doctor for insurance purposes.

A physician who was an Advantage plan provider when a beneficiary checked before signing up during open enrollment (October 15th through December 7th) might not continue as a plan provider for the upcoming year. It's always best to speak with the physician's office manager or billing clerk when considering changing health plans, as they work directly with the paperwork component of the office and can provide accurate information about the insurances they will continue to accept for the upcoming year.

Many Medicare Advantage plans hold down costs by developing contracts with specific nursing homes for rehabilitation rather than to have contracts with many different providers in the community. This might limit the patient's choice of facility for long-term care as well, because it's possible that in order to be accepted he will have to go to a facility that will accept his insurance for rehabilitation and remain there while he applies for a long-term payment source.

Even if the patient asks to go to another nursing home, it's doubtful that this option will be available to him. The Advantage plan has negotiated its rates with other facilities and unless there are extenuating circumstances, it's not likely he'll be able to go to his facility of choice. If the patient refuses to go to a contracted nursing home, his only option might be to discharge home with home healthcare provided by an agency that's contracted with his insurance company. Advantage plan copayment amounts are different than those of traditional Medicare, and rehabilitation admissions in skilled nursing facilities are often much shorter under managed care than those provided under traditional Medicare Part A.

Many nursing homes don't want to accept Advantage plan patients with for long-term care because these plans can be harder to work with; patients might have a difficult time finding a physician who will follow them in the nursing home. Services such as wound care that would otherwise be performed by a physician who comes to the facility might require a painful trip to the doctor. It can also be frustrating when the nursing home changes its contracts to a non-contracted rehabilitation provider, and the patient isn't able to receive the same therapy services as the other patients. Even if the company contracts with the Advantage plan, being enrolled in a Part C plan can limit a nursing home patient's ability to receive the type of rehabilitation services he would normally receive under the Medicare Part B benefit. It's possible that the nursing home will ask patients who have a Part C plan to revert to Original Medicare A&B at the first opportunity.

The Medicare program allows clients to switch between all plan types from October 15th thru December 7th of every year during an *open enrollment period*, with the change being effective January 1st of the following year (example: switching from traditional Medicare to an Advantage plan). Once a patient is enrolled in a plan, it's not likely that he'll be able to switch to a different plan unless there are extenuating circumstances. An example of an extenuating circumstance would be a beneficiary who moves out of the company's service area, or an insurance company going bankrupt. However, if the beneficiary's doctor stops providing services for enrollees in the senior's health insurance plan, this is not considered to be an extenuating circumstance and the patient will have to find another doctor. He will be able to change plans to one in which his doctor participates during the next open enrollment period, but there's no guarantee that his doctor will be able to accept him back as a patient under that plan.

Beneficiaries who have *dual eligibility* (both Medicare and Medicaid) have the opportunity to sign up for special plans that provide extra services to their patients. These patients may change plans as often as they wish, monthly if they want to, in order to receive the services they need. These special needs plans offer additional services to their beneficiaries, such as prescription eyeglasses, dental care and other services. Insurance companies that administer these plans receive additional subsidies from CMS in order to provide a higher level of service to their clients.

Advantage plan providers often try to discourage their patients from making any changes. When a beneficiary moves to another location that isn't served by the Medicare Advantage plan, the provider is supposed to inform him that the plan can't meet his medical needs and refer him to plans in the new area, but this doesn't always happen. Although it doesn't happen very often, some plans refuse to disenroll clients even though they've been notified in writing that a beneficiary has moved out of the service area. It's important to always keep a copy of every letter sent to the insurance company, keep their written replies (and their postmarked envelopes), and note the name and date of any phone call made. In the case of one of my clients, her plan refused her request to revert back to traditional Medicare even though she had moved over 500 miles away. She had to make a formal complaint to CMS to force the plan to make the change. Luckily, she had kept a date stamped letter from them acknowledging they had received her request to change her coverage.

It's possible that the current Advantage plan will refer the patient to a sister plan in the new area, regardless of whether the patient wants to remain on a managed care plan or wishes to revert to Original Medicare A&B. If the plan doesn't make a recommendation, the beneficiary can always ask the agent who signed him up for his previous plan to help. In this case, he'll likely be referred to a plan in the new city that will pay a referral fee to his agent. Everyone has their hand in the pot.

When moving to a new area, the beneficiary can always use the Medicare website to choose a new plan. Transferring to a new plan will help him cancel his previous Advantage plan coverage. It's important to note that the beneficiary doesn't have to continue using an Advantage plan at his new address; he can always choose to revert to Medicare A&B with a Part D prescription plan. He is also able to choose a Medigap plan to cover co-payments and deductibles.

Medicare Advantage plans aren't necessarily a bad choice; they can help to hold down healthcare costs as well as to ensure the safety of their beneficiaries. There are patients with traditional Medicare who go to the doctor and if they don't like what he says, they'll go to another, and then another, until they find one who will say whatever it is they want to hear. This is known in the industry as ***doc shopping.*** Not only is this behavior expensive, it's also possible that the patient could be jeopardizing his health due to lack of care for a condition that requires immediate treatment. The different physicians might write different prescriptions for the same condition, and if the patient accesses multiple pharmacies it's possible that there could be severe medication interactions. Although many states have a database for controlled substances, there is no database that tracks other types of prescriptions at multiple pharmacies. Many Part D providers don't catch these issues, while an Advantage plan case manager can monitor the patient's care, ensuring that there won't be duplications of service. She will do her best to make sure the each patient assigned to her is receiving the medical care that his doctor and the insurance plan believe to be in the patient's best interests.

It's important to understand that the treatment the insurance company authorizes might not be what the physician believes that the patient needs, especially if the treatments are expensive. Some Advantage plans are well known for requiring outpatient care for patients who would recover safer and faster in a facility, even if it creates a hardship for the patient to get back & forth to treatments. A lack of transportation to outpatient services is not considered to be a reason for a patient to remain in a nursing home, although under the traditional Medicare Part A plan, the nursing home stay would probably have been covered. Simply stated, patients with Medicare Part A&B are easier for nursing homes to work with than are those who are insured with Advantage plans.

All Medicare Advantage plans must offer a minimum level of service required by CMS, but many offer plans that include extra services such as dental care or optical care. Some plans offer travel insurance as a part of their package. Because the plans differ so much from each other, it's important to obtain as much information as possible before signing up with a particular company. One way to compare plans is to visit the official Medicare site at www.Medicare.gov and follow the prompts.

Medicare Part D Prescription Drug Programs

Medicare began offering prescription drug coverage in 2006; this program is called *Medicare Part D*. The intent of the plan was to help beneficiaries with their spiraling drug costs because most Medicare recipients either had no prescription drug coverage, or it was very expensive. For those patients taking thousands of dollars of medications each month, the plan was an excellent way to cut back on out-of-pocket costs. But many beneficiaries who were taking very few medications each month felt that the plan wasn't necessary because their Part D premiums cost the same or more than they were paying for their medications alone. Add in co-pays, and it seemed like a waste of money.

There are Part D plans with premiums of less than $15.00 per month, and ones that cost over $100.00 per month. The cheaper plans often don't cover a whole lot of medications until the patient has met a hefty deductible, but all it takes is one illness (not necessarily a hospitalization) to increase medication costs by hundreds, if not thousands, of dollars each month. Since Part D is like all other Medicare plans, it has an open enrollment period that is non-negotiable. If a senior hasn't elected a prescription plan and suddenly develops a need for an expensive prescription, he might have to wait months for open enrollment in order to start his insurance coverage. Sometimes there are prescription discounts through state or county social service programs that might be able to help during the time that there's no coverage, but they don't cover the costs as completely as a Medicare Part D program and there are financial eligibility requirements. Most pharmaceutical companies also offer low-cost programs, but again there are financial eligibility requirements with no guarantee of that the patient will be accepted – and if the medication must be taken immediately (as is true in most cases), the senior is simply out of options. Part D can be viewed like auto insurance; it's important when you really need it, otherwise it's just another unnecessary expense that you wish that you didn't have.

There are many different Part D prescription plans offered across the country; beneficiaries are able to choose a plan with a lower monthly premium and higher out-of-pocket costs or can elect to pay a higher monthly premium for a plan that offers more comprehensive coverage with lower out-of-pocket expenses. The open enrollment period for Part D runs between October 15th and December 7th, with the change taking effect on the first of January. If a Part D plan fails to achieve a 3-star rating three years in a row, the beneficiary will be notified of a ***Special Enrollment Period*** so that he can choose another plan with a higher satisfaction rating.

Just like other Medicare plans, if a beneficiary doesn't enroll in a drug plan when he is first eligible, he will be penalized an extra premium amount for each month he didn't join when he was first eligible to do so. This is the case unless he had a plan that was better or equal to Medicare Part D at the time he was first eligible, such as through a previous employer.

Those beneficiaries who are receiving prescription drug coverage from a past employer or retirement plan will be notified by their insurance company when they are first eligible for Plan D prescription drug coverage. Insurance companies are required to tell their clients if the current plan is equal to or better than the prescription drug coverage offered by Medicare, which allows the senior to choose whether he wants to stay with his current plan or change to Medicare Part D. Be cautious when considering changing plans, because any changes that a beneficiary makes to part of the insurance he receives as part of his retirement plan (such as choosing to participate in Part D) could cause him to lose *all* of the coverage he receives. Once a retirement plan provider drops a customer it's nearly impossible for him to get that coverage back. This is why it's always best to research the risks and benefits of making such a change. If and when a beneficiary decides to drop his retirement insurance and begin using the Part D benefit, he won't be charged any penalties because he was covered under an insurance plan the entire time.

Like other types of Medicare insurance plans, the government doesn't actually provide the Part D insurance. The government (CMS) contracts with many private insurance companies across the country to provide drug coverage for their beneficiaries *at full cost*, rather than using the millions of beneficiaries as leverage to drive down costs – this is as a result of drug and insurance companies successful lobbying efforts. The monthly premium varies according to the plan and company that the beneficiary chooses. CMS also pays various companies and state agencies to monitor the program, which further drives up program costs.

The idea of the Part D prescription coverage is great, although the actual administration of the plan leaves a lot to be desired. There are so many companies competing for patients it can be confusing, and they all have sales staff that bombard beneficiaries with information as to why they believe their plan to be the best. As mentioned before, these sales people probably don't even have knowledge of the plans that other companies offer, they're just trying to make a commission.

Each Part D provider has an extensive ***Formulary***, which is a list of medications that the plan will cover. A formulary helps hold down the provider's costs by providing a less expensive equivalent of many medications. The formulary provides medications that will treat nearly every condition, and if it doesn't carry the specific medication the doctor orders the part D provider will attempt to find an equivalent that will be covered at a lesser cost. This might not be acceptable to the doctor, but in order for the plan to even consider providing a more expensive medication the patient will probably have to try every option the formulary offers. Even if the cheaper medications don't have the desired effect, it's possible that the part D provider will never approve payment for the more expensive medication.

When a doctor has ordered a new medication that isn't on the formulary and the plan instead offers what they believe to be an equivalent, it is possible to make a formal appeal and ask for an *Exception* (the doctor's office will assist with this process). During the appeal process the patient must go without the medication, pay out of pocket, or use the substitute that he is appealing. Some physicians are able to provide samples to their patients that will last during the appeal process, but it's not possible to stock a sample of every medication in their office. Another problem is that drug companies don't provide samples of medications that are available in generic form, and generic medications can cost hundreds of dollars each month.

If they change their formulary during the year, Part D plan providers can't stop paying for an ongoing medication without notifying the patient at least 60 days in advance; most of the time they're required to provide the medication until the end of the calendar year. At that point (open enrollment), the beneficiary will have the opportunity to choose a new drug plan that does cover that medication. If he doesn't want to change plans, he will need to pay the full cost of the prescription from that point forward or use the equivalent offered by the insurance plan.

The original Part D prescription plan idea was supposed to be simple, but in reality the 2014 standard part D plan is quite complicated: the beneficiary pays a maximum deductible of $310.00 out of pocket each calendar year plus co-payments until he and his plan have paid a total of $2,850.00 in medication costs. At that point, he enters the "donut hole" (aka the "coverage gap") where he will have to pay 47.5% of the cost for brand-name prescriptions and 72% of the cost of generics until a total of $6,455.00 has been paid by both him and his Part D provider.

After the beneficiary crawls out of the coverage gap , he enters the part of the plan called *catastrophic* coverage, where he pays a maximum of $2.55 for generics and $6.35 for brand-name prescriptions or 5% of the cost of the medications, whichever is greater. Catastrophic coverage was designed to cover medications for patients who are very sick, although with the cost of medications these days many seniors meet the criteria for this coverage.

The amount the beneficiary is required to pay is referred to as *Cost Sharing*, while the time period where the beneficiary is required to pay the majority of the cost of his prescriptions is called the *donut hole*, or *coverage gap*. There have been some strides toward making medications more affordable; under the new healthcare reform the beneficiary pays a discounted amount during the coverage gap rather than the full cost of the medications and the donut hole will be eliminated completely by the year 2020. However, beneficiaries are still required to pay substantial amounts out-of-pocket for their prescriptions; the 2014 true Out-Of-Pocket (trOOP) costs are $4,550 before the patient is out of the donut hole and begins the catastrophic coverage phase. This is far out of reach for many people.

Low-income beneficiaries might qualify for a program called *"Extra Help,"* which greatly reduces their out-of-pocket costs for prescription medications. The program is available to beneficiaries who live in one of the 50 states or the District of Columbia. The application is refreshingly easy to complete, is offered in larger print so that it's easier for seniors to read the application, and can either be completed on-line at www.Medicare.gov or by mailing the information in. For more information about the Part D Prescription Extra Help Program, visit the Medicare website at www.Medicare.gov, or call Medicare at (800) Medicare.

Medicare beneficiaries who have opted to sign up with Medicare Advantage plans such as HMO's and PPO's almost always have prescription drug coverage wrapped into the Advantage plan and don't need to find a separate provider to meet their prescription drug needs. In most cases, the Medicare computer system won't allow a beneficiary to sign up for Part D while he is signed up for an Advantage plan that includes coverage for medications.

Medicare Part D providers develop contracts with as many local pharmacies as possible in order to remain competitive, and they usually have a contract with a mail-order pharmacy in order to provide three months worth of medications at a reduced out-of-pocket cost to the patient. For the nursing home patient who's paying privately for his room & board, this can mean substantial savings. In most instances the nursing home will require that the medications be "bubble-packed," which means they're placed on a card with see-through compartments that are easily counted. Those patients whose medications are provided by other pharmacies will forward them to the commercial pharmacy that serves the nursing home, and that pharmacy places them in a bubble-pack. The commercial pharmacy will either charge the nursing home or the patient a few dollars for bubble-packing.

There is one other option for medications that has nothing to do with the Medicare program – many pharmacies provide 30-day supplies of over 150 generic medications for $4 per month to anyone, whether or not they have health insurance. This is often less expensive than the Medicare D plan, even with the Extra Help program. It's always best to ask if the pharmacy provides customers with that option, and to check and see if your medications are covered under the $4 prescription plan (some pharmacies charge less for 90-day supplies).

It's important to remember that a medication might not be covered no matter whether or not the doctor has prescribed it. Talk to your doctor to let him know that you're struggling with paying for your medications; he might not realize that you aren't able to afford the copayments and therefore aren't taking the medication. Even if he prefers the more expensive option, he might be able to prescribe something that's affordable rather than to have a healthcare condition go untreated. Doctors aren't always aware of medication issues unless the family tells them they're struggling to find the money to pay for the patient's drug-related costs.

Traveling with Medicare

It's important to understand that when a Medicare beneficiary becomes ill and is admitted to the hospital while on vacation, he will be sent to a nearby nursing home if he requires rehabilitation or skilled nursing services afterward. Medicare Part A and most Part C plans do not pay for a patient to be transported back to his home, nor do they cover the associated travel costs, such as hotel room, meals, and car rentals for family members. This makes it difficult and expensive for the family to remain with the patient, and nearly impossible to bring him home to recuperate.

Many commercial airlines won't allow people on the plane if they appear to be sickly; they can (and often do) refuse to fly anyone who might require medical attention during the flight. Patients who require oxygen must notify the airlines in advance, will need a physician's release and might have to pay a surcharge for their ticket that's separate from the cost of the oxygen; they will also be limited as to where they will be allowed to be seated on the airplane.

There are medical equipment companies who specialize in providing oxygen concentrators for flight-related purposes; it generally takes up to a week to make all of the arrangements in order to ensure that a concentrator will be available to the patient in time for the flight. All of the associated costs must be paid up-front by the patient, and generally aren't reimbursed by health insurance (these costs can easily top $500). Hopefully a social worker can help the patient with these arrangements, but if not it's up to the family to figure out how to get the patient home safely.

There are other accommodations that might need to be made for frail patients who are traveling; even if they don't require supplemental oxygen the airline might require a physician's statement certifying that the patient is fit to travel. In many cases, a wheelchair-bound patient must make arrangements to use an airport-provided wheelchair to get to the plane while his own wheelchair will be treated as checked luggage (with the associated costs). Special arrangements will need to be arranged for any layovers. There are many things to consider when a patient is traveling after being discharged from a facility, much of which must be facilitated by professionals.

A case manager or social worker at the hospital or nursing home might be able to assist in arranging for medical-related travel, but usually the patient or family member has to specifically ask for help with the arrangements. Ask each facility where the patient has been for a copy of your medical records to take home to your primary doctor; don't trust that they will automatically fax your medical records to him. You will need to make a separate request to each provider, because they are only allowed to provide a copy of their own records (example: the nursing home can't provide you with a copy of the hospital's history & physical).

Those patients who are too sick to fly home on a commercial carrier will probably have to wait until they have recovered sufficiently in order to be able to fly commercially or to withstand the drive home. The other option would be to pay for a **Medical Evacuation Carrier (Medivac)**, which can cost tens of thousands of dollars. It is possible to purchase travel insurance to help cover these potentially devastating costs; in most instances travel insurance must be purchased at the time the original travel arrangements are booked. Travel Insurance policies vary depending upon the company, the travel destination, and the type of coverage. Some Medigap policies provide travel insurance; it's always best to verify insurance coverage before leaving rather than to find out there's none when you need it the most. Most insurance agents or travel agents can provide information about travel insurance and it can also be ordered online.

Mrs. Smith suffers a heart attack while she is on vacation with her husband and is admitted to a local hospital for several days. Even though she would prefer going home to recuperate, she is too weak to fly on a commercial airline. As she isn't able to afford the cost of a private plane to fly her home, Mrs. Smith is discharged to a local nursing home for rehabilitation. When she's well enough to fly, she will require oxygen on the plane. Her husband attempts to change their original plane reservations, and finds that there is no refund for the tickets they have purchased. If he stays in town with his wife, Mr. Smith will have to pay the following expenses out-of-pocket:

- New airfare for both Mr. & Mrs. Smith
- Extra charge for oxygen for the plane trip home
- Hotel charges for himself while she recovers
- Extra rental car charges
- Food and miscellaneous expenses

It's important to verify the amount of travel insurance coverage a beneficiary has before traveling far away, or out of the United States. If the beneficiary isn't a well person, it might be best to postpone the trip until he recovers rather than to risk having to deal with a health problem thousands of miles away from home.

Regarding emergency Medivac carriers, Medicare or regular healthcare insurance providers will only pay most of the costs of a Medivac if the patient's needs are so great that they have to be immediately transported to the nearest acute hospital that can provide the necessary level of care. For example, a patient who has been in an accident might be life-flighted from the scene of the accident directly to the nearest trauma center, which might not necessarily be located in the patient's hometown. The patient will have to make arrangements to return to his home when he is discharged, even if it's hundreds or thousands of miles away. For the patient who is unable to fly via commercial airlines, the transportation via Medivac can be so expensive that some families opt to rent a motor home and hire a nurse or nurse's aide to travel with them, then pay for their airfare home. This is cheaper than the cost of a Medivac carrier, although it does take several days to drive cross-country.

Mrs. Smith has a heart attack while she is on vacation with her husband. When they had made their travel arrangements, they paid around $200 for travel insurance. She is admitted to a local hospital for several days; when she is discharged the insurance company makes all of the arrangements and sends a nurse to accompany her on the plane home. Travel insurance pays for all of the extra charges, including hotel accommodations, rental car and airfare for Mr. & Mrs. Smith to return home.

Or: Mrs. Smith becomes sick while she is on vacation, which will require immediate surgery and a long period of recuperation before she is able to fly home in a commercial carrier. She is admitted to a local hospital for the surgery; when she is stable for discharge her travel insurance carrier pays for her to be sent home in a medivac plane and makes arrangements for her admission to a facility near her home. Also covered are the extra hotel accommodations, rental car and airfare for Mr. Smith to return home.

Or: Mrs. Smith becomes sick while she is on vacation; she did not purchase a travel insurance policy. Her husband must pay the extra costs of changing the airplane reservations, renting a hotel room, extra meals and other associated costs. When she is ready to discharge from the hospital, their son flies out and rents a motor home; they hire a nurse's aid to travel with them and fly her home. This adds well over $1,000 in unanticipated costs.

Regardless of whether or not there is travel insurance, it's always a good idea to leave a copy of insurance cards, driver's licenses and any other identification information with a trusted family member at home in case they need to fax it to a hospital or other medical facility.   Preparing for any vacation should also be an occasion to review and update advanced directives such as health care powers of attorney and living wills.

Covered & Non-Covered Items

Like every other insurance plan, Medicare is required to provide certain items that are medically necessary to its beneficiaries. As long as the patient is in a nursing home receiving rehabilitation services, all of his equipment and supply needs are provided by the facility under the daily rate paid by Medicare. After his Medicare benefit has been exhausted, the nursing home must continue to provide for his needs at no additional cost as long as he's eligible for Medicaid. Patients who aren't eligible for Medicaid will have to pay separately for each service, which can add hundreds or thousands of dollars to their monthly bill.

Once a patient is discharged home, he might have a problem paying for certain non-covered items. An item isn't considered to be "medically necessary" merely because a doctor writes a prescription for the item. Medicare doesn't necessarily cover supplemental meals like Ensure®, or nutrition that must be administered via a G-tube (gastrointestinal tube placed directly into the patient's stomach). This is because the patient would need to eat anyway, and Medicare doesn't pay for meals at home. The cost of certain nutrition products can be thousands of dollars each month, an amount that the average senior can't afford to pay. Most Medigap plans don't cover nutritional supplements, although there are some Medicaid programs and private insurance plans that will pay for these products in the patient's home. Quite often patients aren't able to return home because of the associated costs for this type of care.

Medicare will pay for a front-wheeled walker, but only pays a portion of a specialty walker with a seat and brakes (called a four-wheeled walker). Medicare doesn't pay for grab bars in the home, shower chairs, wheelchair lifts & carriers for cars, or other assistive devices. These items are convenient, and they keep a patient safe – but they're not considered to be medically necessary. As with nutritional supplements, there are some Medicaid programs that will pay for various items of equipment. For more information on the Medicaid program in your state, contact your local Medicaid office or the Area Agency on Aging.

Medicare pays for a walker or a wheelchair, but not for both at the same time. Medicare will provide a hospital bed if the patient isn't able to move around in his bed and requires caregiver assistance, although the patient's need must be supported by medical documentation. For the patient who is completely bedbound, Medicare might possibly provide a specialty mattress to help deter decubitus ulcers (bedsores) but does not pay for an egg-crate mattress pad to make the bed more comfortable.

Medicare will not cover the cost of sheets and blankets for the hospital bed, even if the patient doesn't have a bed that size and must make a special trip to the store to purchase these items. Medicare doesn't cover the costs of supplies such as heating pads, under pads, briefs and wipes.

Medicare will pay for oxygen in the form of a concentrator and/or portable bottles in a patient's home, but the patient must qualify by having an oxygen saturation rate of 89% or less on room air. It's common practice for a patient to be removed from oxygen and asked to walk up & down a hallway until he has exerted himself and lowered the oxygen levels in his blood. As long as the reading is at or below 89% the oxygen will be provided, and since a medical chart is considered to be a legal document most medical providers won't generally "fudge" on the numbers to obtain equipment for a patient. Medicare does pay for CPAP and BPAP machines (often used to treat obstructive sleep apnea), diabetic supplies such as glucose monitors, test strips, syringes and needles. Even though Medicare pays for oxygen, it does not pay for the specialty concentrators required by the FAA for air travel. These costs must be paid out of the patient's pocket – and they can be expensive.

Medicare doesn't provide items that can be purchased over the counter such as wrist braces and supports, and in most cases doesn't pay for specialty gel pads for comfort (although it will pay for wheelchair pads for patients who have bedsores). There are many items that Medicare doesn't cover, and if the beneficiary can't afford the cost out-of-pocket he will have to do without. Even if he is low-income and qualifies for Medicaid, most Medicaid programs have their coverage limits.

As a health insurance program, Medicare doesn't pay for blood draws in a patient's home unless the patient is receiving other services from a home health agency. The patient will have to go to his doctor's office or an outpatient laboratory for blood draws, injections, or other types of medical care.

The Medicare program does not pay for access ramps to be built for beneficiaries, even if the patient isn't able to leave the house without the accommodations. There is no provision for bathroom remodeling or specialty walk-in bathtubs. There are often social service programs that will pay for special accommodations for patients who own their homes, but the patients generally have to be very low income in order to qualify. For additional information about social service programs that might pay for accommodations, contact your local Area Agency on Aging or a local medical equipment company.

l.e. green

Medicare.gov Website

The most difficult thing about choosing a Medicare plan that's right for you is finding out enough information about the available options in your area. CMS offers a website that contains all of the information you need in order to make an informed choice as to which plan might best suit your needs. Medicare.gov not only offers a myriad of information about the Medicare program, insurance providers and the different plans available; it also provides the opportunity to either download or order any number of free publications.

The website allows a senior the opportunity to compare and choose prescription plans, secondary (Medigap) plans and Part C Advantage plans while remaining anonymous – which means no high pressure sales pitch from a salesperson whose livelihood depends upon selling you on their health plan. Medicare.gov also offers customers the ability to check the record of nursing homes, hospitals, home health care and hospice providers, locate a doctor and even to make a change of address or order a new Medicare card.

Because everyone doesn't have access to a computer, many senior centers offer volunteers who will help to access the Medicare site and search for information. It's worth calling to find out if the senior center in your town provides this service. The book **Medicare & You** might be able to answer basic questions as well, and is available in both book and e-book forms. It can be ordered online or by calling 1-800-Medicare.

Under the Older American Act, each state also offers a ***State Health Insurance Counseling and Assistance Program (SHIP)*** that provides one-on-one counseling assistance for Medicare beneficiaries. The goal of the program is to provide confidential assistance maneuvering through the system from a specially trained volunteer who isn't affiliated with any specific program and doesn't sell or solicit customers for any company.

Additionally, the Medicare website provides seniors with an area to file complaints and obtain additional information. It's fairly user-friendly, but if a senior doesn't have access to a computer he can always ask his questions directly by calling 1-800-Medicare.

l.e. green

Nursing Home Survey Agencies

State	State Survey Agency	Ombudsman
AL	Alabama Department of Public Health 1-800-356-9596	1-800-243-5463
AK	DHSS of Alaska - DMA Health Facilities Licensing and Certification 1-888-387-9387	1-800-730-6393
AZ	Department of Health Services of Arizona - Assurance and Licensure Division of Long-term Care 1-602-364-2690	1-800-432-4040
AR	Department of Human Services of Arkansas - Office of Long-term Care 1-800-582-4887	1-501-682-2441
CA	Department of Health Services of California - Licensing and Certification Program 1-800-236-9747	1-800-231-4024
CO	Colorado Department of Public Health and Environment 1-303-692-2800	1-800-288-1376
CT	Department of Public Health of Connecticut - Division of Health Systems Regulation 1-860-509-7400	1-866-388-1888
DE	Health and Social Services of Delaware - Division of Long-term Care and Resident Protection 1-877-453-0012	1-800-223-9074
DC	Dept of Health of Washington, D.C. - Health Regulation Admin, Health Care Facilities Division 1-202-724-8800	1-202-434-2140
GA	Department of Human Resources of Georgia - Office of Regulatory Services 1-800-878-6442	1-888-454-5826

FL	Agency for Health Care Administration of Florida 1-888-419-3456	1-888-831-0404
HI	Hawaii Department of Health 1-808-692-7420	1-888-875-9229
ID	Idaho Department of Health and Welfare 1-208-334-6626	1-877-471-2777
IL	Illinois Department of Public Health 1-800-252-4343	1-800-252-8966
IN	Department of Health of Indiana - Long-term Care Division 1-800-246-8909	1-800-622-4484
IA	Department of Inspections and Appeals of Iowa - Health Facilities Division 1-877-686-0027	1-800-532-3213
KS	Kansas Department on Aging 1-800-842-0078	1-877-662-8362
KY	Office of Inspector General of Kentucky 1-502-564-7963	1-800-372-2991
LA	Department of Health and Hospitals of Louisiana - Health Standards Section 1-888-810-1819	1-866-632-0922
ME	Department of Health and Human Services of Maine 1-800-791-4080	1-800-499-0229
MD	Maryland Department of Health and Mental Hygiene 1-877-402-8219	1-800-243-3425
MA	Massachusetts Department of Public Health 1-800-462-5540	1-800-243-4636
MI	Michigan Department of Community Health 1-800-882-6006	1-866-485-9393
MN	Health Facility Complaints and Provider Compliance Division of Minnesota 1-800-369-7994	1-800-657-3591

MS	Mississippi Department of Health 1-866-458-4948	1-800-948-3090
MO	Elder Abuse and Neglect Hotline of Missouri 1-800-392-0210	1-800-309-3282
MT	Department of Health and Human Services of Montana - Quality Assurance, Certification Bureau 1-406-444-2099	1-800-332-2272
NE	Health and Human Services of Nebraska - Regulation and Licensure Credentialing Division 1-402-471-3324	1-800-942-7830
NV	State Health Division of Nevada 1-800-225-3414	1-702-486-3545
NH	Health Facility Administration of New Hampshire 1-800-852-3345	1-800-442-5640
NJ	State Health Insurance Assistance Program (SHIP) 1-800-792-9770	1-877-582-6995
NM	Department of Health of New Mexico - Bureau of Health Facility Licensing and Certification 1-800-752-8649	1-800-432-2080
NY	New York State Department of Health 1-888-201-4563	1-800-342-9871
NC	Division of Nursing Home Licensure 1-800-624-3004	1-919-733-8395
ND	North Dakota Department of Health 1-701-328-2352	1-800-451-8693
OH	Bureau of Long-term Care of Ohio - Quality Assurance 1-800-342-0553	1-800-282-1206
OK	Oklahoma State Department of Health 1-800-747-8419	1-800-211-2116
OR	Seniors and People with Disability 1-800-232-3020	1-800-522-2602

PA	Pennsylvania Department of Health 1-800-254-5164	1-717-783-1550
RI	Rhode Island Department of Health 1-401-222-2566	1-401-785-3340
SC	Department of Health and Environmental Control of South Carolina - Bureau of Certification 1-800-922-6735	1-800-868-9095
SD	South Dakota Department of Health 1-605-773-3356	1-866-854-5465
TN	Tennessee Department of Health 1-800-778-4504	1-877-236-0013
TX	Department of Aging and Disability Services 1-800-458-9858	1-800-252-2412
UT	Dept of Health of Utah - Bureau of Medicare/Medicaid Program-Certification and Resident Assessment 1-800-662-4157	1-877-424-4640
VT	Department of Aging and Independent living 1-800-564-1612	1-800-889-2047
VA	Virginia Center for Quality Health Care Services and Consumer Protection 1-800-955-1819	1-800-938-8885
WA	Dept of Social and Health Services of Washington- Aging and Adult Services Admin-Residential Care 1-800-562-6078	1-800-562-6028
WV	Dept of Health and Human Resources of West Virginia-Office of Health Facility Licensure and Cert 1-800-442-2888	1-877-987-4463
WI	Dept of Health and Family Services of WI-Division of Supportive Living-Bureau of Quality Assurance 1-800-642-6552	1-800-815-0015
WY	Office of Health Quality of Wyoming 1-800-548-1367	1-307-322-5553

Glossary

2567 Form – a form that is used to document a nursing home investigation performed by a state regulating agency. The information on the actual form is more comprehensive than the information posted on the Medicare website.

2-day Notice of Medicare Non-Coverage (NOMNC) – a denial notice that must be given to a patient receiving services under the Medicare benefit 2-days (48 hours) prior to being discharged from that service.

Abuse Coordinator – the nursing home staff member who is responsible for reporting all incidents of suspected abuse to the state and ombudsman's office. While every staff member is a mandated reporter and is required to report suspected abuse, there is always one person designated as the abuse coordinator.

Activities of Daily Living (ADL's) – activities of self-care that people perform on a daily basis, such as bathing, eating, toileting, walking, and dressing themselves.

Acuity – a patient's level of care according to his medical and custodial needs.

Acute Facility – a hospital that provides services such as medical care, surgical services, intensive care units, etc. The care provided in acute facilities is generally short-term care, although there are special Long-Term Acute Care (LTAC) facilities that provide longer term care to patients.

Acute Rehabilitation Facility (ARF) – rehabilitation units or stand-alone facilities that provide three or more hours each day of physical, occupational and/or speech therapies to patients. ARF's provide a higher amount of rehabilitation services than skilled nursing facilities and are reimbursed under the Medicare acute care benefit.

Adult Protective Services (APS) or *Elder Protective Services (EPS)* – a public agency whose mission is to investigate suspected abuse, neglect and exploitation of adult clients, usually 60 years or older.

Advanced Directives – forms that declare the type of care that the patient would prefer to have if he is unable to give consent. Advanced Directives include Living Wills, Durable Powers of Attorney for Health Care, and Medical Treatment plans.

Advantage Plans (Medicare Part C) – insurance coverage offered by private companies as an alternative to Traditional Medicare Parts A&B; these plans use contracted providers and are generally limited to specific coverage areas.

Affinity Fraud – fraud or exploitation that is perpetrated by people that the victim either knows or has grown to know by pretending to have certain things in common. The victim is targeted because they are easy "marks."

Aging Waiver Programs (Medicaid Waiver Programs) – special Medicaid programs that waive certain eligibility criteria in order to provide care in a patient's home, or possibly in an assisted living facility.

Aging-In-Place – the act of remaining at home with assistance rather than moving to another location such as assisted living facility or nursing home.

Aid & Attendance (A&A) – a supplemental income paid to veterans or their families who require personal care and help with ADL's.

Alert & Oriented (A&O) – a generally accepted term for a patient's mental status. A&O times four refers to a patient's awareness of person (who they are), place (where they are), time (the general date), and also the situation at hand. A&O status is not a legal term, and this status can be judged by almost anyone.

AMA (Against Medical Advice) – the act of leaving a medical facility without the doctor's permission.

Ancillary Services – extra services that aren't considered to be a part of the base rate of nursing home placement, such as oxygen, supplies, wheelchairs, etc.

Annual Inspections (State Surveys) – a state conducted annual event in nursing homes or assisted living facilities that consists of chart reviews, patient/staff interviews, kitchen inspections, other physical plant inspections, business office audits, medication audits, and any other review that the state deems necessary to ensure that the facility is operating within the rules and laws required.

Appeal – a formal process that a beneficiary can use to ask that Medicare ***(CMS)*** take another look at a decision that has been made regarding payment for a Medicare-covered service.

Area Agency on Aging (AAA) – agencies whose primary mission is to help older adults and persons with disabilities to live with dignity and provide them with information about caregiving.

Asset Recovery Programs – programs that file liens on the homes of patients whose room & board in a nursing home were paid by the Medicaid program in an attempt to recover some of the monies spent on their care.

Assignment – a term used to describe a medical provider's acceptance of Medicare as a payment source. Those providers who accept assignment can only charge the patient the amount that Medicare approves but doesn't pay, such as copayments and deductibles. Medical providers that don't accept assignment have a limit as to what that they can charge over and above the Medicare approved amounts.

Assisted Living Facility (ALF) – a facility that provides a homelike environment for seniors who aren't able to maintain their independence, but don't have a high enough acuity to require nursing home placement. ALF's are subject to annual inspections in much the same manner as nursing homes and can be small and informal or large facilities.

Attorney in Fact (Healthcare Proxy or *Designee*) – the person named in a power of attorney form to make decisions on behalf of a patient.

Baseline – information about the patient's regular physical condition that is gathered in order to provide the staff/physician with a point of comparison. The baseline can either be his functioning before he was became debilitated, or can refer to his functioning at the time of his admission.

Bedsores (Decubitus Ulcers or *Pressure Sores)* – skin lesions normally caused by pressure from sitting or lying without moving for longer periods of time.

Beneficiaries (Medicare Beneficiaries or *Recipients)* – people who receive insurance from Medicare plans.

Benefit Period – the length of time that a benefit is provided. The SNF Medicare benefit period starts on the day of admission to a facility, and continues until Medicare has not been the payment source for inpatient services for 60 consecutive days. At that point, a new benefit period begins.

BIMS (Brief Interview of Mental Status) – a part of the MDS assessment that is completed by nursing home staff members at regular intervals in order to provide insight about a patient's mental status decline or improvement.

Blister-packs (bubble-packs) – a method of medication storage that makes it easier to keep an accurate count of number of pills left. Most nursing homes require medications in bubble-pack form.

Bubble-packs (blister-packs) – a method of medication storage that makes it easier to keep an accurate count of number of pills left. Most nursing homes require medications in bubble-pack form.

CAA's (Care Area Assessments) – areas of concern that are identified during the MDS process.

C-diff (Clostridium difficile) – a type of bacteria that causes diarrhea and is highly contagious, requiring that the patient be isolated. It is most often associated with the over-prescription of antibiotics.

Capacity – the ability to make informed decisions about one's healthcare.

Care Area Assessments (CAA's) – areas of concern that are identified during the MDS process.

Care Continuum – the term used to describe the coordination between patient care providers, ensuring that there is continuity of care and that the patient's needs are being met.

Care Plan – an individualized plan for a patient who is receiving any type of medical care.

Care Plan Meeting (IDG* or *IDT) – a meeting where the family is able to meet with different staff members to discuss the patient's plan of care and progress in a medical setting.

Care Planning Process – the process of developing an individualized plan of care, using assessments required by CMS, that is designed to meet the patient's needs.

Caregiver Breakdown – the term used to describe the situation that occurs when a caregiver desperately needs a break from providing care to a sick patient.

Case Manager – an employee, usually a registered nurse or social worker, who is employed by a hospital or health plan to monitor patient care and provide assistance with discharge planning.

Catastrophic Coverage – insurance coverage for medications and illnesses that are very expensive.

Centers for Medicare and Medicaid Services (CMS) – the agency that administers the Medicare program and partners with states to provide Medicaid programs at the direction of the United States Department of Health and Human Services. CMS also ensures the standards for nursing homes and monitors the services provided to nursing home residents.

Certified Nursing Assistant (C.N.A.* or *Nursing Aide) – staff member who provides direct care to patients. A C.N.A. course generally takes 6 weeks to complete.

C.N.A (Certified Nursing Assistant* or *Nursing Aide) – staff member who provides direct care to patients. A C. N.A. course generally takes 6 weeks to complete.

Co-mingled Funds – the act of mixing the patient's funds with someone else's. People are often denied Medicaid because of co-mingled funds.

Community Spouse – the spouse of a nursing home patient who remains at home or in the community, rather than in a nursing home.

Competent – a legal term for a patient's ability to make decisions. People are considered to be competent unless a judge determines otherwise.

Conservator – a person or entity legally appointed by the courts to manage a patient's money. The same person can also be appointed as guardian over his person to make decisions on the patient's behalf.

Continuity of Care – the term used to describe the way that care is administered as the patient is transferred from facility to facility, or from one hospital unit to other parts of the hospital.

Cost Sharing – the amount(s) that a Medicare beneficiary must pay out of his own pocket, often referred to as copayments.

Coverage Gap – a period of time where there is little or no payment for services until certain criteria are met. An example of a coverage gap is the *Donut Hole* for *Medicare Part D*.

Custodial Care – a type of care that is provided to meet the Activities of Daily Living for a patient. Examples of ADL's are bathing, eating, toileting, walking, etc.

Decubitus Ulcers (Bed Sores or Pressure Sores) – skin lesions normally caused by pressure from sitting or lying without moving for longer periods of time.

Deficit Reduction Act of 2006 (DRA) – an Act of Congress that affected Medicaid eligibility by limiting certain transfers of assets. The Act itself is confusing and it's best to consult an elder law attorney to determine whether a patient is affected by the DRA.

Deficiencies – the term for problems found by a state survey team. Deficiencies are identified on the 2567 Form.

Denial Letter – a form that is sent out to a person who is being denied benefits or assistance. The denial letter provides the applicant with information as to the method of appealing the decision.

Department of Health and Human Services, United States (HHS) – the branch of the U.S. Government that governs the *Medicare* & *Medicaid* programs.

Determination – a formal decision that is made as to whether a service (or bill) will be covered under the beneficiary's health insurance plan.

Determination Letter – (Medicare Summary Notice or MSN, Explanation of Benefits or EOB) – a letter that is sent out to beneficiaries to notify them as to the amounts that their health insurance will cover for services provided.

Designee – also known as a Healthcare Proxy, this is the person assigned in a power of attorney form to make decisions.

Director of Nursing (D.O.N.) or ***Director of Nursing Services (D.N.S.)*** – the nurse who coordinates and supervises all of the nurses in a medical facility.

Discharge Plan – a plan for a patient's care and destination upon his discharge from a facility. A discharge plan is developed by the doctor, patient, family member, and a social worker or case manager in order to ensure that the patient's needs will be met at the time of discharge. Discharge plans can be safe or unsafe depending upon the situation.

D.M.E. (Durable Medical Equipment) – medical equipment that can be reused such as walkers, wheelchairs, hospital beds, etc.

Do Not Resuscitate Order (DNR) – a physician's order that directs the medical staff to allow the patient to die a natural death rather than to have heroic measures applied, such as CPR, IV fluids and antibiotics, placement on a ventilator, etc.

Doc Shopping – a term used for patients who visit many physicians hoping to be told what they want to hear. Doc shopping is also a way to obtain narcotics, because most physicians don't have the ability to verify what medications have been prescribed by other physicians.

Donut Hole (Coverage Gap) – the term used to describe the gap in the ***Medicare D*** program when medications aren't covered; the donut hole is in the process of being phased out.

D.O.N. (Director of Nursing or ***Director of Nursing Services D.N.S.)*** – the nurse who coordinates and supervises all of the nurses in a medical facility.

D.N.S. (Director of Nursing Services or ***Director of Nursing D.O.N.)*** – the nurse who coordinates and supervises all of the nurses in a medical facility.

D.P.O.A. (Durable Power of Attorney) – a type of advanced directive that designates the person who is able to make decisions on a patient's behalf after he no longer has the capacity to act on his own.

DRA (Deficit Reduction Act of 2006) – an Act of Congress that affected Medicaid eligibility by limiting certain transfers of assets. The Act itself is confusing and it's best to consult an elder law attorney to determine whether a patient is affected by the DRA.

Drug Seeking Behaviors – the act of requesting medications for pain that doesn't exist, or is greater than the patient's need. Some medical professionals will accuse patients of such behaviors and refuse to give medications.

Dual Eligibility – refers to low-income patients who have both Medicare and Medicaid coverage for health insurance.

Durable Medical Equipment (D.M.E.) medical equipment that can be reused such as walkers, wheelchairs, hospital beds, etc.

Durable Power of Attorney for Health Care (DPOA) – a type of advanced directive that designates the person who is able to make decisions on a patient's behalf.

Durable Provision – a clause included in a power of attorney for health care that states that the document continues to remain in effect after a patient no longer has the capacity to make his own decisions.

E.C.F. (Extended Care Facility) – a professionally staffed nursing home that provides 24-hour care to patients. An extended care facility might also provide skilled nursing services and/or physical, occupational and speech therapies.

Elder Protective Services (EPS or Adult Protective Services APS) – a public agency whose mission is to investigate suspected abuse, neglect and exploitation of adult clients, usually 60 years or older.

E-kit (Emergency kit) – a locked or sealed container that contains emergency medications. Many nursing homes have e-kits available.

Elder Law – the type of law practiced by attorneys who specialize in issues specific to the elderly, including Medicaid eligibility.

Elective Procedures – treatments recommended by the doctor that aren't considered to be life-threatening at the time. Many elective procedures need to be authorized by the patient's insurance company before the treatments have started.

Emergency Room – a hospital unit staffed by physicians 24 hours per day, 7 days per week, that provides emergency services to patients.

Emergency Medical Technicians (EMTs) – personnel that are trained as first responders to administer emergency medical care to a patient wherever he's located. EMTs usually stabilize a patient before they are transported to the hospital emergency room.

E.M.T.s (Emergency Medical Technicians) – personnel that are trained as first responders to administer emergency medical care to a patient wherever he's located. EMTs usually stabilize a patient before they are transported to the hospital emergency room.

E.O.B. (Explanation of Benefits, Medicare Summary Notice* or *MSN,* or *Determination Letter) – a letter that is sent out to beneficiaries to notify them as to the amount that their health insurance will cover for services provided.

End-of-Life Care (Palliative Care, Hospice Care, Terminal Care) – a type of comfort care provided to patients; hospice patients receive palliative (non-aggressive) care designed to make them comfortable, but not to extend their lives.

Exception – a formal appeal that can be used to ask a Part D Provider to cover a medication that isn't on their formulary. Exceptions need to be justified by the doctor and are approved on a case-by-case basis.

Executor (Executrix) – a person legally appointed to follow the wishes of a deceased person regarding the distribution of his property. An executor can be named by the deceased in his will, or can be appointed by the court.

Exit Interview – a formal meeting at the end of a state survey or complaint investigation, where the outcome and recommendations are discussed with the facility representatives.

Explanation of Benefits* – (*EOB, Medicare Summary Notice* or *MSN, Determination Letter) – a letter that is sent out to beneficiaries to notify them as to the amount that their health insurance will cover for services provided.

Extra Help – a program offered by Medicare that reduces the out-of-pocket cost of medications for Medicare Part D prescription drug plan beneficiaries.

Extended Care Facility (ECF) – a professionally staffed nursing home that provides 24-hour care to patients. An extended care facility might also provide skilled nursing services and/or physical, occupational and speech therapies.

Face Sheet – a form that contains all of the patient's demographic information, including social security number, date of birth, mortuary of choice, insurance information, next-of-kin, and the person who is financially responsible.

Filial Responsibility laws – laws that impose a duty upon adult children for the support of their impoverished parents. In some states, filial responsibility extends to other relatives as well.

Financial Power of Attorney (General Power of Attorney) – a form that designates the person who is able to make financial decisions on behalf of a patient.

Formulary – a list of medications that an insurance company will provide to its clients; formularies are a way of holding down costs because the companies negotiate a discount with the pharmaceutical manufacturer.

G.A. (General Assistance) – a financial-based program that assists people who aren't working and need help paying for housing.

G.I.P. (General Inpatient Care) – a level of care provided to a hospice patient in a skilled nursing facility, hospice inpatient unit or hospital.

General Assistance (G.A.) – a financial-based program that assists people who aren't working and need help paying for housing.

General Inpatient Care (G.I.P.) – a level of care provided to a hospice patient in a skilled nursing facility, hospice inpatient unit or hospital.

General Power of Attorney (Financial Power of Attorney) – a type of advanced directive that designates the person who is able to make decisions on a patient's behalf.

Geri-chair – an adjustable reclining chair on wheels that provides patients with positioning choices. These chairs are used in many medical settings and can be viewed as a restraint.

Gifting – the act of giving away a patient's money or otherwise hiding it with the goal of the patient becoming eligible for Medicaid.

Greyhound Therapy – the act of sending a patient by bus to another city or state in order to alleviate the facility from setting up aftercare services. This is unethical, but it happens all of the time and unless providers are careless, they're rarely caught.

Group Homes – smaller assisted living facilities that provide a homelike environment for seniors who aren't able to maintain their independence, but don't have a high enough acuity to qualify for nursing home placement.

Guaranteed Issue Rights (Medigap Protections) – the right to purchase a Medigap insurance policy (policy choices might be limited) without regard to pre-existing conditions at the same price that would have been charged during the Medigap open enrollment period.

Guardian – a person legally appointed by a judge to manage the personal matters or physical care of a patient. There are often public agencies that can be appointed, and fees will be assessed for those patients with the ability to pay.

Guardian ad litem – a person who has been court appointed to conduct an independent investigation on behalf of a patient in order to make recommendations to the court as to what might be in his best interests.

H&P (History & Physical) – a patient assessment completed by a physician that addresses the patient's medical history, current diagnoses, medications, and any test results that affect the patient's plan of care.

H.H.S. (Department of Health and Human Services, United States) – the branch of the U.S. Government that governs the ***Medicare*** & ***Medicaid*** programs.

Health and Human Services, United States Department of (H.H.S.) the branch of the U.S. Government that governs the ***Medicare*** & ***Medicaid*** programs.

Health Maintenance Organization (H.M.O.) – a company that contracts with medical providers of all types in a specific service area to administer medical care to its members.

History & Physical (H&P) – a patient assessment completed by a physician that addresses the patient's medical history, current diagnoses, medications, and any test results that affect the patient's plan of care.

H.M.O. (Health Maintenance Organization) – a company that contracts with medical providers of all types in a specific service area to administer medical care to its members.

Home Health Care – a type of medical care provided to Medicare beneficiaries in their homes.

Homebound – the status of a patient who is unable to leave the home unless it is for necessary medical care.

Hospice Care (Palliative Care, Terminal Care, End-of-Life Care) – a type of comfort care provided to patients; hospice patients receive palliative (non-aggressive) care designed to make them comfortable, but not to extend their lives.

Hospitalist – a physician who acts as the primary doctor and coordinates the patient's care while he is in the hospital.

I.A.D.L.'s (Instrumental Activities of Daily Living) – activities of self-care that people perform on a regular basis including shopping, housekeeping, meal preparation, managing finances, etc.

I.D.G. (Interdisciplinary Group or I.D.T. Interdisciplinary Team) – a group containing a representative of each of the disciplines that provide care to patients in medical facilities.

I.D.T. (Interdisciplinary Team or I.D.G. Interdisciplinary Group) – a group containing a representative of each of the disciplines that provide care to patients in medical facilities.

In-Home Care – light housekeeping and personal care (non-medical) services provided to patients who require assistance to remain in the home.

Income Cap Trusts (Qualified Income Trusts, or *Miller Trusts)* – a type of trust account that is set up to reduce a nursing home patient's income to an amount that allows him to become eligible for Medicaid.

Inpatient Level of Care – a higher level of care provided to hospice patients on a short-term basis in nursing homes or hospice inpatient units.

Inpatient Unit (I.P.U.) – a stand-alone facility that provides services to hospice patients.

Institutional Medicaid (Long-term or *Nursing Home Medicaid)* – a federally subsidized program that pays for the room & board of low-income patients in nursing homes.

Instrumental Activities of Daily Living (IADL's) – activities of self-care that people perform on a regular basis including shopping, housekeeping, meal preparation, managing finances, etc.

Interdisciplinary Group or *Team (IDG/IDT)* – a group containing a representative of each of the disciplines that provide care to patients in medical facilities.

I.P.U. (Inpatient Unit) – a stand-alone facility that provides services to hospice patients.

Last Will & Testament (Will) – a document that a person completes designating how and to whom his property will be distributed after he dies.

Legal Guardian – a person appointed by the courts to make decisions for someone who is no longer mentally competent to do so himself.

Level of Care – a description of the amount of service a patient receives, often associated with nursing home placement or hospice care.

Licensed Practical Nurse (L.P.N. or *L.V.N. Licensed Vocational Nurse)* – a classification of nurse that possesses less education than registered nurses (generally 12 months); they are limited as to the treatments they provide.

Licensed Vocational Nurse (L.P.N. or *L.P.N. Licensed Practical Nurse)* – a classification of nurse that possesses less education than registered nurses (generally 12 months); they are limited as to the treatments they provide.

Liquid Assets – assets that are easily converted to cash, such as bank accounts, investments, non-residential property, etc.

Living Will – a form that a person completes to advise medical providers as to type of care he would prefer if & when he has no likelihood of recovery.

Local Contact Agencies – local agencies that are federally mandated to assist patients in discharging from nursing homes to less restrictive environments.

Long-Term Acute Care hospitals (LTAC's) – hospitals designated to provide complex medical care to patients on a long-term basis.

Long-term Care (Custodial Care) – the general term for services provided in a nursing home to a person who is unable to participate in some or all of his Activities of Daily Living (ADL's).

Long-term Care Insurance – a type of private insurance that pays for custodial care in a nursing home. Some policies also pay for care in the home, or in an assisted living facility.

Long-term Medicaid (Institutional or Nursing Home Medicaid) – a federally subsidized program that pays for the room & board of low-income patients in nursing homes.

Look-back Period – the time period that Medicaid can "look back" into a patient's finances to determine eligibility for payment of nursing home placement.

L.P.N. (Licensed Practical Nurse or L.V.N. Licensed Vocational Nurse) – a classification of nurse that possesses less education than registered nurses (generally 12 months); they are limited as to the treatments they provide.

L.T.A.C. (Long-Term Acute Care hospitals) – hospitals designated to provide complex medical care to patients on a long-term basis.

L.V.N. (Licensed Vocational Nurse or L.P.N. Licensed Practical Nurse) – a classification of nurse that possesses less education than registered nurses (generally 12 months); they are limited as to the treatments they provide.

M.A.C.'s (Medicare Administrative Contractors) – private insurance companies that assist the government in administering the Medicare program by evaluating insurance claims and determining which claims will be paid.

M.A.R. (Medication Administration Record) – the chart or book in a nursing home or facility that documents the patient's medications, doses, times administered, etc.

Managed Care – the type of care provided by a Health Maintenance Organization (HMO) or Preferred Provider Organization (PPO) that is designed to hold down costs while delivering quality care.

Mandated Reporter – every nursing home employee is required by law to report any suspected patient abuse or neglect. The report may be filed with the facility abuse coordinator or the state agency charged with protecting seniors.

Material Safety Data Sheets (M.S.D.S.) – binders held in facilities that contain information about every chemical used in a medical facility, including what to do if the product is ingested.

M.D.S (Minimum Data Set) – an assessment form that is completed by a nursing home when the patient enters the facility, and at regular intervals afterward depending upon the patient's payment source.

Medicaid – federally subsidized medical insurance provided to low-income patients. Medicaid can either be primary insurance, act as a secondary insurance to Medicare, or pay for a patient's room & board in a nursing home.

Medicaid Waiver (Aging Waiver) Programs – special Medicaid programs that waive certain eligibility criteria in order to provide care in a patient's home, or possibly in an assisted living facility.

Medical Savings Accounts (M.S.A.'s) – plans that offer coverage to Medicare beneficiaries that deposits money into a Medical Savings account to be used for the patient's health care costs.

Medical Treatment Plan – a contract that a doctor completes with a patient that agrees upon a plan of care in case the patient has no likelihood of recovery.

Medical Necessity – the term used to describe a patient's need for services that must be supported by the documentation provided by hospitals, doctors, nursing homes and other providers.

Medicare – the government sponsored healthcare program offered to retirees and people who are disabled.

Medicare.gov – the official website that provides information about Medicare-related issues including nursing homes, hospitals, home health, hospice, etc.

Medicare Administrative Contractors (M.A.C.'s) – private insurance companies that assist the government in administering the Medicare program by evaluating insurance claims and determining which claims will be paid.

Medicare Part A Hospitalization – insurance coverage of hospital costs offered by Medicare and most often combined with Part B.

Medicare Part B Medical Coverage – insurance coverage of non-hospital medical costs offered by Medicare, most often combined with Part A.

Medicare Part C Advantage Plans – insurance coverage offered by private companies as an alternative to traditional Medicare Parts A&B using contracted providers and are limited to specific coverage areas.

Medicare Part D Prescription Drug Coverage – insurance coverage that is offered by Medicare to help offset the costs of prescription drugs.

Medicare & You – the name of the official government handbook that explains the Medicare program and is sent out to Medicare beneficiaries every year.

Medicare Rights – an explanation of the rights of every Medicare beneficiary that can be found on the website Medicare.gov.

Medicare Select Plans – Medicare supplements (Medigap policies) that utilize contracted providers to cover the cost of copayments and deductibles.

Medicare Summary Notice – (MSN, Determination Letter, Explanation of Benefits or ***EOB)*** – a letter that is sent out to beneficiaries to notify them as to the amounts that their Medicare insurance will cover for services provided.

Medicare Supplements (Medigap policies) – insurance polices that pay some or all of the charges that Medicare approves but doesn't pay, including copayments and deductibles.

Medication Administration Record (M.A.R.) – the chart or book in a nursing home or facility that documents the patient's medications, doses, times administered, etc.

Medigap Policies (Medicare supplements) – insurance polices that pay some or all of the charges that Medicare approves but doesn't pay, including copayments and deductibles.

Medigap Protection (Guaranteed Issue Rights) – the right to purchase a Medigap insurance policy (policy choices might be limited) without regard to pre-existing conditions at the same price that would have been charged during the Medigap open enrollment period.

Medivac – emergency medical transportation by airplane or helicopter.

Methicillin, or ***Multi-drug Resistant Staphylococcus Aureus (M.R.S.A.)*** – a type of bacterium that is responsible for infections that are difficult to treat, especially for patients with weakened immune systems. MRSA infections often create the need for patients to be isolated from other residents.

Miller Trusts (Income Cap Trusts or ***Qualified Income Trusts)*** – named after the 1990 Colorado Case Miller v. Ibarra, a type of trust account that is set up to reduce a nursing home patient's income to an amount that allows him to become eligible for Medicaid.

Minimum Data Set (M.D.S.) – an assessment form that is completed by a nursing home when the patient enters the facility, and at regular intervals afterward depending upon the patient's payment source.

M.R.S.A. (Methicillin, or Multi-drug Resistant Staphylococcus Aureus) – a type of bacterium that is responsible for infections that are difficult to treat, especially for patients with weakened immune systems. MRSA infections often create the need for patients to be isolated from other residents.

M.S.A.'s (Medical Savings Accounts) – plans that offer coverage to Medicare beneficiaries that deposits money into a Medical Savings account to be used for the patient's health care costs.

M.S.D.S. (Material Safety Data Sheets) – binders held in facilities that contain information about every chemical used in a medical facility, including what to do if the product is ingested.

MSN – (Medicare Summary Notice, Determination Letter, Explanation of Benefits or EOB) – a letter that is sent out to beneficiaries to notify them as to the amounts that their Medicare insurance will cover for services provided.

Multi-drug or Methicillin, Resistant Staphylococcus Aureus (M.R.S.A.) – a type of bacterium that is responsible for infections that are difficult to treat, especially for patients with weakened immune systems. MRSA infections often create the need for patients to be isolated from other residents.

N.O.M.N.C. (Notice of Medicare Non-Coverage) – a denial notice that must be given to a patient receiving services under the Medicare benefit 2-days (48 hours) prior to being discharged from that service.

Notice of Medicare Non-Coverage (N.O.M.N.C.) – a denial notice that must be given to a patient receiving services under the Medicare benefit 2-days (48 hours) prior to being discharged from that service.

Nursing Aides (C.N.A. or Certified Nursing Assistant) – staff members who provide direct care to patients; a C.N.A. course generally takes 6 weeks to complete.

Nursing Home Medicaid (Institutional or Long-term Medicaid) – a federally subsidized program that pays for the room & board of low-income patients in nursing homes.

O^2 sats (oxygen saturation rate) – the percentage of oxygen in the blood.

Olmstead Decision (1999) – a court decision mandating that patients who are able to discharge from a nursing home to a less restrictive environment must be given the opportunity to do so.

Ombudsman – a person or agency federally mandated to advocate for nursing home patients.

Open Enrollment – a time period when Medicare beneficiaries can change plans without being penalized.

Original (Traditional) Medicare Plan – a combination of Medicare Parts A & B, this is an insurance plan that allows the freedom of choice for patients regarding their medical care.

Oxygen Concentrator – a machine that oxygenates air for patients using electricity or battery power, and can be used in a medical or home-based setting.

Palliative Care (Hospice Care, Terminal Care, End-of-Life Care) – a type of comfort care provided to patients; hospice patients receive palliative (non-aggressive) care designed to make them comfortable, but not to extend their lives.

P.A.S.R.R. (Pre Admission Screening and Resident Review) – a screening that determines whether a patient is mentally ill and/or appropriate to be admitted into a nursing home.

Passing Medications (passing meds or med pass) – the term used for the period of time when nurses are administering medications to the patients.

Patient Dumping – a term used for inappropriate patient discharges from a facility, although families can also dump patients onto medical facilities when they can't (or won't) care for the patient.

Patient Health Questionnaire (PHQ-9) – an assessment included in the MDS assessment that is transmitted to CMS at regular intervals.

Patient Liability (Share of Cost) – the amount that a patient must pay from his monthly income to a nursing home before Medicaid or another financial aid program pays the remainder.

Patient Trust Fund – a savings account that the nursing home is federally mandated to provide for each patient who resides in a nursing home.

Payee – a term for the person who has been appointed by the Social Security Administration to manage a patient's retirement or disability benefits.

P.C.P. (Primary Care Provider) – a physician who provides a patient's primary care.

"Pender" – a slang term for an applicant who's awaiting a decision to be made as to whether or not he's eligible for Medicaid.

"Pending" Medicaid – the period of time that a Medicaid application is awaiting a determination as to whether it will be approved or denied.

Personal Needs Allowance – the amount of money a Medicaid patient is allowed to keep to pay for personal items.

PHQ-9 (Patient Health Questionnaire) – an assessment included in the MDS assessment that is transmitted to CMS at regular intervals.

Plan of Care – an individualized plan for a patient who is receiving any type of medical care.

Plateau – a term used to describe the point in a patient's therapy when he has progressed to the point that he is no longer able to get any stronger.

P.O.A. (Power of Attorney) – a form that designates the person who is able to make decisions on behalf of a patient; can be medical or general (financial) in nature.

P.P.O. (Preferred Provider Organization) – a type of managed care insurance plan that contracts with providers to provide service to members, but also allow members the opportunity to see non-contracted providers at a higher out-of-pocket cost.

Pre Admission Screening and Resident Review (P.A.S.R.R.) – a screening that determines whether a patient is mentally ill and/or appropriate to be admitted into a nursing home.

Pressure Sores (Bed Sores or Decubitus Ulcers) – skin lesions normally caused by pressure from sitting or lying without moving for longer periods of time.

Preferred Provider Organization (P.P.O.) – a type of managed care insurance plan that contracts with providers to provide service to members, but also allow members the opportunity to see non-contracted providers at a higher out-of-pocket cost.

Primary Care Provider (P.C.P.) – a physician who provides the primary care for a patient.

Private Fee-for-Service Plans – companies that offer private insurance to Medicare beneficiaries.

Private Pay – the name for the payment the nursing home receives when the patient pays for his nursing home costs out-of-pocket.

PRN – medical terminology for "as needed." It comes from the Latin term "pro re nata."

Proxy (Attorney-in-Fact* or *Designee) – the person assigned by a power of attorney form to make decisions.

Psychotropic Medications – a group of medications designed to affect a patient's mind, mood, or behavior and are used to treat mental or emotional disorders.

Public Guardian – a public agency appointed by a judge to manage the financial matters or physical care of a patient, or both.

Q.M.B. (Qualified Medicare Beneficiaries) – a program offered by Medicaid that acts as a Medigap Policy for lower-income beneficiaries.

Qualified Income Trust (Income Cap Trusts*, or *Miller Trusts) – a type of trust account that is set up to reduce a nursing home patient's income to an amount that allows him to become eligible for Medicaid.

Qualified Medicare Beneficiaries (Q.M.B.) – a program offered by Medicaid that acts as a Medigap Policy for lower-income beneficiaries.

Railroad Retirement Board – a federal agency that administers a separate social security and Medicare program for railroad workers.

Range-of-Motion – exercises usually performed by therapists or specially trained staff members with the goal of working joints to their full potential, thereby decreasing pain and stiffness.

Recipients (Medicare Recipients* or *Beneficiaries) – patients who receive insurance coverage from Medicare.

Registered Nurse (R.N.) – a nurse that possesses at least a two-year education.

Rehabilitation Services – services provided in a variety of settings to patients to return them to the highest level of functioning that they are able to attain.

Representative Payee – a term for the person who has been appointed by the Social Security Administration to manage a patient's retirement or disability benefits.

Respite Care – a type of care that provides a short term rest (respite) to a caregiver, and can be provided in the patient's home, or an institutional setting such as assisted living facility, nursing home, or hospice inpatient unit.

Restorative Therapy – therapy designed to keep a patient at his highest level of functioning that is provided by a specially trained nurse's aide under the direction of a licensed therapist.

Resource Utilization Group (R.U.G.) Rates – the complicated payment system used by Medicare to pay for skilled services in a nursing home.

Revoke – to withdraw permission.

Right to Self-Determination – the term used to describe that a patient has the right to make choices and decisions on his own behalf.

Room & Board – also referred to as custodial care, this is a type of general care that is provided to meet the activities of daily living for a nursing home patient.

R.N. (Registered Nurse) – a nurse that possesses at least a two-year education.

R.U.G. (Resource Utilization Group) Rates – the complicated payment system used by Medicare to pay for skilled services in a nursing home.

R.S.D.I. – the Social Security amount that is paid monthly to people who are retired or disabled. RSDI stands for Retirement, Survivors, and Disability Insurance.

Scrubbing Charts – the process of changing or removing documentation to help a nursing home pass an inspection. This behavior is illegal, but hard to prove.

S.E.P. (Special Enrollment Period) – a special enrollment period offered by Medicare when a Part C or Part D plan provider fails to achieve a 3-star rating three years in a row. A beneficiary will be notified if he qualifies for a ***Special Enrollment Period*** so that he can choose to elect another plan with a higher satisfaction rating

Share of Cost (Patient Liability) – the amount that a patient must pay from his monthly income to a nursing home before Medicaid or another financial aid program pays the remainder.

SHIP (State Health Insurance Counseling and Assistance Program) – a federally funded program that provides Medicare information to seniors via specially trained volunteers.

S.F.F. (Special Focus Facilities) – a designation for nursing homes with a history of quality issues so egregious that they are in danger of losing their Medicare and Medicaid certification and payment. Because of the added costs of monitoring such facilities, there is only enough funding for monitoring of approximately 140 of the nearly 16,000 skilled nursing facilities that exist in the United States.

Skilled Services – refers to medically necessary services provided by licensed staff members such as Registered Nurses, Physical Therapists, Occupational Therapists or Speech Therapists.

Skilled Nursing Facility (S.N.F.) – a nursing home that provides medically necessary skilled services to patients on an inpatient basis because they generally can't be provided in a less restrictive setting.

S.L.M.B. (Specified Low-income Medicare Beneficiaries) – a program administered by Medicaid that pays the Part B premiums for lower income beneficiaries with limited assets.

S.N.F. (Skilled Nursing Facility) – a nursing home that provides medically necessary skilled services to patients on an inpatient basis because they generally can't be provided in a less restrictive setting.

Social Security Administration (S.S.A.) – the government agency that administers Social Security benefits, Supplemental Security Income (SSI) and determines eligibility for the Medicare program.

Social Security Income (R.S.D.I.) – the amount that is paid monthly to people who are retired or disabled. RSDI stands for Retirement, Survivors and Disability Insurance.

Special Enrollment Period (S.E.P.) – a special enrollment period offered by Medicare when a Part C or Part D plan provider fails to achieve a 3-star rating three years in a row. A beneficiary will be notified if he qualifies for a ***Special Enrollment Period*** so that he can choose to elect another plan with a higher satisfaction rating.

Special Focus Facilities (S.F.F.) – a designation for nursing homes with a history of quality issues so egregious that they are in danger of losing their Medicare and Medicaid certification and payment.

Special Needs Plans – insurance plans operated by private companies that provide extra services with certain chronic diseases and other specialized health needs; recipients often have both Medicare and Medicaid and are often in nursing homes.

Specified Low-income Medicare Beneficiaries (S.L.M.B.) – a program administered by Medicaid that pays the Part B premiums for lower income beneficiaries with limited assets.

Spend-down – the act of spending assets to become eligible for institutional Medicaid, although some states also allow a patient to make payment to the traditional Medicaid program in order to become eligible for the program to pay ongoing medical bills.

Spousal Impoverishment – a rule that allows a "community" spouse to keep some or all of a nursing home patient's income and at least half of the common assets, while allowing the patient's room & board to be paid by Medicaid.

S.S.A. (Social Security Administration) – the government agency that administers Social Security benefits, Supplemental Security Income (SSI) and determines eligibility for the Medicare program.

S.S.I. (Supplemental Security Income) – a program that provides additional income to very low-income seniors with less than $2,000 in assets. SSI recipients are automatically eligible for Medicaid.

State Health Insurance Counseling and Assistance Program (SHIP) – a federally funded program that provides Medicare information to seniors via specially trained volunteers.

State Surveys (Annual Inspections) – a state conducted annual event in nursing homes that consists of chart reviews, patient/staff interviews, kitchen inspections, other physical plant inspections, business office audits, medication audits, and any other review that the state deems necessary to ensure that the facility is operating within the rules and laws required.

Stipend – a minimal, non-taxable wage paid to lower income seniors or other volunteers to provide services to various agencies.

Supplemental Security Income (S.S.I.) – a program that provides additional income to very low-income seniors with less than $2,000 in assets. SSI recipients are automatically eligible for Medicaid.

Telephone Order (T/O) – a physician's order that is given over the telephone. T/O's are recorded on special order forms and sent to the doctor for his signature.

Terminal Care (Palliative Care, Hospice Care, End-of-Life Care) – a type of comfort care provided to patients; hospice patients receive palliative (non-aggressive) care designed to make them comfortable, but not to extend their lives.

(T/O) Telephone Order – a physician's order that is given over the telephone. T/O's are recorded on special order forms and sent to the doctor for his signature.

Traditional (Original) Medicare Plan – a combination of Medicare Parts A, B, & D, this is an insurance plan that allows the freedom of choice for patients regarding their medical care.

Transdermal Patches – patches filled with medication that are administered by adhering the patch to the skin and transmitting the medication into the bloodstream.

TRICARE – a health insurance plan offered to civilians and retired members of the military.

United States Department of Health and Human Services (HHS) – the department of the U.S. Government that governs healthcare programs such as Medicare & Medicaid.

Up-coding – the act of manipulating billing codes in order to bill at a higher rate. Depending upon the type of up-coding, this can be considered fraud.

Verifications – paperwork that provides proof of the information that a Medicaid applicant claims to be true. Bank statements, car registrations, etc. are types of verifications.

Will (Last Will & Testament) – a document that a person completes that designates how and to whom his property will be distributed after he dies.

Work-up – a term used to describe the process of completing diagnostic tests on a patient in order to find a diagnosis, and to hopefully develop a treatment plan.

Wound Vac – vacuum assisted closure (VAC) for a wound that provides negative pressure wound therapy, essentially vacuuming fluids and bacteria out of a wound that allows it to heal more quickly.

l.e. green

Acknowledgements

This book was written over the course of several years, and I couldn't have done it without the support of my friends and family. I'd like to thank Jack, Rosie, Karli, Terilyn, and Alexis for their unwavering love and support. Julie, who put up with my absences for a long, long time. Stan and Johnna, who have helped me in so many ways, I can't even count. Finally, to Patrick, who provided excellent editing skills, thank you for all of your assistance. I appreciate each and every one of you.

l.e. green

About the Author

l.e. green has worked as a social worker in the medical field for more than 24 years. She has specialized in the areas of Geriatrics, Medicare & Medicaid. l.e. is the proud step-mother of two wonderful young adults and lives in the mountains of the Southwest with her various animals.

l.e. green

Made in the USA
Charleston, SC
01 July 2014